WHAT DOES YOUR DOCTOR LOOK LIKE

Naked?

WHAT DOES YOUR DOCTOR LOOK LIKE

Naked?

YOUR GUIDE TO OPTIMUM HEALTH

J. WARREN WILLEY II

TATE PUBLISHING & *Enterprises*

Note for Librarians: a cataloguing record for this book that includes Dewey Decimal Classification and US Library of Congress numbers is available from the Library and Archives of Canada. The complete cataloguing record can be obtained from their online database at: www.collectionscanada.ca/amicus/index–e.html. ISBN 1–4120–3696–8. Printed in Victoria, BC, Canada

Published by Tate Publishing & Enterprises, LLC
127 E. Trade Center Terrace | Mustang, Oklahoma 73064 USA
1.888.361.9473 | www.tatepublishing.com

Tate Publishing is committed to excellence in the publishing industry. The company reflects the philosophy established by the founders, based on Psalm 68:11,
"The Lord gave the word and great was the company of those who published it."

Book design copyright © 2008 by Tate Publishing, LLC. All rights reserved.
Interior design by Lindsay B. Behrens

Published in the United States of America

ISBN: 978-1-60462-878-4
1. Health & Fitness: Healthy Living   2. Exercise & Weight Loss
08.06.09

Dedication

The basis of medicine is sympathy and the desire to help others, and whatever is done with this end must be called medicine.

Frank Payne

What Does Your Doctor Look Like Naked? Your Guide to Optimal Health was a lot of fun to write. I have written on a number of topics in the past, including a medically related textbook, but this one just flowed out. It was the easiest thing for me to write to date. This was due to my wife, Dari. Her daily encouragement during some tough years consisting of long hours, bad moods, and fatigue was essential as I simultaneously mastered the information available in this book and built my medical practice. I therefore want to dedicate this book and all its information to my loving wife. She is my gift from God, my best friend, and my partner in life.

I must also give credit to God, as nothing is possible without Him, and everything is possible through Him. True joy and optimal spiritual health, though not discussed in detail in this book, are as essential as anything in this book. I encourage everyone reading to look up and not around when facing life's problems and challenges. May I suggest reading Rick Warren's book entitled *The Purpose Driven Life*, as it provides a forty–day progression toward optimal spiritual health, which, as I stated before, is essential in optimal health!

The eating plans outlined in this book are dedicated to all my previous and current clients. Together we have forged the information through trial and error, with clients often placing themselves in the position of the proverbial lab rat so I, the mad scientist, could try a new idea or thought. To them I graciously bow and say a heartfelt thank you.

> "In treating a patient, let your first thought be to strengthen his natural vitality."
>
> —Rhazes

Table of Contents

Pre—Introduction, Introduction 9

Chapter One
How This Book and Program Came About 15

Chapter Two
What Is a Doctor of Osteopathic Medicine (D.O.)? 25

Chapter Three
Understanding the Process of "Disease" 27

Chapter Four
Understanding the Process of "Health" 35

Chapter Five
Age—Management Medicine 42

Chapter Six
Hormone Replacement Therapy General Information 55

Chapter Seven
Hormone Replacement Therapy in Women 63

Chapter Eight
Hormone Replacement Therapy in Men 68

Chapter Nine
**The Fallacy of Scale Weight: Understanding
Body Composition** 76

Chapter Ten
Understanding Objective and Subjective Data Tracking . . . 81

Chapter Eleven
Wonderment 86

Chapter Twelve
Those Who Have Done It and Now Are Doing It 93

Chapter Thirteen
Developing an Understanding of Food. 101

Chapter Fourteen
Food Timing. 114

Chapter Fifteen
The Free Window 122

Chapter Sixteen
Eating Plans. 129

Chapter Seventeen
Holiday and Vacation Meal Planning and Eating. 149

Chapter Eighteen
**The Importance of Exercise, or Developing
an Exercise Routine**. 155

Chapter Nineteen
Progression Through Roadblocks, Walls, and Plateaus 164

Appendix I
Food Lists 172

Appendix II
Preventative Medicine Screening 460

Appendix III
Glycemic Index. 466

Appendix IV
Aerobic/Fat–Burning Program 471

Appendix V
Resistance–Training Program. 475

Appendix VI
Supplement Recommendations. 484

Appendix VII
Optimal Style of Eating 486

Appendix VIII
Frequently Asked Questions 488

Appendix IX
How to Contact Dr. Willey 494

Index. 496

Pre–Introduction, Introduction

The title of this book is not meant to conjure up visions of your primary care doctor, or your cardiologist, or, for that matter, any of your health care providers. It is designed to make you think.

The answer to the question *What Does Your Doctor Look Like Naked?* will become apparent as you read the book. You will begin to "see" the answer as you delve into the heart of the subject matter. At the end, I will elucidate the answer in more detail. I would encourage you "skip to the end to see how it ends" readers out there to wait, although, in all honesty, reading the end may give you some perspective and understanding of what's in between.

Time for It

One more thing before I get to the real introduction. One of the most common excuses I hear from people who are literally avoiding ultimate health is the old "I do not have the time for it" justification. I know you've heard the "We are all given twenty–four hours a day, yada, yada, yada" one, so I am not even going to go there. What I want you to think about is this:

How much time do you have for disease?

Let's take a simple illustration: You are a "young" 51–ish–year–old. Your work is busy, your oldest is getting married in a few months, and so forth and so on—I am sure you could fill in a hundred–plus more examples. Then, out of nowhere, you suffer a minor stroke, most likely due to your lifestyle, damaging food choices, and lack of exercise. By the way, you lucked out because it was only minor (i.e. you lived), and not only did you get to the Emergency Room in time, but the head neurologist at the hospital was standing there. She treated you immediately and effectively, but you still had some residual effects, including weakness on your right side, a mild face droop on the left side, difficulty swallowing, and mild cognitive impairment.

Now let's talk about time again. The average time it takes to rehab from this unfortunate event will likely be from eight months to a year, and that is, again, if you are one of the lucky ones. In the meantime, you will miss work, be less productive, and, due to the droop on one side of your face, hate having your picture taken at your daughter's wedding. Your new "busy schedule" will include trips to the speech therapist three times a week, to the physical therapist two to three times a week, and to your doctor at least once every few weeks. You will be on medications with expected side effects and will generally wake up each day in a conundrum, thanking God for sparing you while, at the same time, asking, "Why did this happen?" Time for some quick math: Let's be really generous and say it takes eight months of effort to get you back as close to "normal" as you will be again. That is approximately 5,760 hours. Instead of spending 5,760 hours *fixing* something, let's take that same time frame and work backward: Let's pretend you spent thirty minutes a day preparing foods to nourish and fuel your system properly throughout the day. Then let's add in sixty minutes of exercise three times a week. That is 6.5 hours a week you spend on yourself in the attainment of ultimate health. The same number of hours that you spent on disease could have gone to 18.5 years of proper eating and exercise to *prevent* the stroke. This brings me to my second point:

If you think health costs money, try disease!

Continuing with our example of a stroke, strokes are the leading cause of disability in the United States and the third leading cause of death. According to the American Heart Association,[1] in 2005, the estimated direct and indirect cost of coronary vascular disease, in which stroke is included, is $393.5 billion dollars. Hopefully we have identified and put to rest some of the most common excuses that may pop up while you are obtaining ultimate health. Remember the society we live in. We are *reactive, not proactive*! Health care providers, or, as it should be phrased, "Disease care providers" make their living getting people nonsymptomatic. They do not, in most cases, help people find health, as defined in Chapter 4 of this book. They, and the entire medical, pharmacological, and "health" industry make money off disease. On a daily basis, I see people who really need to get healthy, but have nowhere to turn. We are so focused on disease that true health has taken a backseat.

Many people get a placebo effect from medical advances and technology. I cannot tell you the number of times I have had clients either directly or indirectly refer to the fact that technology will save them, no matter what their lifestyles do to them. Quick fact for you: All technology does is increase the price of disease care. True, *health care* is more cost effective, productive, and a lot less invasive! Our entire paradigm has to shift! This is but one of the objectives of this book and its title. Health needs to be practiced, not just preached!

"There is nothing more tragic than a sick doctor."

-George Bernard Shaw

The Real Introduction

I recently walked down the health, nutrition, and fitness aisles at Barnes and Noble with my wife and daughter. I could not believe the amount of stuff! (I am thinking of another word here…) I feel I have somewhat of a handle on what I am doing in the health and fitness field. I am able to recognize good from bad, yet I must admit a feeling of being totally overwhelmed! How is anyone able to decipher all this stuff? I am truly amazed at how many "health experts" there are out there. What makes a "health expert" anyway? A medical degree? A certificate? The way they look? Supplement sales? (I will quickly step off my soapbox, for now…)

I decided then and there that I wanted this book to be different—simple, refined, and functional. Good information without the hype. That is why it is not as thick as a doorstop, or as wordy as a state senator's pre–election speech. My goal is not to compete with all of these other big programs. Every one of them works for someone. None of them work for everyone. This one has the information that *can* work for everyone. It is self–structured, with simple objective and subjective tracking systems, and has the information you need to advance. Three steps forward and two steps back is okay. Improvement is *never* a straight line. It is a process of forward, sideways, up and down, and occasionally backward. That, in my mind is a–okay, because it is still movement. Complacency is the death of any issue.

Do not be resistant to change, especially where your health is concerned. Initially, efforts to improve your standard of living may leave you feeling fatigued, headachy, etc. This is not what all the hype out there tells you, yet it is something I have seen almost universally in those starting to make the *right change* with the incorporation of diet and exercise into a lifestyle agenda. The body needs to adjust to what you are doing (sort of a "detox," if you will).

Complacency Is the Death of Any Issue

The plan outlined and the facts presented in *What Does Your Doctor Look Like Naked?* are foundational and scientific, without bias of previously held standards or ideas. My hope is that you will take the program as outlined, follow the style and suggestions as closely as possible, but still conform it to fit you. Health is a process. It does not occur in thirty days, twelve weeks, or any other time frame marketing may boast. It is a gradual improvement on the current condition. Improvement starts with education and understanding. This program will not drown you in the esoteric. It will not look or become official by the breadth of the writing or the repetition of information found at so many other sites. This is not written to show you how much I know. It was constructed to be short, concise, and to the point, providing usable information for now and for the future.

The process of health needs to be renewed daily. You must want to be healthy, decide to be healthy, make an effort to be healthy, and persist in being healthy. You will not *get* that ideal body from this book. You can, however, *develop* your ideal body with the information in this book. The majority of the information found in this book is a summary of my medical practice for the last eight years. The program I mention throughout the book is called *The Optimal Health Program.* I am in the developmental stages of bringing this plan to the office of every doctor willing to add diet and exercise to his or her health care regimen. Currently, I am involved in urgent care medicine, as I feel this is the appropriate foundation from which to launch this concept. My goal? That mainstream medicine will utilize the basics such as good eating and exercise in their daily interactions with patients. The program is in continual development. My goal with *the Optimal Health Program* is to provide the right information at the right time to all who are after optimal health. I have had the good fortune of being *very* successful with nearly all of my clients because of our personal interaction and accountability, and because of the outline of information found in this book. I feel that this book is but a picture in time of where the *Optimal Health Program* is now. Life, being very dynamic and ever evolving, allows changes, additions, and deletions from the program almost daily. The more people I work with, the more I learn, the more the plan changes. I hope this book will give you the basis for further knowledge in the quest for optimal health, optimal weight, and optimal living. Please let me know if you have any recommendations, thoughts, or ideas. I love the interaction of multiple minds on a particular subject. The best way to contact me is via e–mail at doc@pocatellopicc.com. I look forward to your input.

Chapter One

How This Book and
Program Came About

How did this book come about? Who am I and what do I do? By way of introduction, I felt it important to discuss the program with each and every one of you reading. Ignoring the obvious incongruity of the previous statement, I did what I thought would be as close to a personal interview as possible and actually had a tape of an initial introductory visit to my clinic transcribed. The following is the initial discussion between a new client and myself.

Dr. Willey: "Let me start off by telling you a little bit about The Optimal Health Program and myself. I'm a board–certified Osteopathic Physician. I am board certified with the American Board of Family Practice and the American Board of Holistic Medicine. My area of expertise is nutritional and exercise medicine, with an emphasis on preventative medicine. My interest in medicine in general and my practice of education, utilizing food and exercise in particular, stem from a sickly childhood. I had asthma, was on a number of drugs, and had what I considered a large part of my childhood limited by the fact that I could not breathe. From my earliest memories, stemming most likely from the repetitive visits to the doctor, I wanted to be a physician. Being less than optimally active, I was a rather pale and skinny kid until my father started me on a weight–lifting program in our basement. From that time on, my health on all levels started to improve. I began reading everything I could get my hands on concerning nutrition, exercise, and the effects of muscle mass on appearance and health. A short time later, I was offered a personal training job at the local gym. I have maintained that designation for over twenty years. As a matter of fact, the only real jobs I have ever had (other than my paper route as a child and a one–summer stint with the city mowing lawns) are personal training and medical care.

"After high school I attended Colorado State University, initially as a pre–med and microbiology major. I was active in the pre–med club and had the opportunity to work with a few physicians as part of the program. I became disenchanted, however, with what I saw occurring. My years of personal training and the many clients whose health I had the opportunity to help improve and optimize reinforced the fact that the basis of *any health* program is twofold: movement and fuel.

"It was disheartening to see health care providers not talking about diet and exercise, much less prescribing it. I asked one doctor I followed about diet and exercise and why he did not discuss that with his patients. His reply: "There is no time for that, and besides, no one listens if you do." I was dumbfounded! Was this the practice of *health care* I wanted to get involved with? It then occurred to me: We in the modern world are used to the practice of *disease care*. I decided then and there that I was not going to spend that much money and that much time training to do that.

"I was clinically depressed. I had always wanted to be a *health care provider*, not a *disease treater.* So, in response, I dropped out of the pre–med program, dropped out of microbiology, and started an exercise physiology program with an emphasis on nutrition, knowing that I would eventually be teaching people how to truly take care of themselves with diet and exercise.

"My plans naturally progressed to pursuing a graduate degree in exercise and nutritional science. The area of study that intrigued me most was the effect of resistance training and food on disease states, specifically the chronic diseases such as cardiovascular disease, obesity, and diabetes. That's when I came across the osteopathic medical field. Do you know what an osteopath is?"

Client: "I have heard the term, but am not familiar with it."

Dr. Willey: "An osteopath (DO) and an allopath (MD) have very similar training. Entrance requirements are similar, and the actual schooling process is the same other than the fact that osteopaths are trained in musculoskeletal medicine, also termed manual medicine. I can do a similar type of manipulation or adjustment as chiropractors, although our techniques are different. I was initially impressed with the fact that the whole person was involved in this kind of medicine.

"The musculoskeletal system was recognized as a major contributor to health, both preventative and curative. One thing in particular I enjoyed about the osteopathic profession was the fact we became hands–on physicians from day one. I always wanted to be a doctor, and the osteopathic program gave me everything I had hoped for.

"From osteopathic school I went on to The Mayo Clinic for a thirty–six–month residency program in Family Medicine. Following some time in Arizona, I moved to Colorado and started The Fitness Medicine Clinic, a full service age–management clinic that utilizes the power of nutrition and exercise in the quest and attainment of Ultimate Health. My practice was somewhat limiting due to the fact that it was a fee–for–service arrangement and restricted my preaching of truth and righteousness in the power of eating and exercise. I wanted to reach everyone. My thoughts and energy then turned to urgent, or walk–in, medicine. I learned as much as I could about the practice of urgent care and decided that was the vehicle that would take proper eating and exercise to the masses."

Client: "That's awesome and very impressive! Were you able to maintain your health and physique during all of that?"

Dr. Willey: "Yes, I was. Though my physique changed on occasion and in accordance with my schedule, I was exercising, eating right, and trying to learn as much as possible about the effects of nutrition, food, food timing, and movement on the prevention of the common ailments *regrettably and falsely* associated with aging. I have learned to use food as my medicine, and I use exercise as my medicine primary and first line in every intervention I undertake. If I need to write a prescription for an antibiotic for example, I'll do it, but overall it's teaching movement and fuel.

"Now a little bit about what I do now. There are many levels to my practice based on your goals, your needs, and what you want to do. My personal goal with each and every person I work with is to help her understand how her body works, her relationship with food, and her relationship with all the other variables in her life that make her, *her*! I do that with a very detailed initial evaluation. It consists of about ten pages of information for you to fill out so I can learn as much as I can about you. We then do a full physical, multiple body measurements, such as lean mass, percentage body fat, heart rate recovery, grip strength, etc. We get into detail about you, because everything around you, work, driving to work, your family life, spirituality, everything has to do with who you are, and we try to get to the heart of each. I utilize food and exercise in helping you accomplish what you want to do with your health and your body, but other variables will interplay. We try to cover those so we can utilize them to our benefit or understand when they are impeding progress.

"One of my first objectives with clients is to teach them to view *food as a drug.* When we sit back and think about it, we realize the truth in this statement. We have all had a food that made us feel good, or gave us an upset stomach, or made us feel tired. In every sense of the word, food is a drug. Understanding how food acts like a drug is a powerful tool to have. It applies to body goals, weight/fat loss, and lean mass gain. Whatever your goals may be, changing your paradigm about food in this manner will allow you something you have truly never had previously: the power to choose. Food then becomes an instrument, a tool in your toolbox, to utilize and control to help you do what you want to do. Looking at it this way allows you to develop an understanding of consequences related to choices (and thereby actions). This is something you *learn* while following the eating plans. My goal is to make you reliant upon no one, especially me. I want to teach you how to do it and then have you only use a doctor or a specialist when necessary. Overall, if you understand how your body works, how your body stays and maintains health, and how you can continually improve on that health, you can make it a continuous process. That is a very broad overview of my practice. Is there anything in particular that you are interested in?"

Client: "Well, I have similar goals in mind. With my age, I am starting to hit that wall. I can tell my hormones have started changing and my body is changing…all in ways I do not like."

Dr. Willey: "How old are you, may I ask?"

Client: "Forty–nine in another month. I have parents with dementia, heart problems, diabetes, and overall poor health. Now I know they lived a very different lifestyle than I, but I'm very fearful of those things. And I know that there have got to be things that I can do today that are going to benefit me when I am eighty."

Dr. Willey: "Very wise."

Client: "The anti–aging, hormone balance, and fueling the body with food are very intriguing. I would like to be doing something right, but I know I don't do things right. I take Synthroid for my thyroid daily, but it seems like weight has always been a problem for me. And that is probably my focus in here. I'm tired of doing all the things that I do and never getting to where I need to be.

"As far as my weight management is concerned, I don't necessarily eat healthily. I just did a popular program, as they have these ridiculous weight–loss centers all over the place. I did lose twenty pounds, but I quickly put twenty–plus pounds back on. I did that through monitored supplements, and I didn't understand, and still don't know, what that did for me. My heart was racing and there was something that told me, 'This really isn't good.' I was diligent with it for four months, and I dropped twenty pounds. But I couldn't stomach some things. I didn't understand what they were doing to my body. For example, they put you on a one thousand–calories–a–day diet. I don't think that is the proper amount of calories. I mean, you lose a lot of weight really quickly, but your body is tired. I felt worse when I was doing that diet, and I kept telling them, 'I'm really hungry. I don't think I'm getting enough calories.' They would add about fifty calories more. Then they said, 'Have some more protein and that should help your hunger.' It didn't. I knew I was not getting enough calories. I felt terrible, and still do even though I have been off of it for three months."

Dr. Willey: "It is so unfortunate. And you are so right. One of the biggest flaws with all the programs out there is that they focus on scale weight. That is one of the first things that I will emphasize to you. You have got to differentiate fat loss from lean muscle mass.

"I could easily put you on an eating program and guarantee that you will drop thirty pounds in thirty days without the use of ephedrine–based products or counterfeit foods like all these programs out there are dependant on. The problem is that twenty–five of those pounds would be muscle mass. By doing so, we literally destroy your metabolic system. For every pound of muscle that you gain, you, to a great extent, increase your metabolism. The programs out there make themselves look good by dropping scale weight, but the majority of it is lean mass. It takes but a few calories to burn one pound of muscle, which is the last thing we want. In comparison, it takes 3500 calories to burn one pound of fat, which is obviously what we are after. Low–calorie dieting supports muscle loss.

"Calories are something that we want to control, but if you are physiologically hungry all day, that is your body telling you that the muscle is getting used and you have to listen to that. One area where I differ from other programs is I help you to determine true success. We will use objective and subjective data tracking to actually *see* the changes and improvements. I encourage weekly to bi–weekly body composition measurements, and I teach you how to do them as well. As a matter of fact, I partnered with a personal trainer who used to work for me, and we wrote a booklet that comes with a measurement caliper for you to learn how to do it yourself (See Appendix IX: How to Contact Dr. Willey). This way you are able to follow *true* changes and make adjustments accordingly.

"Our goal together and your goal long term should always be to *increase lean mass*. I don't write diets for weight loss. I quit that about ten years ago after writing diets for years prior to that. I found that when we focus on your lean mass and your overall health, fat loss is a side effect. It always happens, because our bodies have a place where they like to be, but we are survivalists by nature. Thinking in terms of our ancestors, our great, great, great–grandfathers, who used to roam the plains out there hunting and gathering, would eat a large meal and then they wouldn't get to eat for a long time. Their bodies knew that, so they stored fat. So the first thing that your body does when you are on a calorie deficit is save the fat and burn the muscle. The body is planning on being hungry later. We have to pull what I call metabolic trickery. We have to teach the body that muscle should be left alone. We do that with types of food we eat, when we eat, and with the proper supplements. Then we provide it with an appropriate amount of fat in the diet and an adequate amount of calories. This tricks the system into utilizing that extra energy source, fat, while it is maintaining or building lean mass, which, again, increases your metabolism. So here is the paradigm that our so–called conventional wisdom squawks at: Your goal with fat loss should not be weight loss; it should be muscle gain!

"This is the basis of my program, and the reason for the long–term success of those who have utilized it. It is likely hard to imagine that my goal for you with this program will be to gain muscle."

Client: "Yeah! I should say! That seems to go against what I have been told in the past."

Dr. Willey: "That is the paradigm that we have to shift, and that is why we don't worry about scale weight. Imagine us putting five pounds of muscle on you in the next three months. With your increase in muscle mass, you're burning extra calories everyday just sitting around. That means while you are at work, enjoying a movie, or taking a break, you are burning fat! Add those additional calories over a week's time, and you end up burning a whopping amount of extra calories a week just by putting on more muscle! That can equal a lot of extra ice cream cones or chocolate bars! That is what makes it real life! That is how people like me can stay under ten percent body fat year–round. My lean mass and knowledge of food lets me do whatever I want, whenever I want.

"But, again, it involves an understanding of food and its effects, always being prepared, and food timing. Let me give you another example: This coming Saturday my wife and I are planning a big date together. We are going out, and I plan on eating whatever I want. The way I get away with it is I prep my body for it. I know what my body needs to do before I eat this way and then how to allow my body to recover from it. My night out, as it turns out, actually benefits me. I actually gain lean mass by indulging myself. That is where I want you to be as well. That is what this program will allow you to do. My goal is for you to feel good, strong, and energetic and no longer feel fatigued and hungry. All this and the ability to indulge in a piece of chocolate!

"People are going to ask, 'What the heck are you doing? How can you eat that and still look so good and be healthy?' You have it figured out, and you have learned how your body works.

"As humans, we all have a physiological foundation that we need to follow, a law, if you will. Once that law has been met, the rest becomes individualized for every single person. Everybody is different. That is why certain variables come into play in some but not in others. Variables like stress, workload, cravings, and goals make you different from the last client. That is why I teach you to track objective and subjective data sets to help you learn about you."

Client: "What are objective and subjective data, and how do I use them?"

Dr. Willey: "Objective data includes body composition, the lean mass versus the fat mass, cholesterol levels, blood pressure, heart rate response, etc. But there is something that is even more important than that, your subjective data. This includes things such as, how are you feeling? How is your energy? How are you sleeping? How is your sex life? How are your moods?

"What you learn from this becomes ingrained in your daily life. You will know that at ten o'clock in the morning your body needs X amount of protein, X amount of fat, X amount of carbs from different sources for optimum functioning, both then and the following day. That is the secret that makes this a *longevity program*, both in the sense that you can do it the rest of your life, but also that the optimal health you achieve will help your chances at longevity."

Client: "It sounds like my chances of failure, especially in the long run, are lessened with this program. Is that your experience?"

Dr. Willey: "Yes! You can come off the program, but once you've increased that lean mass, you will literally have to work to gain that unwanted and excess fat again. You would have to wait for your metabolism to slow back down before you would start gaining fat, which could take months. That is an important thing because usually you don't let yourself go for months after you learn this. That, again, is what makes it long term."

Client: "It sounds like part of success is the fact that this program allows me to become educated about how my body works and it eventually becomes habit forming. It's a real life change, and that is exactly what I want."

Dr. Willey: "Exactly."

Client: "This is precisely what I have been looking for. Real life. Real answers, based on *me!* Where do I sign…"

Chapter Two

What Is a Doctor of Osteopathic Medicine (D.O.)?

Adapted from American Osteopathic Association Web Sight: http:// www.aoa–net.org

If you're like most people, you've been going to a doctor ever since you were born, and perhaps were not aware whether you were seeing a D.O. (osteopathic physician) or an M.D. (allopathic physician). You may not even be aware that there are two types of complete physicians in the United States. The fact is, both D.O.s and M.D.s are fully qualified physicians licensed to perform surgery and prescribe medication in all fifty states. Is there any difference between these two kinds of doctors? Yes. And no.

D.O.s and M.D.s are alike in many ways:

Applicants to both D.O. and M.D. colleges typically have a four-year undergraduate degree with an emphasis on scientific courses.

Both D.O.s and M.D.s complete four years of basic medical education.

After medical school, both D.O.s and M.D.s can choose to practice in a specialty area of medicine—such as psychiatry, surgery, or obstetrics—after completing a residency program, which requires an additional two to six years of training.

Both D.O.s and M.D.s must pass comparable state licensing examinations.

D.O.s and M.D.s both practice in fully accredited and licensed health care facilities.

D.O.s comprise a separate, yet equal branch of American medical care. Together, D.O.s and M.D.s enhance the state of care available in America.

D.O.s bring something extra to medicine: Osteopathic medical schools emphasize training students to be primary care physicians.

D.O.s practice a "whole person" approach to medicine. Instead of just treating specific symptoms or illnesses, they assess the overall health of their patients including home and work environments. Osteopathic physicians focus on preventive health care.

D.O.s receive extra training in the musculoskeletal system— your body's interconnected system of nerves, muscles, and bones that make up two–thirds of its body mass. This training provides osteopathic physicians with a better understanding of the ways that an injury or illness in one part of your body can affect another.

Osteopathic manipulative treatment (OMT) is incorporated in the training and practice of osteopathic physicians. With OMT, osteopathic physicians use their hands to diagnose injury and illness and to encourage your body's natural tendency toward good health. By combining all other medical procedures with OMT, D.O.s offer their patients the most!

Chapter Three

Understanding the Process of "Disease"

Disease never happens. I have gotten myself in trouble with this statement on a number of occasions, from arguments with other doctors to deep metaphysical discussions with ingenious friends. It is my firm belief that disease is a process, one that can be intervened, interrupted, stopped, and, in some cases, reversed. We have control over most noncongenital and accidental conditions, especially the age– and lifestyle–related situations such as diabetes, cardiovascular disease, osteoporosis, osteoarthritis, obesity, etc. It never just materializes because your number came up or you drew the short stick. Health and disease are processes. Disease has a course of action just as health does. It develops for a reason. Of course, it is multifaceted, has many variables, and combines a number of causes, some of which are out of our control. But, in most instances, it does not just "come about."

Disease Never *Happens*

Let me explain with an example: Motor vehicle accidents "happen." You have no control over them (ignoring the fact that it may be your fault). People do not wake up one day and decide to get a head injury or lose a limb in a car accident. A car accident is an event that causes disease.

Your chosen lifestyle is a process that causes disease. In other words, it "happens" over time and due to your influence. Placing blame on the multitude of possibilities out there without first looking in the mirror is a (no pun intended) grave mistake. You have control over disease! It is not in your doctor's control; it is not your mother's fault. You are the biggest piece of the "disease process pie." With this chapter, I hope to explain what disease really is. I also hope to point out some very common misnomers in our thinking and our medical philosophy. Let's start with the definition of disease:

> Disease via *Merriam-Webster* is defined as: *Obsolete*: Trouble. A condition of the living animal or plant body or of one of its parts that impairs normal functioning: sickness, malady. A harmful development.

This definition states it all. First of all, disease is *trouble*. No kidding. Next: *A condition of the living animal or plant body or of one of its parts that impairs normal functioning.* Right on the money, jocko. It impairs *normal* functioning at any level, be it cellular, such as the development of a small pre–cancerous polyp in the colon, or large scale like the ability to think following a stroke. And finally: *A harmful development.* Key word here: *Development.* It does not say a harmful event, indicating it just happened, but a harmful development. Disease is a progression of events that advances to an outcome.

So where have we gone wrong in our thinking? Why, when I have had the unfortunate experience of telling someone they have a disease, do they and their family members and friends ask me, "What caused it?" as if to say, "What event that I had no control over did this to me?" To answer this, I am going to need someone who is much better with the English language and verbiage than I to explain, but let me give you my two cents.

Throughout time, from our great, great ancestors and even earlier, across all spans of culture and societies, disease and, therefore, health have been "released," or given to another for safekeeping and control. In most societies, the religious leader was also the medicine man. This wise sage was seen as mystical in power and connected to unseen influences that controlled sickness and health. Our ancestors gave the power of health and disease over to another person. We still do the same today. Why this occurs, I cannot say. My guess would be that the pain suffered on all levels by all involved was better dealt with by disassociation, but that is beyond this writing.

In our modern society, that shamanistic view of the doctor is still present. I have been in continual amazement of this fact since I started personal training twenty–plus years ago. People of all backgrounds, influence, and financial status turn their health over to someone else. As a medical student and a resident physician, I used to sit and watch patients give all control to their doctor. Doctors and health care providers are to blame as well. On a number of occasions I have seen desperate people with all sorts of ailments begging the doctor to help them with their condition. The health care provider starts to puff up; his chest expands and his chin is thrust toward the ceiling as he follows the desperate plea with the characteristic response: "I will make you feel better..." "I will cure your high blood pressure..." "I will save you..." Big mistake.

I have had a number of smart, well–educated people look me right in the eyes and tell me they trust me to, for example, lower their blood pressure. "Wait a minute," I am quick to respond. "It is not *my* blood pressure that needs fixing. It is yours! Why don't I help you understand the cause and the process of treatment, and then *you* treat your *own* blood pressure. That might involve a prescription medication that I write for you, but that is only one variable in the treatment approach *you* will be taking."

After an initial "deer in the headlights" look, reality sinks in. It is their problem, not mine. I am their health care consultant, not a shaman. Only on a rare occasion will I put face paint on and dance around a client…

The take–home message is this: Do not relinquish control of your health to anyone! It is yours for the keeping! As the old marriage adage states, "In sickness and health, till death do you part."

The Natural Progression of Disease

Now that you understand that disease is a process and you are in control of that process, let's discuss the natural progression of disease. Using breast cancer as our example, let's walk through a simplistic view of its progression (see Table 3–1 for a schematic representation of the following). Breast cancer starts at the cellular level; we can call this the biological onset. The actual cause of the microscopic cellular change is multifactorial. Let's say our cancer sufferer is overly fat, has a diet high in charred meats, drinks a lot of alcohol, and smokes—all proven risk factors for breast cancer. These lifestyle choices have set the stage for a cellular change to take place within her breast. Now we have some time pass where the cellular changes are starting to proliferate. Lifestyle conditions have rendered the immune system defenseless against the microscopic change and it starts to grow. We get to a point where early disease detection is possible via preventative screens such as mammography. However, our fine example ignores the suggestions of her doctor and decides she can skip the ol' mammogram because it is somewhat time consuming and painful. At this point, if our example had had a screening test, we might have caught the disease in a state where it could have been immediately identified and rectified. But, as stated earlier, "that takes too much time and hassle," so we can follow the continued course.

After the stage when early disease detection was/is possible, more time passes and we get to the clinical diagnosis stage. This occurs when her microscopic changes are now big enough to cause a mass in the breast. Had our example been doing monthly self–screening exams, she might have caught it at this stage. She did not, and more time passes. The mass is quite noticeable and she is having a bloody nipple discharge. At this point, she goes to her doctor, and a clinical diagnosis of breast cancer is made. We then have another time frame until an eventual outcome takes place, being either medical intervention for a hopeful conclusion, or death.

Box 3-1 Schematic representation of the course of disease[1]

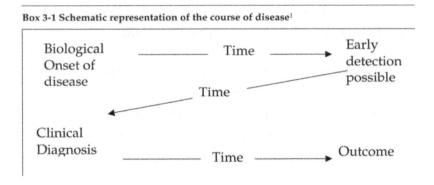

This is the natural progression of disease, and it can be applied to almost all of the chronic "age related" diseases. I use this example to make yet another point: Using our breast cancer example, our patient had a number of opportunities to intervene and make a potential difference in the outcome. To review them:

- Lifestyle factors
- Change diet and eat healthy
- Decrease alcohol intake
- Quit smoking
- Exercise daily
- Get screening mammography as directed by doctor
- Do self–screening breast exams
- Become aware of other potential "out of your control" risk factors, such as genetic predisposition (see below), age and family history, and estrogen exposure

I am by no means stating that all disease is preventable or avoidable. It does occur, but we must recall the *power* we have to influence it! We are part of the equation. In most cases, it is not all luck of the draw or chance. It is not up to our doctors or anyone else to do something about it. We are responsible for our own wellbeing!

Genetic Predisposition vs. Determinism

In the Pre–Introduction/Introduction, I mentioned the true price of technology and the placebo comfort that many people feel from medical advances. One area of concern I would like to tie in is inherited disease, and from the technological side, genetic testing. Genetic testing and inherited disease that we "obtain" from our parents can be both a false comfort and/or a false fear. Let me explain: I have been a passive and active observer of people's beliefs and reactions to disease states and diagnoses all my life. One thing seems to be prevalent in that search for an answer to the difficult question, "Why do I have this disease?" and that's *blame placing*. I mentioned this under different circumstances above, but the message is the same: You have some control of your health! False comfort comes in the form of avoidance of disease if no one in your family has had it. False fear sets in when someone in your family has a condition and you sit back (in fear) and wait for it.

We all, to some degree or another, look to our parents in anticipation of our eventual outcome. It is ingrained. Is there some truth to it? Yes, but not enough to sit and watch it play out. In the medical world, we are taught from the beginning to get a detailed family history and apply that information in risk assessment of our patients. But let me emphasize something here: This is not a finger–pointing exercise. We are wrong to assume that because our parents had something we are bound and destined to get it. We may be at greater risk to get it, but this is different from us *needing* to get it. This brings me to a common speech in my clinic: the difference between genetic determinism and genetic predisposition.

Determinism in general, genetic determinism specifically, removes all forms of control for the involved participant. It also removes all accountability. If your father passed on from a fatal heart attack at age forty–eight, you will not necessarily die of a heart attack at age forty–eight. You may be more inclined to have heart disease in your late forties, but your father's premature death is not necessarily a death sentence for you.

In western medicine we think in a deterministic way: If X, then Y. No questions asked. No wavering allowed. Cold=virus. Your mother had diabetes=you're going to get diabetes. This is deterministic, without any input from you. It is also a common excuse I hear for not exercising or eating right. The Vikings played out the same scenario—"Eat, drink, and be merry, for tomorrow we die!" Now, of course, this did not and does not always come to pass, but it is essential to understanding the process of disease and health that you grasp the real control you have over it.

I like to think in terms of genetic predisposition. This returns control to the participant, i.e. you. If your father had a fatal heart attack at age forty–eight, then yes, you are predisposed (at a greater risk), but you are still a part of the equation. You have a say in whether or not you, too, will suffer a heart attack at age forty–eight. When we change our thinking to involve the potentialities and all the variables that are included, especially the ones we have control over, we have taken control of the process of disease and started to rein it in. You have taken control and not relinquished it to your doctor, chance, your parents' inevitabilities, or any other power. In this case, realizing the *potential* for heart disease may encourage you to exercise more, eat right, and get regular screening exams. In other words, you have become an active part of the equation; you have made the choice not to be deterministic and let other factors govern you. You have taken charge and control.

Inherited potential ties right in to technology and other medical advances, such as genetic testing. I feel there is a danger in our current state of technology. The thought of putting it to practical and everyday usage is misleading. It allows for the process of disease to become an uncontrolled *event*, one that will happen with or without our influence. This is a serious mistake, a part of the rising cost of health care, and, on an individual level, a factor in the speed of the disease process.

In brief, this was a review of the disease process and a few of the potential influences we have on that process. I will say it until I am blue in the face and write about it until my hands fall off—*we control our health, and we control our disease*. In the next chapter, we will review the process of health and the amazing control we have over it as well.

Who controls *your* health? Who controls *your* disease?

Chapter Four

Understanding the Process of "Health"

Your decision to live healthier, lose weight, and get stronger is a process that has already begun. There are stages of change that we use in medicine that help us gauge where someone may be in terms of generating or constructing change in their lives. Used most commonly for smoking cessation, these stages help us determine if someone is ready for the intervention we are prescribing. The stages of change were developed by James o. Prochaska, Ph.D., and Carlo C. DiClemente, Ph.D., at the Texas Research Institute of Mental Sciences. The stages of change are precontemplation, contemplation, preparation, action, maintenance, and extinction. Precontemplation is the stage at which there is no intention to change behavior in the near future. Many individuals in this stage are unaware, or under-aware, that they may have a problem. For example, someone walks by this book in the bookstore and comments on the interesting title, but states to herself that she does not need to read it, as, "I have no medical problems and am on no drugs, so I do not need to read it."

Contemplation is the stage at which people are aware that a problem exists and are seriously thinking about overcoming it but have not yet made a commitment to take action. In our example, that same person in this stage would walk by the book, pick it up, think about it (knowing she needs to do something for her health), but make no commitment to do so. Preparation is a stage that unites intention and behavioral measures. Persons in this stage are intending to take action in the next thirty days and have unsuccessfully taken action in the past year. In our example, that same person in this stage would walk by the book, pick it up, buy it, and plan to read it within the month.

Action is the stage in which individuals modify their behavior and environment in order to overcome their problem(s) or lack of accomplishment. Action involves the most obvious behavioral changes and requires a commitment of time and energy.

Maintenance is the stage in which people work to prevent relapse and consolidate the gains attained during their action stage.

Extinction is the stage I hope to get you to with this book, the stage where a previous unhealthy lifestyle will never return, and complete confidence that you can manage without fear of relapse is obtained.

Table 4-1: Stages of Change

Precontemplation – You have no intention of taking steps toward ultimate health.
Contemplation – You do intend to take action in near future.
Preparation – You intend to take action within the next thirty days and have taken some behavioral steps in this direction.
Action – You have changed evident behavior. You are on the path toward ultimate health.
Maintenance – You have changed your lifestyle and are living healthy for more than six months.
Extinction – Previous unhealthy lifestyle will never return, and there is complete confidence that you can manage without fear of relapse.

By reading this book, you are likely in the contemplation stage, preparation stage, action stage, possibly even in the maintenance stage, looking for further support to your actions, or in the extinction stage, looking for some other viewpoint. If you have attempted, without success, to get a handle on your health in the past, discouragement can be present even though you are in a later stage of change. With all the different training systems, diets, and supplements out there, it is difficult to judge what really works and what does not.

This program's attitude is clear and simple: Commit to a healthy lifestyle and stick with it. Evaluate your progress and position regularly and make adjustments based on your needs and results. Expect to make consistent and measurable improvements. Each person's level of commitment (intensity, amount of time, resource allocation, etc.) will vary and will impact how quickly results occur, but everyone should see and feel results.

In my practice, I commonly ask my clients the definition of health. Though the responses are varied, one common consideration usually comes out (and I quote): "Health is not needing to see a doctor or take drugs." Talk about a misinformed concept. This, in my opinion, is a product of mass marketing and our current *disease care system* (See Chapter 3). This is not, I repeat, is not the definition of health! Health in *your* new system of thinking is "a continuing process of *transformation*, both physical and mental, that allows your body and mind to take the next step into maximal living by decreasing the chance of disease, thereby increasing the chance of enjoyment."

There are many very decent self–help books out there on emotional, spiritual, family, financial, and cognitive health. The primary focus of this book, however, is what I would consider the *basis* of any age–management program and/or health–attainment information. In my experience, and barring physical limitations, maximum health is not attainable without the following. Once the process of The Optimal Health Program has been understood, these two variables are what we will spend the most time modifying to help you obtain maximum health. You have the most control over these variables. Day–to–day decisions and long–term lifestyle modification for the continued process of health maximization include these two factors. To what am I referring? *Movement and fuel!* (Also known as exercise and nutrition, including supplementation.)

One more definition of health: Enjoying life to the fullest on all levels imaginable. This includes physical, emotional, spiritual, family involvement, financially, and cognitively with the vigor and vitality you crave and desire! This is the goal for each and every one of you. This is my personal goal as well!

Unfortunately, in the past the process of health has always been viewed as an event. One of the more popular books out there that I give kudos to for changing so many lives fails to point out that twelve weeks of change does not equal permanent success. Health is not an event. It is a process that takes time to occur and time to maintain. Just as we learned in the previous chapter that disease is a process, health is even more so. We have a paradigm about healthy people that has to change as well. Our vision, possibly a bit severe, of a "health nut" is that of a vegetarian who exercises four hours a day, sleeps twelve hours a day, and meditates the rest of the time. As some good friends of mine like to say, "If it is worth doing, it is worth doing in excess!" This addictive personality trait is not shared by all of us.

Health is *not* an event. It is a process...

When you change your thinking from "I am *now* healthy" or "I need to *get* healthy" to "I am in the *process* of health," a number of things occur on many levels. I would like to focus on four of them.

1. *Time and Effort.* First and foremost is the fact that you realize that time and effort are involved. Health does not just happen.

2. *Freedom and Choices.* Secondly, it allows you to live life! When the lifestyle is in place for ultimate health, extremes are only visited for a short while—never lived out. What I mean by this is you may go on a weeklong, two–hour–a–day exercise kick, or you may go on a daylong binge–eating session that puts one of the Krispy Kreme donut facilities out of business for the day. Both are okay (though not recommended). The process allows you to *get out of the extreme* and *back to the lifestyle* that allows ultimate health! I get asked all the time how it is possible for me to stay in top body–building shape year round. Guess what? I don't! I fluctuate with the best of them out there. Overall, however, I am healthy, and my lifestyle keeps me that way. I love getting caught by one of my clients at a pizza joint eating to my heart's content. What this demonstrates is that real life happens, and I like pizza. I can continue to enjoy pizza because the process of health is not dependent on one or two events. When the big picture is looked at, the forest through the trees, if you will, health is a daily objective.

3. *"Stuff" Happens.* The third thing that tends to happen when the process is understood is the "I blew it, and that's okay" realization, especially for us all or nothing types. If you continue to look at health as an event and you have a slipup, let's say you miss a meal during the day and on the drive home are so hungry that after you get a ticket from a police officer for reckless driv-

ing and road rage, you stop at a fast–food hamburger establishment and eat twelve super–sized double cheeseburgers. The all–or–nothing types would then say "what the heck" and go home and binge some more, eventually turning our one time full–bore effort toward health into a full–bore effort to get sick. The *process* of health lets an occasional slipup go by practically unnoticed and definitely without any adverse effect on the body.

4. *Understanding Multiple Factors Involved in Health.* The fourth thing that happens when the process of health is understood is a realization that the process has a large number of variables. There is not, I repeat *not* a pill for it, nor is there a magic exercise device, or a screening exam, or a hormone, or a surgery, or a specialist. The process is multifaceted and involves a number of variables. These range from the obvious nutritional and exercise variables to family issues, emotional wellbeing, spiritual concerns, history, and day–to–day events. Understanding health as a process allows individuals more acuity in all that is involved and gives us power over the variables we can control (i.e. diet and exercise), as well as a better understanding of the variables over which we have less control (i.e. world events/stresses). The process occurs when we realize the control we have over it. One thing I suggest everyone do is to start keeping track of a few variables. Learn about yourself. It is all about modification, or adjusting what you do to make it more effective. What caused you to fall off the proverbial wagon of your eating program? What emotions accompany hunger? When you are feeling fatigued, what foods might be involved? The accompanying eating and exercise program gives you control over two very important and effective variables. However, they are not the end all. Understanding that health is a process is really everything you

need to know to master your own personal health maximization program.

Maximal health starts when you become happy with who you are and the life choices you make. Anyone who tries to pursue physical perfection as the main foundation for his or her life is doomed to failure. No level of fitness, no amount of body transformation will make you become a "whole" person unless you are continually working on your inner being as well. Achieving maximal health and your best body will enhance your life and can bring about dramatic changes in your emotional, spiritual, and intellectual life.

It's about working smarter, not necessarily harder. In writing for a number of publications, specifically for the exercise crowd, I end every article with a simple statement: *Train with your brain.* Knowledge, as has been and will be emphasized throughout this book, is the cornerstone to any health process. As we continue with the next chapter on age–management medicine, I feel it is important to emphasize once again that there are many variables influencing our day–to–day lives. This includes health, and this includes disease. I treat my patients with their health in mind, not their disease. Eating and exercise is the cornerstone of every visit in my office, be it for a cold or cough or for weight loss. It is a conviction I believe in, not, in my personal viewpoint, to live forever, but truly better today. It takes into account many of the variables that affect daily living, which, in turn, affect how long you live. It also raises the crucial question that you must ask yourself throughout this book:

What does your doctor look like naked?

Chapter Five

Age–Management Medicine

For centuries, humans have looked for a way to extend and improve life, from the gods of ancient Greece to the well–known Ponce de Leon and his quest for the fountain of youth. Futile as it was, it set in motion today's true "health movement," and the pursuit of longevity began to actually work. Two–thirds of *all* people in the history of the world who lived past the age of sixty–five are alive today! We are becoming an ageless society. To name a few well–known people (as of December 2002): Actress/Singer Lena Horn, age eighty–five; Mick Jagger of the Rolling Stones, age sixty; Tony Bennett, age seventy–seven; Sandra Day O'Conner, age seventy–three. These people are in their prime! What makes them different from you?

Before we go further, I think it is important to define "old age." Without utilizing *Webster's*, we all envision a defining example of "old age." The classic archetype is of an elderly person sitting in a living room chair, wearing a burgundy cardigan sweater, slightly hunched over with one arm in his lap and the other arm supported by a cane, with a small dog sitting faithfully at his feet in what appears to be a long, tedious wait for death. This, my friends, *is not* what I have in mind. My vision of later years, and hopefully yours following your application of the information in this book, is one of vitality, vigor, and pride, taking on the world with all four limbs without fear of disease or limitation. I envision finally spending the money and wisdom that I worked so hard for on my loved ones and myself, living life to the fullest, on my terms, within my control. This, my dedicated reader, is "old age." And this is obtainable at any chronological starting point with the information provided here.

Age–management medicine is the application of any therapy or modality that delivers very early detection, prevention, treatment, or reversal of age–related dysfunction and disease.[1] It is the utilization of cutting–edge technologies to detect, prevent, and treat aging–related diseases. It is scientific, evidence based, and well documented in peer–reviewed journals. It is based on nutrition and exercise, with supplements and pharmaceuticals being a close second. It is not reliant on human growth hormone therapy, nor is it a type of alternative medicine. Age–management medicine thus enhances the *quality* and extends the quantity of the human lifespan.[1] This program has its foundations in age–management medicine, the truest form of preventative medicine. This patient–controlled intervention *will* change, challenge, and improve your life!

So, can I really influence how I age? It is demonstrated by a number of studies[2–51] that we have the power to directly affect the way we age. I have condensed all the information out there into what I consider the five most effective modalities: nutrition, supplementation, exercise, stress reduction, and preventative screening. Before we delve into your future, it is important to understand the "normal" aging process. As we get "wiser," it is held by our current medical standards that some inevitable events take place. Our society has been overrun with common ailments *regrettably and falsely* associated with aging! Each of these changes and their associated interventions will be reviewed under specific subtitles.

Nutrition

Due to our current diet standards, or lack thereof, we have a propensity for the following to take place: increased body fat, decreased lean mass (I will interchange muscle mass with lean mass throughout the book), increased cardiovascular disease, osteoporosis (or loss of bone mass), type–II diabetes, increased fatigue, and a general increase in chronic diseases, including cancer.

With nutritional intervention, like the program offered here, the above to–be–anticipated changes never take place! A proper, focused eating plan with goals and

What Defines Old?

In the Late 1800s, Baron Otto Von Bismark of Germany set up the first pension plan for government employees. This was to start at age sixty-five. Hence, our chronological definition of old age. Wisest in the business sense, one fact was ignored: the average life expectancy at the time was forty-five years...

limited intake, as well as a thorough understanding of the consequences of foods, allows us to avoid all of the above "inevitabilities." As a matter of fact, research tells us that a good eating plan will have the following effect: decreased body fat, increased lean mass, decreased heart disease, decreased stroke risk, diabetes prevention, increased energy, and decreased risk of chronic diseases. In other words, your eating is one of the most powerful interventions you have in your ultimate health and wellbeing!

TABLE 5-1: Nutrition and Influenced Aging

Normal Aging	Influenced Aging
Increase in body fat	Decrease in body fat
Decreased lean mass	Increased lean mass
Osteoporosis	Strong, healthy bones
Insulin resistance/Type II diabetes	Strong, healthy bones
Increased cardiovascular disease	Decreased heart disease and strokes
Fatigue with daily living	Increased energy
Chronic diseases	Decreased chronic disease

Exercise

I remember sitting in medical school listening to a lecture on the diseases associated with aging. A term was brought up that to this day, and from my experience, does not make any sense. The term was *sarcopenia*, and it was defined as the associated loss of lean muscle mass that (and I quote) "inevitably occurs with aging." This made no sense to me. I had trained a number of "older" clients who made spectacular gains in their lean mass, even into their seventies. What was this disease state my professor was talking about? I feel this disease state is purely a function of not moving! It does not inevitably occur with aging. Some other to–be–anticipated problems associated with aging (that went hand in hand with loss of lean muscle mass) are increased body fat, decreased heart function, increased falls/loss of balance, decreased cognitive function, and an increase in all chronic diseases. What is one of the best ways to prevent all of the above? Exercise. Specifically, resistance training or weight lifting. By increasing lean muscle mass, we decrease body fat, improve cardiac function, lower blood pressure, improve cognitive and psychological wellbeing, and prevent chronic disease. Exercise is one of the most vital components of the age management system!

Table 5-2: Exercise and Influenced Aging

Normal Aging	Influenced Aging
Sarcopenia	Increased lean mass
Increase in body fat	Decreased in body fat
Decreased heart function	Improved cardiac function
Increased loss of balance and falls	Decreased falls
Decreased cognitive function	Improved cognitive and psychological well-being
Chronic diseases	Prevents chronic disease
Fatigue with daily living	Increased energy

Supplementation

As I mentioned under Nutrition, our current diet standards are insufficient for optimal living. Even following the American Dietetics Association (ADA) suggestions for optimal food intake, it is my and many other authors' opinion that we still are far behind the eight ball when it comes to truly optimal intake. Supplements are essential for health attainment and living. They can be used to complement good nutritional intake or be utilized as mediators in a specific function, for example, sugar modification. Utilizing supplements such as cinnamon and chromium picolinate, we can change the way sugars are processed and utilized in our bodies.

With the normal aging process, we see a lack of essential vitamins and minerals and a lack of disease–preventing antioxidants.

We undergo metabolic changes that make supplements essential for optimum functioning. Due to our busy schedules, or whatever reason, we miss meals, which may be replaced with meal–replacement supplements.

Supplementation allows us to correct all the above. It also allows us to use concentrated food sources, herbs, minerals, etc., to our advantage in our pursuit of health. Without supplementation, none of us would be able to get *optimum* amounts of certain nutrients. It would be both physiologically and financially unfeasible.

Table 5-3: Supplementation and Influenced Aging

Normal Aging	Influenced Aging
Lack of essential vitamins and minerals	Adequate supply of disease preventing and modifying: vitamins, minerals, antioxidants, and amino acids
Lack of disease preventing antioxidants	
	Utilizing supplements as powerful modulators of metabolic function
	Adequate nutritional intake in any situation (meal replacements)
Metabolic changes	
Missed meals	

Stress Reduction

Many studies and reports have touted the negative effect of stress on the body. [52–58] From heart attacks to increased cancer risk, stress is dangerous. As we age, the predominant thought is that we lessen our stress. The kids have moved away, we no longer have to deal with the daily grind of work, etc. In my experience, however, the opposite is true. If you feel you have been immune to the effects or speed of the world around you, think again. The same pressures still have an impact and, more importantly, take a toll on the body. In the normal aging process, a few areas in particular come to mind: increased stress over your health status, the fear of disease, the fear of daily activities (be it due to weakness, inability to cope in situations, or any of a myriad of other worries), and one very important fact, the inability to handle or modify the stress we are under. Influenced aging specifically alters a large majority of the effects of stress on you. When you focus on doing everything you can to prevent disease (i.e., this book!), and you exercise and eat right to develop strength in daily activities, you increase your body's ability to handle/modify stress and stressors. You are able to ward off and even be a major factor in treating your own disease. The simple knowledge of doing all you can do is stress reduction in and of itself. Use stress to your benefit; do not let it be used against you!

Again, there is a lot of information out there on "how to," including how to relieve stress. Some of the simplest yet most effective tools I have found to work in my practice, other than diet and exercise, include the following:

1. Laugh! Nothing is healthier or more stress relieving than to let the gut roll, especially at yourself. If you do not, the result will be someone else laughing at you.

2. Avoid procrastination. When something comes up, take care of it!

3. Go with the flow. Life begins now...and now...and now... (Get my point?) Use the past to learn from and the future to anticipate. Stressing about either only prevents you from enjoying the present.

4. Practice wonderment! Read Chapter 11 once a week!

5. Practice Balance. Make time for friends, family, self, socializing, work, etc. Equilibrium in life means leaving no stone unturned. Take time to just sit and relax, spend some quality time alone. Cultivate outside interests.

6. Just say no! Nancy Reagan said it best. Do not try to please everyone. By doing so, you please no one and kill yourself in the process!

7. Slow down! Life will pass you by.

8. Develop a support group. Have close friends or family who act as consultants for any and all projects you undertake, including the attainment of ultimate health. These people are also quick to point out the "truth of our critics." Objective eyes are nice to see through.

9. Avoid perfectionism. We perfectionists are a setup for failure. When you make a mistake, learn from it and go on. Focusing on it only will cause more to occur.

10. Eat right and exercise. Did I mention this one before? My point is...well, you know!

Table 5-4: Stress Reduction

Normal Aging	Influenced Aging
Increased stress of health status	Doing everything to prevent disease
Fear of daily activities	Daily strength in activities
Inability to handle/modify stress	Ability to handle/modify stress
Fear of disease	Ability to ward off disease if present
	Knowledge of 'doing all you can do'

Preventative Medicine

Medicine has advanced more in the last few decades than in the centuries before. Though we have a predominantly reactive system, there are more and more opportunities for a proactive approach to early disease detection. I must emphasize: No matter whether you undergo all the expensive tests and screening exams available, and whether or not they find anything, the basis of this program still applies. You must have a foundational base in real health. All future endeavors, be they interventional (for example, to treat a "find" on a screening exam) or not, can be improved with eating right and exercising. Just because you pass a screening test does not mean you're clear until the next test, which brings me to my next point. If there is one thing all screening tests do, it's set you up for more tests. Let me rephrase that: There are risks in screening exams! You probably have not heard that one before. I am not in any way, shape, or form telling you not to do screening tests. I am, however, going to review some of the good ones out there, and Appendix II has current recommendations from the United States Preventative Service Task Force. But, like the rest of this book, optimal health first involves knowledge!

The definition of a screening exam is the use of diagnostic tests or procedures to a symptom–free person for purposes of dividing them into two groups: the haves and the have–nots. With our understanding of the natural progression of disease, as discussed in Chapter 3, it becomes possible to attempt intervention with a screening exam to try to thwart disease. Sounds simple. Sounds logical. Unfortunately, screening tests have a number of hidden problems that remain relatively unknown even in the medical community. We will review those in a minute. Let's start with some of the benefits of screening exams:

1. Improving prognosis. Prognosis means the prediction or forecast of how a disease might turn out. You are likely to have a better outcome by detecting disease at its early stages.

2. Less radical treatment. When you catch a disease in its early stages, you are likely to need less invasive and therefore less–expensive forms of treatment. It is much easier to remove a polyp during a colonoscopy than to remove a part of the colon later.

3. Resource savings. This follows benefit two, as stated above: Colonoscopies are much less expensive than open surgeries, hospital stays, anesthesia, rehabilitation, etc.

4. Reassurance from negative results. We all feel better when the doc gives us a clean bill of health.

"An ounce of prevention is worth a pound of cure," as everyone's grandmother used to say. Wisdom at its best! As I stated earlier, however, preventative screening is not the end all of answers. You cannot go about life as you please without paying attention to diet and exercise and the other health modalities we are discussing in this book and hope your doctor, if you decide to even see one, catches a problem before it wreaks havoc. Even those of us who follow detailed screening and preventative recommendations need to be aware of potential flaws in the system.

There are *risks* with screening exams!

Two of the biggest problems come in the form of false–positive tests and false–negative tests. A false–positive test is a result that indicates something is there when, in reality, it is not. In other words, the test states you have cancer when, in reality, you do not. This sets you up for unneeded anxiety, fear, and anger. It automatically labels you as someone who has this condition, and that "label" may be hard to shake for the rest of your life (especially with insurance companies). It sets you up for additional tests and possibly even a treatment protocol, such as surgery, being implemented when it is not needed. A false–negative test tells us that nothing is there when, in fact, something *is* there. This will provide false reassurance and allow you to go about your business without being concerned with potential smoldering problems.

At the risk of sounding as if I am focusing on the downside of screening exams, I would like to discuss two more biases that are present when doing screening examinations:[59]

1.   Lead–time Bias

A lead–time bias states that screened individuals do not necessarily live longer; they just have the potential to know about their disease longer. This is assuming that nothing can be done about the disease found on screening. A lot of debate occurs in the medical ethics world due to the lead–time bias. Knowing about disease (or even the potential of it) can be as devastating, if not more so, to the patient than the disease itself, especially in the light of false positives.

2. Length–time Bias

When a length–time bias is present, it will demonstrate longer survival in some diseases, but not others. This is due to the fact that a length–time bias selects for patients (and therefore diseases) with the best prognosis. Screening programs appear to improve survival when they actually only select patients with the best prognoses. Aggressive diseases like lung cancer are harder to detect early because of the aggressive nature of the disease. Slower–acting diseases, such as most cases of prostate cancer, are detected more easily because of their slow or non–aggressive nature.

I am reviewing these things because I do not want you to hang your hat on screening tests. Some are very good, others need more research, and others stink. My primary point is the following: Use screening exams with caution. Screening is an important part of an optimal health program, but you still need to eat right, take your supplements, and exercise. Do not rely on your doctor, another health care provider, or screening exams to catch your disease before it gets you.

In Appendix II, I have listed the current preventative recommendations as put forth by the United States Preventative Services Task Force. They pick good and bad tests based on what I reviewed above and a number of different testing modalities for each test. Some of the newer screening exams, such as the heart scan or virtual colonoscopy, are not covered here. Do your research before you plunge into one of these. They are expensive and have not proven themselves as of yet.

The above information on what I call age–management medicine is, in my opinion, the cutting edge of optimal health. By incorporating nutrition, exercise, supplementation, stress reduction, and preventative medicine, you have taken charge of your health and are on the path to optimal health attainment and maintenance. I will spend a few more chapters on another hot topic in anti–aging, and that is hormone therapy. Following that, we will get to the how–to in true age–management technology—understanding and developing eating plans and a movement, or exercise, program!

Chapter Six

Hormone Replacement
Therapy General Information

Hormone replacement has been a long time medical practice/procedure, and, until recently, it was used almost exclusively by women. Proper balancing of hormones has become a standard in anti–aging medicine. The human body and all of its functions are in some way or another affected, changed, modified, or controlled by hormones. There is even evidence of gene regulation and expression being altered by the influence of hormones. You have over one hundred different hormones active in your body at any one time. Hormones are involved with everything from bone growth, as is very apparent in children and teenagers, to muscle growth and tone, fat loss, and even the production of body heat. Hormonal health is unequivocally involved in total health. The influence of nutrition and exercise on the powerhouses of the body is evident in a number of different situations. The way we eat and the amount of exercise we do directly influences our hormones. One simple example in understanding that this is the following: After a good bout of exercise, your mood is improved, your feeling of overall wellbeing is better, and you are better prepared to handle the stresses of the day. All of this is due to the associated hormonal changes that take place with exercise. That is why my primary prescription, if you will, in this program is nutrition and exercise.

Before getting deeper into the hormone issue, it is important to clarify *hormone replacement* from *hormone misuse*, particularly in men. Unfortunately, the media has put a bad light on hormone usage due to its immediate connotations with the use of anabolic steroids in sports. Remember the Ben Johnson story in the 1988 Olympic Games? Let's differentiate: Hormone replacement is the act of bringing the levels of hormones back to a *physiological level* of an average thirty– to thirty–five–year–old, in hopes of deriving all the benefits of health and wellness from said levels. Hormone misuse is the procedure of taking hormones *beyond physiological levels* in hopes of improving performance.

What has become apparent is the affiliation of hormonal changes, generally a decrease in amounts, with a propensity for disease states, not to mention missing optimum function, as we age. As I said earlier, proper balancing of hormones, in terms of replacement, has become a standard in anti–aging medicine. Some would argue that this is a natural decline and should be viewed as a normal part of aging. I must respond with the following statement, using the same fallacy in logic: You do not need to change the oil in your car, because its decline is a natural occurrence of driving. Ridiculous in my mind, but unfortunately, a prevailing notion.

In my practice, we use *natural hormone replacement therapy* or *bio–identical hormone replacement*. Natural hormone replacement therapy utilizes hormones that look exactly like the hormones your body produces or used to produce. Though derived by a process of chemistry or from plant sources, particularly soy and wild yam, they are impossible for your body to distinguish from their own (See Table 6–1). Synthetic hormones "look" different from your body's natural hormones, but are close enough in appearance to stimulate the hormone receptors to elicit a response. The natural hormones include estrone (E1), estradiol (E2), estriol (E3), progesterone, testosterone, DHEA (dehydroepiandrosterone), pregnenolone, and androstenedione. In humans, the estrogens are primarily composed of ten to twenty percent estrone (E1), ten to twenty percent estradiol (E2), and sixty to eighty percent estriol (E3). By comparison, Premarin (a synthetic hormone (see below)) is composed of five to nineteen percent estradiol (and others), seventy–five to eighty percent estrone, and six to fifteen percent equilin (specific to a horse (see Chapter 7)).

TABLE 6-1: Natural vs. Synthetic Hormones

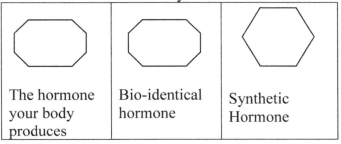

The hormone your body produces	Bio-identical hormone	Synthetic Hormone

With the numerous hormones in the body and the effect each has on different individuals, it is beyond the scope of this book to detail each and every one. In Table 6–2, I have provided a list of some of the most common hormones that a competent anti–aging physician can help you optimize. Of note, in the table you may find a lot of crossover of actions. This is not a typographical error. This is meant to demonstrate the importance of hormone balance, as all the hormones have interchangeable roles and mechanisms responsible for everyday living and activities. This chart is not all–inclusive either, as more detail is beyond the scope of this book.

We will focus on a few of the hormones that I feel can have a good amount of sway on overall health and function, particularly weight management. The hormones we will review in more detail are the sex hormones: testosterone, estrogen, and progesterone. I will break this down further in terms of male– and female–hormone replacement so it becomes a little more specific to each reader (see Chapters 7 and 8).

Utilizing Hormone Replacement

Natural hormones are prescription medications. There are a number of health care providers out there who claim to help your hormones with all sorts of plant derivatives, herbs, and procedures. To some extent, some of this stuff may work through symptom control. However, overall optimization of hormone replacement takes an individual skilled in diagnosis and treatment of hormone deficiency, followed by proper hormone replacement. This is not a simple task. Though we all follow some basic laws of physiology, individualization is key. One, or even two, simple answers generally do not exist. The physician you choose to help you optimize your hormones must not only understand them, but, more importantly, he or she must understand you. This, as I am sure you know, does not occur in a ten–minute office visit. I have helped some with their hormonal regimens in as little as a one to two hours of consultation, while others have taken multiple visits, multiple adjustments, and multiple attempts at finding what works for them. Simply put, there is no simple answer or single approach to hormone–replacement therapy. More importantly, it must be realized that one cannot successfully treat hormone imbalances with hormones alone. As this book contends, it is a combination of understanding the multiple factors and influences that make each and every one of us unique individuals, controlling for and modifying food intake, and a proper balance of movement.

The decision to use hormone–replacement therapy is an individual one. It is based on the individual's particular goals and potential risks. The (generalized) goals of natural HRT are to (1) alleviate the symptoms caused by the natural decrease in production of hormones by the body, (2) replace the hormones to an extent to provide positive benefits, (3) bring the body back to normal hormonal balance, and (4) imitate the body's natural pattern as much as possible.

Table 6-2: Hormones an age-management physician can work with:

Name	Primary Function
Melatonin	The sleep hormone; helps you fall asleep, maintain good sleep and then causes you to wake. It creates the "biological clock" that regulates your days and nights. It also is a powerful antioxidant, protecting against heart disease and cancer by its abilities to "grab" free radicals. It acts as a muscle relaxant and lowers blood pressure.
Growth Hormone	As the name indicates, hGH is involved in growth in childhood and adolescence. In the adult it is responsible for muscle tone, bone integrity, organ protection, immune system preservation, energy and endurance while awake, restful sleep at night, skin integrity, a feeling of well-being, and helps with fat loss.
Thyroid Hormones (T3 and T4)	The primary acting thyroid hormone is T3, or triiodothyronine. It is involved with metabolic rate, heat and cold regulation, regulation of blood flow, responsiveness of mind and thought, prevention of dry hair and hair loss, and is involved with a number of other physiologic functions.
DHEA	Precursor to a number of hormones in the body including testosterone and estradiol. Energy booster, mood improver, increases sex drive in women, helps with memory enhancement.
Cortisol	The "stress hormone"; helps the body deal with stress. Also functions as an appetite stimulator, increases energy, and aids digestion. It is a strong anti-

	inflammatory and pain controller and is an immune system enhancer.
Aldosterone	Controls blood pressure when standing, elevates blood pressure when under stress.
ACTH	Controls adrenal secretion of the anti-stress hormones. It is vital in memory, specifically visual memory. It has calming effects, helps tan the skin, and prevents hair loss.
Calcitonin	Improves the strength of bones, helps your body deal with stress, mild control over the effect of inflammation.
Estrogen	Primary female hormone. Gives female sexual characteristics, including breasts, body shape, etc. Involved in pregnancy and menstruation. Keeps the skin smooth and unwrinkled. Prevents excessive hair growth. Keeps the vagina moist. Aids in sexual stimulation in women. Aids the immune system and impedes bone loss. Men need it, too, as it aids in sex drive and fertility.
Progesterone	Very important hormone during pregnancy. During the second half of the menstrual cycle, it causes the buildup of tissue in the uterus (caused by estrogen) to shed (menstruation). It is important for good, restful sleep and has a calming effect by reducing anxiety and worry.
Testosterone	Primary male hormone. Stimulates sex drive in men and women, reduces the risk of heart disease, builds and maintains muscle tone, stimulates the growth of hair. Provides a

	baseline sense of well-being, prevents depression and anxiety, and fights fatigue. It provides an awareness of confidence and self-esteem and prevents excessive reaction to situations. It aids sleep and tightens up the skin.
Pregnenolone	Precursor hormone for all the adrenal and sex hormones. Very high concentration in the brain and exceptionally important in memory and brain function. Also some involvement in fighting fatigue and depression.
Vasopressin	Aids in water preservation at night and prevents excessive bleeding in case of injury. Promotes memory and concentration.

Chapter Seven

Hormone Replacement Therapy in Women

Women have very well known and well–documented hormonal changes throughout their lifetimes. This is very obvious in women who are going through menopause. The changes the female body goes through as hormones decrease are numerous (See Tables 7–1 and 7–2.). In the year 2000, an estimated twenty million women became menopausal in the United States. Obviously, this is a subject that all of us, in one way or another, will have to deal with. Before going any further, it is important to distinguish two definitions: Estrogen replacement therapy (ERT) involves treatment using a number of different estrogens that are available; hormone replacement therapy (HRT) involves a combination of hormones, including estrogens, progesterone, and even androgens (testosterone).

TABLE 7-1: Symptoms Associated with a
Decrease in Estrogen

Anxiety	Depression
Dry skin	Headache
Heart palpitations	Hot flashes
Inability to reach orgasm	Lack of menstruation
Memory loss	Mood swings
Night sweats	Painful intercourse
Shortness of breath	Sleep disorders
Vaginal dryness	Vaginal shrinkage
Yeast infections	Others

TABLE 7-2: Symptoms Associated with a
Decrease in Progesterone

Acne	Asthma
Anxiety	Bloating
Cramps	Depression
Early menstruation	Emotional swings
Food cravings	Fuzzy thinking
Headache	Inability to concentrate
Insomnia	Irritability
Low libido	Moodiness
Painful breasts	Painful joints
Swollen breasts	Weight gain

Until recently, the only choice offered to women for ERT was Premarin, a hormone derived from the urine of pregnant mares (Pre – pregnant, Marin – mare, also called a conjugated equine estrogen). This synthetic hormone was at one time the most commonly prescribed medication in the United States. For progesterone replacement, the common surrogate is medroxyprogesterone acetate, a synthetic Progestin. Notice I have to differentiate Progesterone (natural) from Progestin (synthetic), a very important distinction when talking to your doctor (See Table 7–3 on The Woman's Health Initiative).

Unfortunately, current female hormone replacement therapy fails to take individual needs, backgrounds, and lifestyles into consideration. In many situations, women are offered a one–size–fits–all therapy when they approach their medical doctor for information on ERT. Hormones, and therefore hormonal response, are a very individual issue. Adequate time for adjustment and implementation are essential in finding an ideal amount not only to (and for example) control symptoms associated with hormonal loss, but also to ensure optimal health. The following is a quick review of the sex hormones, their actions, particularly in women, and a few of the signs and symptoms associated with deficiency. Recall, as I stated earlier, this list is neither all–inclusive, nor is it indicative of exacting deficiencies. In other words, *all* symptoms listed can (and always do) have multiple causes and etiologies. As I stated in the section on understanding disease, nothing ever has one cause; nothing can ever be isolated to one reason. (See Chapter 3, Understanding the Process of Disease)

Hormone replacement *must* be individualized!

Estrogens

The estrogens are responsible for normal growth and development of female sex organs, maintenance of secondary sex characteristics, promoting the proliferation and growth of specific cells in the body, protection against bone loss, and protection against heart disease. Without adequate estrogen, you may have male pattern hair distribution (loss on the head, gain on the body and face), vaginal dryness, fatigue, depression, and all the associated symptoms of menopause.

Progesterone

Progesterone is important for promoting the shed of the uterine lining during menstruation, is necessary for maintaining pregnancy (maintains the uterine lining and decreases uterine contractions), prepares the breasts for lactation (milk production and secretion), increases bone mass and density, and is metabolized to other active hormones. With insufficient levels of progesterone, one could have painful breasts and stomach bloating before menstruation and increased general anxiety and irritability. In my experience, women who are low in progesterone have a tendency for increased lower–body weight in the legs and stomach area and mild water retention in the hands and face.

Testosterone

Testosterone serves to enhance sex drive (libido), provide protection for the heart, enhance bone building, and improve energy level and mental alertness. It is also responsible for muscle growth and tone and aids in fat loss. Without it you may have decreased sexual desire, depression, fatigue, and low self–confidence. Memory and cognitive function may decrease, and the skin may look dry and pale. I have found in my practice that very low–dose testosterone replacement, when called for, greatly benefits a woman's everyday life. Energy as needed for daily events or sexual activities is greatly improved, as is her general sense of well–being.

Table 7-3: The Woman's Health Initiative

Hormone replacement, particularly estrogen replacement, has come under a lot of fire recently with the *Woman's Health Initiative*. This study was, in my opinion, somewhat flawed in its design and therefore in its results. Let me explain: First of all, the women who participated in the study did not fit the "normal" criteria of women seeking estrogen replacement; two thirds of the participants were older than sixty, and most were first-time hormone users. This differs from common practice, as most women who seek hormone replacement therapy are in their forties or early fifties. This is also a set up for the negative findings of the study including increased risk of blood clots, increased heart disease, and cancer. Women of this age, who have stopped producing natural hormones, are already at increased risk for all of the above conditions. Therefore, the study's finding of increased risk of these things can be partly attributed to the age of the woman involved with the study. The study also should be called the "Premarin and Provera Study," as these were the only two hormones utilized. The authors unfortunately labeled all hormone replacement as potentially dangerous when they should have labeled Premarin and Provera as potentially dangerous. Had they had a bio-identical hormone group, I think the findings would have been different. In summary, coupling the demographics of the women involved in the study (older than sixty, not pre-screened for disease) and the type of hormone used (synthetic and horse derived), this study, as it applies to the use of bio-identical hormones, is not valid and should not be used as a reference point for discussion.

Chapter Eight

Hormone Replacement
Therapy in Men

In the last chapter we reviewed menopause, that "life change" our mothers, grandmothers, wives, and daughters are subjected to in their lifetimes. However, not many people are familiar with the male menopause called *andropause*. This is a relatively new term in the medical and lay literature to define what happens to a man as he ages in relation to testosterone, the predominant male hormone. Andropause also involves a number of other hormonal, physiological, chemical, and psychosocial changes, but our discussion will focus on testosterone replacement. There is still some disagreement within the medical community as to whether this condition (and therefore treatment) actually exists. In this simple review, we will take the "in favor of" side and limit our discussion to the symptoms and treatment of andropause in relation to hormone replacement therapy, specifically testosterone. It is of interest that a number of ancient peoples, including Indians, Greeks, and Egyptians were aware that extracts of animal testes could be used to promote virility, potency, and vigor in men. Also of note, testosterone was the first hormone to be discovered, yet its overall role is still not completely defined.

Andropause is a natural reduction of androgens levels in the aging male. Andropause is similar to menopause in women without the obvious onset like the cessation of menstruation. The decreased levels of androgens may lead to distressing signs and symptoms for some men. The signs of andropause are loss of muscle mass, osteopenia, dry skin, insulin resistance, and visceral obesity. Other symptoms include tiredness, fatigue, mood change (depression), irritability, and sexual dysfunction, including decreased libido, erectile dysfunction, and an overall decreased quality of life.

So the next logical question is: Does testosterone decrease with age? A number of studies have shown that it does.[11–14] Bio–available testosterone and total testosterone can actually start decreasing in men's middle to late twenties!

The incidence and prevalence of andropause is increasing in the aging male population. In 2004, an estimated two to four million American men had andropause, and only five percent of those men were treated.[16] In 2002, the Massachusetts Male Aging Study[17] estimated an incidence of 481,000 new cases of androgen deficiency per year. The study was a large population based, random–samples cohort using 1709 men, ages forty to seventy, investigating the age-related trends of androgen levels in this age group.

Most men, however, begin to experience deleterious changes in their bodies somewhere between the ages of thirty and fifty–five. In the past, we attributed it to "growing old." A lot of information now points to changes in the levels of hormones that the body produces that help influence these changes. That is not to say that keeping the hormone levels at their youthful peak will prevent aging, but that some of the subjective and objective changes we see with aging may be related to this natural decrease in circulating hormones. Unlike changes females undergo at the start of and during menopause, such as the ceasing of menstruation, the symptoms of andropause tend to come on slower and more gradual. These signs and symptoms are quite impressive and are listed in Table 8–1.

Testosterone levels begin to decrease for a number of reasons. These include a decrease in the number of cells that produce testosterone and an increase in a protein called sex hormone binding globulin (SHBG), resulting in greater binding of testosterone with less of the free or "active" testosterone available for the body's use.

There is also a higher relative amount of estrogen, the predominant female hormone, with less testosterone being produced. This can be caused by an increase in aromatase activity (the hormone that converts testosterone to estrogen) partly due to the increase in fat that occurs with "normal" aging, as fatty tissue contains more aromatase activity than lean tissue. Alteration in liver function, zinc deficiencies and/or vitamin C deficiencies, obesity, and overuse of alcohol also add to the problem. A number of drug–induced estrogen imbalances can occur, and the ingestion of estrogen–enhanced food or environmental substances also contributes to the rise. This increase in estrogen can cause a change in fat distribution, a decrease in lean mass, breast development, and an enlarged prostate.

TABLE 8-1: Symptoms Associated with a
Decrease in Testosterone

Fatigue	Nervousness, anxiety, and irritability
Poor sleep quality or insomnia	Aches and pains
Body fat gain, particularly abdominal weight gain	Bone deterioration
Lean muscle deterioration and loss of strength	Hair loss
Decreased libido (sex drive)	Wrinkling and drying of the skin
Erectile dysfunction and reduced potency and/or penile size	Memory problems
Decreased ejaculatory force and volume	Depression
Reduced motivation	Increased apathy

Other effects of aging that we see include increasing amounts of heart disease, type–II diabetes, dementia, and other age–related conditions. While all of these have other causative factors, including diet, activity level, etc., the steady decline of testosterone is implicated as well.[1–10]

As early as 1944, data indicated a correlation between the above–mentioned symptoms and hormonal changes.[15] Men also experience psychosocial symptoms as they enter this stage of their lives. These range from death of family members, in particular their parents, to workplace and life–goal opportunities decreasing. Retirement becomes imminent. Friends and acquaintances develop diseases. These psychosocial events can add to the depression and reduced motivation experienced with a decrease in testosterone levels. These issues are very important not only to realize but also to equate with one's ability to handle them, and I have found that testosterone replacement aids men during this time in their lives.

Many men experience mild versions of andropause and, just as in the case with some women, some go through "the change" totally unscathed.

One method of treating the hormonal aspect of andropause is similar to that for women, natural hormone replacement therapy. In my opinion, the future will dictate hormone replacement therapy as commonly for men as it now does for women.

Hormones and, therefore, hormonal response are a very individual issue. Adequate time for adjustment and implementation are essential in finding an ideal amount not only to control symptoms associated with hormonal loss, but also to ensure optimal health.

There is no evidence that natural testosterone stimulates the development of prostate cancer, and, to my knowledge, there has been no relationship established between endogenous testosterone and benign prostate hyperplasia (BPH) and prostate cancer.[16] However, there *is* a contraindication to natural testosterone replacement therapy *in the presence* of prostate cancer.

Testosterone deficiency has been implicated in accounting for a number of the symptoms listed in Table 8–1. Again, it is beyond the scope of this book to delve into great detail, but I would like to review a few more medically related examples:

Blood Pressure[5]

In one study, researchers tested 1,132 men thirty to seventy–nine years of age. Those with hypertension, categorically defined as systolic blood pressure (top number) greater than 160 mmHg and/or diastolic blood pressure (bottom number) greater than 95 mmHg, had significantly lower testosterone levels than non–hypertensive patients. This demonstrates an inverse relationship between testosterone and blood pressure (people with low testosterone had higher blood pressure).

Brain Function[4]

Short–term testosterone supplementation improves spatial functions and verbal memory in healthy older men, according to a report published in the *Journal of Neurology*. Twenty–five healthy men, fifty to eighty years of age, received a six–week course of weekly placebo or testosterone (100 mg) injections. Spatial memory, spatial ability, and verbal memory were significantly improved in the testosterone group compared to their baseline cognitive function and the cognitive function of the placebo group. This study also demonstrated an increase in estradiol (a type of estrogen) in the treatment group, and the researchers commented on the fact that it is difficult to tell if this hormone or the testosterone was responsible for the noted improvements.

Heart Disease[3, 10]

One study demonstrated that a decrease in testosterone levels with age is associated with potentially unfavorable changes in blood lipids. Triglycerides, an independent risk factor for heart disease, were higher, and HDL cholesterol (the good cholesterol) was lower.

Body Composition[1, 6, 8]

Studies have shown that testosterone treatment was followed by a decrease of visceral fat mass, as measured by computerized tomography (CT scan), without a change in body mass, subcutaneous fat mass, or lean body mass. Other studies have demonstrated that men with increased abdominal obesity (yet another risk factor for cardiac disease) have lower testosterone levels than men without central obesity.

Other medical improvements with testosterone therapy include a decrease in insulin resistance, improved blood sugar, a decrease in serum cholesterol,[6] increase in bone density,[10] and sleep improvement.[2]

Insulin Resistance

Testosterone is an important regulator in insulin sensitivity, and low levels of testosterone have been observed in men with diabetes, metabolic syndrome, insulin resistance, and coronary artery disease (CAD). A study of metabolic syndrome showed that men with testosterone levels in the lower third were 1.7 to 2.8 times more likely to have metabolic syndrome.[19,20] The association between low testosterone and insulin resistance is mediated by obesity and visceral adipose tissue in non–diabetic men.[19] Another study found that testosterone levels and glycosylated hemoglobin levels are inversely related.[21] Low testosterone levels may be an independent risk factor for the development of diabetes, and it has been shown that low ranges within the normal range of free and total testosterone were associated with diabetes, independent of adiposity.[22]

Improvements in the other andropause symptoms mentioned (sex drive, depression, skin changes, etc.) also occur with testosterone replacement, as has been noted in a number of well–designed studies.

There are, of course, risks involved with therapeutic testosterone replacement (as with any medication), and these need to be discussed and reviewed on an individual basis with a physician trained in this area.

Most of the available evidence suggests that testosterone replacement is potentially beneficial to aging men, particularly in the areas of bone density and body composition. However, the amount and longevity of the beneficial effects are not yet known.[10]

Table 8–2 is the St. Louis University Androgen Deficiency in Aging Male (ADAM) Questionnaire.[18] If you are male and, after reading this chapter, feel you may have andropause, fill out this questionnaire and take it to your physician or health care provider to discuss possible intervention.

Table 8-2: ADAM Questionnaire

St. Louis University Androgen Deficiency in Aging Male (ADAM) 18 Questionnaire:
A positive screen for hypogonadism includes a "Yes" response to numbers 1 and 7 or any other 3 questions.

1. Do you have a decrease in libido (sex drive)?
2. Do you have a lack of energy?
3. Do you have a decrease in strength and/or endurance?
4. Have you lost height?
5. Have you noticed a decreased enjoyment of life?
6. Are you sad and/or grumpy?
7. Are your erections less strong?
8. Have you noticed a recent deterioration in your ability to play sports?
9. Are you falling asleep after dinner?
10. Has there been a recent deterioration in your work performance?

Chapter Nine

The Fallacy of Scale Weight: Understanding Body Composition

My wish is that everyone reading this book or adjusting their weight in general would understand the problems associated with the *dreaded scale*. I can recall my mother being very upset that the scale "can lie so often without conscience." Even in her jest, she hit it right on the head. Scale weight is misleading, uninformative, and essentially a terrible way to judge the accuracy or strength of any weight–adjustment program. I believe it is crucial for you to stay focused on lean mass gain and fat loss, *not* weight loss.

Our current paradigm dictates that the scale weight changes, whether from fat, water, or lean mass. Unfortunately, this thinking is flawed because what you are losing is more important than how much you are losing. The word "loss" in and of itself has negative connotations. I do not know about you, but I get rather moody when I lose something, from car keys to that to–do list I lost in the pile on my desk. Forget about losing weight and start focusing on *gaining* lean mass. *Gain? Did he just say gain?* Yes I did! Focus on gaining muscle, because that is what burns the fat! Doesn't gaining something sound and feel better than losing something?

Lean mass makes up a majority of your metabolism: For every pound of lean mass you put on from the time you start your optimal health program, you greatly increase your metabolic engine. You burn more calories just sitting there! In the same sense, every pound of lean mass you lose results in a large number of calories a day you are not burning. These programs that claim thirty pounds in thirty days can help you lose thirty pounds of scale weight. Unfortunately, however, and to their extreme discredit, ninety percent of that scale weight loss will be lean mass. It goes without saying, based on the above information, that by doing this you have destroyed your metabolism. The disservice to you is literally criminal! That is why we have such severe diet "yo–yos" out there. Lose twenty, gain thirty, lose fifteen, gain twenty–five…As you can see, there is a continual and gradual *increase* in your scale weight (all of which is fat with this type of fluctuation) and the source for extreme prejudice with all current diet programs. What scale weight fails to recognize is lean mass versus fat mass. Your goal, from the time you finish this sentence, should be to focus on body composition and a continual *increase* in lean mass. The side effect of increasing lean mass is automatic…fat falls off!

Doesn't gaining something sound and feel better than losing something?

To better help you understand this point, I will briefly review body composition and the measurement of fat and lean mass.

The evaluation of body composition permits quantification of the major structural components of the body: muscle, bone, and fat. Body fat testing not only determines what (approximate) percentage of total mass is fat, but also gives the amount of lean mass available. Since muscle makes up the greatest percentage of lean mass, it is a good indication of how much muscle comprises a body.

Body fat testing has many implications, associations, and undertones. Utilization can be for medical purposes—by a physician monitoring progress of a rigorous diet and exercise program, or inquiry by an athlete to help direct performance– or appearance–enhancing efforts. There are many options available for the inquisitive mind and body in the determination of body composition. I have found, through years of experience, that skin–fold assessments are not only the least expensive, but also one of the most accurate in the determination of change. Let me repeat that: the determination of *change!* In other words, the total number does not matter and should not be focused on. Part of our definition of health, as you recall, is a continuing process of transformation or positive change. This is one of my primary goals with this book: empowering you to continually improve.

Unfortunately, our present system utilizes height–weight tables and body mass index (BMI) to determine if a person is "overweight." Such methods do not provide any information about the relative composition or quality of an individual's body. The term "overweight" only refers to body mass in excess of some standard, usually the average body mass for a given stature. Being above average or not ideal by height–weight charts does not dictate whether or not you need to go on a weight–loss program. For example, as I write this information, I am fifty–six pounds "overweight" in terms of my insurance company's height/weight tables (5' 8" and 210 pounds where they say I should weight 154 pounds...) and my BMI is 32 (anything greater than 30 is considered obese). Here is what they fail to account for: My percentage body fat is currently eight percent, placing my lean mass at 193.2 pounds and my fat mass at 16.8 pounds. Determination of body composition is a much better way to actually see what your body consists of: Are you fat or just heavy? To better understand body composition, it is important to understand the difference between lean body mass and fat mass as it relates to total composition of the human body.

Essential Fat and Storage Fat

The total amount of body fat exists in two storage sites. The first site, called *essential fat*, is the fat stored in the marrow of bones, heart, lungs, liver, spleen, kidneys, intestines, muscles, brain, and spinal cord. This fat is required for normal physiological functioning (i.e. life). In the female, this fat includes sex–specific fat or sex–characteristic fat. It is not known if this particular fat is expendable or serves as reserve storage. The second storage site is termed *storage fat*. This is the popular fat that accumulates in adipose (fatty) tissue. This "nutritional reserve" includes fatty tissue that protects organs and the fat located directly under the skin. The proportion of storage fat is very similar in males and females (average twelve percent in men and fifteen percent in women), while the amount of essential fat is approximately four times higher in women. This is most likely needed for childbearing and hormone–related functions.

Lean Body Mass

For purposes of this book, lean body mass will be viewed as muscle and bone. Lean body mass does not necessarily indicate fat–free mass. Lean body mass contains a small percentage of fat (roughly three percent) within the central nervous system (brain and spinal cord), marrow of bones, and internal organs. It should be everyone's goal to increase or, at a minimum, to maintain their lean mass weight. In this book, we will use "lean mass" interchangeably with "muscle." Remember that for every pound of muscle you put on, your body burns a number of extra calories per day.

Forget about weight *loss!* Focus on muscle *gain!*

Why keep track? Keeping track of your progress, specifically gains and losses, is one of the most important keys to health renovation. This area is often overlooked because it seems confusing, time consuming, or too technical to learn and accurately track. In my experience, I have found that those who take the time to learn how to measure and monitor their results have better and more consistent results than those who do not. Do not overlook the importance of *objectively* measuring your progress!

While I consider it essential for everyone who is after optimal health and fat loss to track their body composition with an accepted measuring device, I chose not to include one with this book. They are available, however, with detailed instructions. Just contact my office and I will send you skin calipers and an instruction manual (See Appendix IX, How to Contact Dr. Willey). Until then, the following chapter provides you with a weekly measuring chart that will help you track to important data sets: Objective Measurements and Subjective Input.

Chapter Ten

Understanding Objective and Subjective Data Tracking

When I meet with a client in a one–on–one situation, we follow any and every variable we can to ensure our efforts are progressing in a positive way. We use two broad categories for this purpose: Objective and Subjective Data. Objective Data is information that is impartial or independent of the user's frame of mind or input. This would include blood pressure, cholesterol levels, body composition (lean mass and fat mass), scale weight (*if* used correctly), cardiovascular endurance, muscle strength, blood sugar, etc. Subjective Data is information that *is* biased or inclined by the user's state of mind or perception. This set of data includes energy levels, cognitive abilities, moods, hunger, how one is sleeping, sexual vigor, and satisfaction, etc. It is important to realize that there is some crossover between the two areas. For our purposes, and as you achieve health maximization, categorizing them with the following chart will help you literally *see* results and then make appropriate changes/adjustments.

Keeping Track

The chart provided allows you to see subjective and objective facts to help you track your progress toward optimal health. I would suggest you make a copy of the chart and fill it out *once a week* for as long as you need to. This is provided for three primary reasons: 1) to give you the ability to *see* changes taking place; 2) to give you a framework to look back on and utilize as a tool for future use and program design; and finally 3) to get you in the habit of tracking yourself with more reliable data than the scale. In the *Objective* portion of the tracking chart, we will use *four* of the primary objective data marks. These include clothes fitting differently, scale weight, cardiovascular endurance, and muscle strength. Other sets of data, such as blood pressure, cholesterol levels, and blood sugar, though very important to track (and I would encourage you to do so with your medical professional), will not be followed here. It has been my experience with hundreds of patients whom I have had the good fortune to track all of the above that seeing changes in these four standards helps the other health measures change for the better as well! The *Subjective* result section includes what I have experienced to be the "big eight." There are eight subjective questions that tie directly into optimal health. I encourage each one of you to utilize the information you keep track of in the future to help you to make adjustments and life changes that will keep you on a continual progression of positive change.

Following the Algorithm

As you view the chart, you will see a simple *yes* and *no* tracking system. The progression is simple: If you have at least *two* yes answers for the objective section and *four* yes answers for the subjective section, you will need to advance your diet by adding one to your Eating Variable and determining your new dietary caloric intake (reviewed in detail in Chapter 16). The Eating Variable is a number I have established to help you find your average daily caloric needs and will differ based on your amount of exercise and progress.

If you do not answer two objective and four subjective questions with a yes, you need to use the back of the chart to Reevaluate and Review (our version of R and R). To reevaluate your program means to look at the previous week and determine a few simple facts: 1) Did I follow the eating program at least eighty percent of the time (this includes food timing, suggested amounts, etc.)? 2) Did I plan my food intake according to my schedule? 3) Did I exercise to the best of my abilities and as often as suggested? 4) Were there any confounding variables that I did not account for (e.g., stress, illness, etc.)?

If you answer no to any one of these questions, Reevaluate and Review the previous week's eating and exercise and try to determine what may have altered your course. Be honest with yourself. No one is looking, and the only one you'll be cheating is yourself. After doing this, recalculate your daily caloric need using the equations in Table 16–3.

Once you have mastered this manner of gauging yourself and your quest for optimal health, the meticulous part of filling out the chart can lessen. I would suggest, however, that you keep it up. As the old saying goes: If you fail to plan, you plan to fail. Part of your quest for optimum health involves staying on top of things and planning for the future. I have found this is done best by reviewing the past. History does repeat itself. We will cover more of this topic in Chapter 19, Progression Through Roadblocks, Walls, and Plateaus. Review the charts and keep them in mind as you start to gain an understanding of the material following.

Table 10-1: *What Does Your Doctor Look Like Naked?*
Optimal Health Tracking Chart

Directions:
Circle the most appropriate answer to the provided question.
If you have two yes answers for the objective section and
four yes answersfor the subjective section, continue with the
program as directed. If you do not, use the back of the chart
to reevaluate and review.

OBJECTIVE DATA

My clothes are starting to fit me differently.	YES	NO
My scale weight is changing in the direction I want.	YES	NO
My cardiovascular endurance is improving.	YES	NO
My strength has improved.	YES	NO

If you answered yes to two or more,
continue program as directed.

SUBJECTIVE DATA

I feel better overall.	YES	NO
I am sleeping well.	YES	NO
I am thinking with good clarity.	YES	NO
My mood is improved.	YES	NO
My outlook on my health is better.	YES	NO
I have more energy.	YES	NO
I am satisfied with my food intake.	YES	NO
I am enjoying life.	YES	NO

If you answered yes to four or more,
continue program as directed.

Reevaluate and Review

Did I follow the program at least 80% of the time?	YES	NO
Did I exercise to the best of my abilities and according to the schedule?	YES	NO
Did I Schedule my food intake according to my schedule every day?	YES	NO
Were there any confounding variables that I did not account for (e.g., stress, illness, etc.)?	YES	NO

If you answer no to any one of these questions, Reevaluate and Review the previous week's eating and exercise and try to determine what may have altered your course.

Be honest with yourself, no one is looking, and the only one you'd be cheating is yourself. After doing this, recalculate your daily caloric need using the equations in Table 16-3.

Chapter Eleven

Wonderment

I have learned more about life by observing children than I ever did by reflecting upon the writings of philosophers.

G.K. Chesterton

I have memorized the movie *Shrek* by DreamWorks. I am not kidding. I know the entire movie, line for line, scene by scene. I find myself quoting lines from the movie that have relevance in my everyday life. Not just once in a while either, but all the time. I often chuckle when I respond to a question using one of the many aphorisms. No one else, except possibly my wife, knows why I am laughing. I do. That movie kills me (in the "roll over and laugh to the point of tears and joy" sense, that is).

Let me explain my passion for "Monkey." Those of you who have experienced this movie know that Shrek is an ogre, a "terrifying" one at that (per his own words). So why did I just call him Monkey? That is part of my explanation. For the last year, since my daughter was about sixteen months old, she has been fascinated to the point of perpetual awe with Shrek. Shrek, in her little mind, is the spitting image of a stuffed monkey her uncle gave her a few months prior to her interest in watching movies. Therefore, when she wants to visit with Shrek, she asks my wife or me for "monkey." Now on to my fascination.

Let me provide you with a nightly scenario that occurs at my house. After I come home from work or the gym, my wife, my daughter, and I eat dinner. We then wrestle around the house, play outside on the slide or swing, or discuss in detail all the many toys my daughter has. Once fatigue starts to set in on my daughter, long after it has afflicted me, by the way, she gets a deliberate grin on her face. Her eyes go to the top and left side of her head as if she is in deep thought, she tilts her head sideways, getting as close as possible to my face, and says, in the most irresistible whisper, "Monkey… watch Monkey?"

> "…the most powerful tool in the longevity and health quest—the art and practice of Wonderment!"

Obviously armed with the knowledge that Dad is a big sucker, this development occurs every night. And in the same manner, Dad, being the big sucker, sits and watches *Shrek* with her nightly.

That is how I have memorized *Shrek*. But let me explain what is happening on a slightly deeper level. My daughter has demonstrated the most powerful tool in the longevity and health quest—the art and practice of Wonderment. Every night, without fail, I watch my daughter's eyes widen, her face elongate as her lips purse, each time the dragon makes its first appearance in the movie. It is as if it is happening for the first time, again, and again, and again…She fails to see the monotony of the action. She has not succumbed to the acquired boredom we all master as we age. The true fascination that we have that first time is not lost with her. She finds joy in the mundane, excitement in the repetitive. She has Wonderment. This is applicable for every scene in the movie. Now I, too, look for the dragon's appearance with a sort of fearful joy. I, too, am thrilled to see the princess beat up the robbers in the woods. I, too, feel the pain when "Monkey is crying." Wonderment has set in.

We have covered a large number of topics so far in this book. All have dealt with and involved the attainment and/or maintenance of optimal health. None, however, are as important as this chapter.

I initially intended for this chapter to be at the beginning of the book. Actually, in retrospect, it should be a book in and of itself, not due to the amount of content, but the true importance of this topic. I will not pretend to be an expert in the area of optimal mental and emotional health and function. There are a number of self–help books available for delving further into the topic. I will, however, count myself as an authority in practice, in my own life and in the viewing of thousands of patients' lives. Hence the reason for this chapter: Ultimate Health is not possible without Wonderment.

An admission before I start: So far this book has been written on twenty–plus years of schooling, reading, studying, and experience. This chapter came to light, and the power of Wonderment was sealed in my life, with the birth of my daughter, Madilyn. In the last two years, she has taught me more than all the schooling, books, and degrees ever could. She has given me the reason for life itself and, for the first time, an understanding of unconditional love.

G.K. Chesterton, a well–known early last century writer (1874–1936), once declared that he learned more about life by observing children than he ever did by reflecting upon the writings of philosophers. He was right. The ability for us "adults" to view life through the eyes of a child can be one of the most powerful tools in the quest for ultimate health as defined by this book. One argument I come up against when this statement is acknowledged is that health and disease are not topics of children. I agree. As Ravi Zacharias, one of my favorite Christian apologists, states in his short writing entitled

The Romance of Enchantment: "Exhilaration alone is not sufficient to find lasting fulfillment. Yet undeniably, wonder plays a role in satisfying our hunger for meaning. What I am arguing is that for a child, meaning is gained by her recognition of the awe–inspiring reality that surrounds her life."

Our quest for ultimate health and the steps it takes to understand the process (see Chapter 4), be it weight loss, lean mass gain, defeating food cravings, or whatever strides need to take place, the ability to see the big picture and enjoy the mundane must be factored in. Failure and disappointment occur when boredom sets in. When the mundane overpowers you, the setup has occurred and the *process of disease* begins.

Wonderment is the act of amazement, awe, and wonder. Synonyms for this verb include astonishment, amazement, bewilderment, fascination, surprise, and stupefaction. In simplistic terms, and in relevance to this book and the achievement of ultimate health, it is: The need to find the everyday, the mundane, the ordinary, in a new light of mystery, enthrallment, and enrapture.

At one time, and in a number of our memories, we were amazed at the simplest of things: a sunrise or sunset, the crashing of waves on a rocky shore, how good food tastes, the smell of our parents' clothes. These once were (and should be) amazing things, enthralling and capturing.

My daughter demonstrates Wonderment every day. The ceiling cap that a ceiling fan would connect to above my bed *does* look like the moon! Walking up stairs *is* an amazing thing! The ability to sit at the table with Mom and Dad *is* quite the honor and thrilling to no end! Seeing a horse and all its majestic curves and shapes, with a concealed power that can be felt in its presence, *is* one of the coolest things I can think of. This is Wonderment. And this must be obtained to achieve ultimate health.

One issue in the process of ultimate health is the monotony that seems to overpower people while they work at it. Exercising every day, eating right every day—just saying it sounds boring, and I am an addict! One way to truly prevent boredom from setting in is Wonderment. Find a thrill in the everyday. Look for it, look hard and deep. It is there, just muddied by the pressures and stress of life.

Why do we lose wonderment?

H.L. Mencken said, "The problem with life is not that it's a tragedy, but that it's a bore." As I have explained in previous chapters, I am not by any means a wise sage or philosopher. I am, however, an observer. Dealing with people one on one, as I do in my practice, I have come to learn a commonality in just about everyone I see. Part of health is joy and Wonderment. Translating what I see and hear in my practice and then having the opportunity to watch my daughter live life, I see an immense contrast. People have lost wonderment. Why? Again, as an observer, I feel it is the everyday stresses and demands that overpower our vision and senses and place us in the daily grind of survival. Stress, jobs, relationships, money issues, etc.—all of these things become horse blinders. Our vision and outlook are narrowed. We focus on the next paycheck, the current problems at work, the future…you name it, whatever your personal *raison d'tre*, it has consumed you and taken your wonder with it. It has happened to me and still does happen to me. It happens to us all. So what can we do about it? How do you get that powerful anti–aging tool back and put it to use?

Obtaining and Maintaining Wonderment

First and foremost in the quest for Wonderment is the realization that nothing matters yet everything is important. That's right. Nothing matters. Everything eventually burns. Your house, your car, your bills, and your money, all of it one day will be of no use to you. What am I saying here? Perspective. Gain perspective. If you were stripped of all worldly goods, both assets and liabilities, what's left? I will tell you what's left: health, family, friends, relationships, and a beautiful world to live in—green grass, majestic mountains, inspiring sunrises, awesome storms, beauty in everything you can behold. Even man-made beauty in skyscrapers, large bridges, and computers is wonderful. The ability to obtain Wonderment is right outside your door. Look for it. Get inspired by it. Become awestruck by it all around you. Everything within earshot, eyesight, or touch deserves it.

Wonderment can also be obtained by searching out *God*. As I mentioned in the dedication, true joy and optimal spiritual health, though not discussed in detail in this book, are as essential as any portion of this book. Look up and not around when facing life's problems and challenges. May I, once again, suggest reading Rick Warren's book entitled *The Purpose Driven Life*, as it provides a forty–day progression toward optimal spiritual health, which, as I stated before, is essential in optimal health!

Become amazed by simple things. Think of the mechanisms at work every time you take a step—balance, joint movement, environmental awareness, timed muscle contraction, blood flow, nerves signaling. What an amazing thing!

Become amazed by simple things!

Think what it took to build the building you are sitting in right now. Think of the sky. How high is it? Why is it blue? There are, of course, answers to many of life's questions, but that is part of the problem. Let an astrophysicist tell you how high the sky is, yet maintain your Wonderment.

That brings me to my next point: Question *everything*! Nothing should ever fear questions. No government, idea, religion, person, place, or thing.

Become like a child. Let simple things amaze you. So you know the mechanisms of air travel, look at the size of a 747 and be amazed that that thing can even get off the ground! The best way to become childlike in your outlook on life, in my opinion, is to start hanging around them. Why do you think grandparents love their grandbabies? Because of the family heritage? Maybe. That would be the boring answer, the answer of someone lacking Wonderment. I think it is because they bring back Wonderment, joy, simplicity, and thoughtfulness. Youth is restored when youth is sought.

I cannot stress enough to my clients or to you, the reader: Your quest for ultimate and lasting health will be stopped in its tracks unless Wonderment is allowed back into your life. It crept away, now go and grab it back and hold on to it! Get up tomorrow and do it again. Seek it out daily. Your body, your mind, your emotions, your family, and friends will all thank you for it!

Ultimate and true health will be lacking without it!

Table 11-1: Simple Steps to Wonderment

Look up, *not* around
Question Everything.
Become amazed by simple things.
Find some children to play with.
Gain perspective—nothing is worth not being happy and healthy!
KISS principle of life: Keep It Simple, Smarty!

Chapter Twelve

Those Who Have Done It
and Now Are Doing It

I have had the honor and privilege of caring for hundreds of people who are looking for true health and life improvement. The concepts defined in this book have been constantly refined and molded to work for everyone who puts their heart, mind, and time into it. I am going to review a few typical clients who have put this program into practice and application. Though they spent a short time with me, they started a lifetime of knowledge, understanding of consequences, and the power to obtain and persevere in health maximization.

Jim and Jane

History
A personal trainer friend of mine introduced Jim and Jane to my practice. They were each fifty–five years old at the time we began working together. They had no major medical problems, but were frustrated with the lack of progress they had experienced in their attempts to get healthy. They stated their overall reasons for consultation with me were to 1) feel better, 2) increase energy, 3) reduce weight (stating they had a lot of trouble in past), and 4) improve their immune systems after a recent bout with colds and flu–like symptoms.

Intervention

Our intervention was exactly as this book dictates. We started with a specific dietary, supplemental, and exercise intervention/treatment based on current likes and dislikes, goals, history of previous attempts, and schedules. We utilized the same supplemental intervention that this book suggests, and I helped Jim and Jane to understand the power of food as a medicine or drug (see Chapter 13, Developing an Understanding of Food). I had the privilege of seeing them weekly for subjective evaluations and objective measurements to ensure progress and ease of use and to stay one step ahead of the dreaded monotony. They each, in turn, learned how to make adjustments to their programs to continuously "shock the system" and never allow their bodies to conform to their current intervention.

Results

Our results, very representative of this program, were outstanding in every sense of the word (See the chart below). Jim was sleeping better, had more energy than he knew what to do with, and told me, "I feel better now than I can ever remember feeling!" Jane was equally successful. She experienced improved energy, a general and consistent sense of wellbeing, and most notable to her, *no illness*, not even a headache, following the start of the program!

Table 12-1: Jim's and Jane's Results

JIM			JANE		
Objective Measure	Start date	12 weeks later	Objective Measure	Start date	12 weeks later
Scale Weight	176 lbs.	166 lbs.	Scale Weight	148 lbs.	135 lbs.
Fat %	21.7%	9.9%	Fat %	37.5%	27.4%
Fat lbs.	38.192 lbs.	16.434 lbs.	Fat lbs.	55.5 lbs.	36.99 lbs.
Lean Mass	137.81 lbs.	149.57 lbs.	Lean Mass	92.5 lbs.	98.01 lbs.

Larry

History

Larry is a very pleasant fifty–four–year–old male who came to me for a totally different reason. He had a long and tenuous history of severe and debilitating headaches and had recently suffered a severe exacerbation following a motor vehicle accident. On presentation he was on multiple drugs and medications, and he was seeing a *number* of health care providers, including medical doctors, chiropractors, massage therapists, physical therapists, etc. He was experiencing little to no relief from his headaches, despite these efforts.

Intervention

We started with the basic premise and concepts found in this book. Following a thorough review of Larry's medical records, personal history, and inventory, and an examination to rule out "hidden" causes of his symptoms, we started by changing his eating patterns, utilizing the information found in this book with a slight twist to it. I utilized a simple elimination diet that consisted of removing known food allergens that may have been involved with his symptoms. We then incorporated exercise and movement therapy that involved a combination of resistance training and cardiovascular exercises. I started him on essential vitamins and antioxidants, hormone replacement therapy, as well as food directed to treat his symptoms and the underlying cause of his symptoms. One area of great importance was helping Larry to learn techniques of stress reduction and control, involving little more than simple lifestyle modification with the incorporation of exercise and a *planned* eating schedule. Once we started seeing results, we began slowly tapering him off his current medications. (Only attempt this under medical supervision for any conditions you may have.)

Results

Larry did fantastically! He eventually got off all of his maintenance medications! Larry had a notable fat/weight loss and an unbelievable increase in his energy and vitality. His general sense of wellbeing greatly improved, and he noted positive changes at work, including increased productivity and pride. He became knowledgeable about foods and other "things" that trigger headaches, as well as how to use food in the prevention of headaches. He obtained a "body and mind education" that will give him the power to control symptoms and maintain Health Maximization for the rest of his life!

Vicky

History

Vicky is a forty–two–year–old motivated self–employed go–getter who is a classic example of someone who succeeded, but not by the current standards. She made drastic changes in her body composition, size, shape, and energy levels; however, her scale weight hardly moved (see Chapter 9, The Fallacy of Scale Weight: Understanding Body Composition). She had/has minimal medical problems, but has had a tough time with eating and getting any results from exercise prior to meeting with me. Her goals were to develop whole body health, get her metabolism moving, firm up, and learn more about her body. She had read, and then attempted, a number of diet programs, but was at a loss as to why they did or did not work.

Intervention

We started with the basics, developing an understanding of whole body health. Her initial eating program taught her to eat active carbohydrates in the morning, following exercise, and to slowly decrease them throughout the day. Dinner consisted of lean meats, green vegetables, and salads. She ate smaller, more frequent meals, and started to get the good feeling of being properly hydrated. As we worked together, she developed an understanding of how her body was reacting toward foods and the importance of food timing (See Chapter 14).

Results

If one were to simply look at scale weight, Vicky did terribly! Her scale weight only changed, with some minor fluctuations in between, three pounds in fourteen weeks. Her percent body fat, however, went from 37.4% to 23.7%! None of her clothes fit, she was firm, and, in her words, she "looked stunning in a sleeveless evening gown!"

I have the honor of calling Vicky my friend now, as our families have gotten together on a more social basis. She is ever in hot pursuit of learning and the quest for that elusive understanding of why her body responds to food the way it does.

Lonni

History

What a great gal. Lonni came to me after she saw a picture of herself on a holiday occasion with her family. She was (and I quote) "disgusted." She was a classic chronic exerciser, but admitted that the "whole picture of health is elusive." She had what I call the typical American eating plan: no breakfast, chips and crackers when she walked by them during the day, and a large dinner late in the evening, usually at a restaurant. Starting at 5'4" and 181 pounds, she measured in at thirty–five percent body fat.

Intervention

Lonni and I started out with a simple eating plan, focusing on the *how–to* versus the *whats*. She learned to eat a good breakfast following her exercise and to eat regularly scheduled snacks, and she slowly learned to decrease her active carb intake throughout the day. She also learned to eat at home once in a while, but when she could not, dinner consisted of lean meats and salads as early in the evening as possible.

We also changed her exercise schedule. She learned to train smarter, not harder. By drastically cutting back the amount of time she spent exercising, she made rapid improvements in strength and endurance, and in her favorite sport, tennis.

Results

Lonni was one whose scale weight followed her fat. She dropped forty pounds of scale weight in four months. Her lean mass took a hit initially, but with modifications to her exercise program to include more weight lifting and less aerobics, she was able to maintain her muscle. Her percentage body fat fell below twenty, and she dropped from a size sixteen to a size four!

DB

History
DB was referred to me by a personal trainer due to his elevated triglyceride levels. He had numbers ranging from seven hundred to eight hundred, and despite the attempts of numerous doctors, he never got it lower than four hundred. He also had borderline blood pressure issues that he was watching closely, as he was told he would likely need medication at some point. DB was an avid bodybuilder and weight lifter who had followed the sport with great enthusiasm, but, as he put it, never really figured it out. He also had some complaints of shoulder pain and some sporadic shortness of breath, which he attributed to allergies. Other than high lipid levels, his medical history was relatively free of problems.

Intervention
DB was provided an initial eating program that, contrary to *all* he was told in the past, actually included fat. He undertook the *style* of eating that we will review in detail in Chapters 14–17, and, like Lonni, started exercising smarter, not harder.

Results
DB dropped an incredible fifteen–plus percent body fat! In his words, he has now "got it"! Understanding the style of eating and the process of health enabled him to accomplish goals only dreamed about in the past. As for his lipid problem, I will let the numbers speak for themselves. (PS: no medication!)

Table 12-2: DB's Lab Work

Date	Total Cholesterol	Triglycerides	HDL	CRP - HS (marker of inflammation)
3/11/03	263	738	43	0.26 mg/dl
6/12/03	198	136	42	0.13 mg/dl

In my goal to keep this book as concise as possible, I will limit the examples I use to the above. Some of those reading this may be Larrys or Vickys and/or DBs. If not, the concepts are the same. In the next chapter we get to the heart of the matter, *Developing an Understanding of Food*. To truly understand optimal health, the previous chapters were essential…one might say your appetizers. Now for the main course…(Pun intended!)

Chapter Thirteen

Developing an Understanding of Food

The title of this chapter says it all. Endurance and knowledge, without reliance on a quick fix or a gimmick program, are the way to sustained weight optimization. The key to any health maximization or optimization program is the fuel you utilize for your body. Just as you would never think of putting water in the gas tank of your automobile, you should not put anything but the best into your system. You have to think of food in terms of consequences. Just as putting water in your gas tank would have a very dire set of consequences, so does putting less than optimal food into your system. This does not mean you can *never* eat a treat or something less than ideal. Quite the opposite. When you have conditioned your body for optimal health by learning *how* to eat instead of focusing on *what* to eat and thereby increased your lean mass (thus increasing your metabolism), you have the opportunity to eat what you please without affecting your progress (refer to the definition of health in Chapter 4).

Act in Haste, Repent at Leisure...

A brief, though I hold my tongue, proclamation of one of the biggest charades ever perpetrated by the food/marketing industry: low fat and diet food. Never in the history of man has a more criminal act been pulled on the masses. Simple question: Why are obesity and all its associated diseases so prevalent with all the low fat and diet foods out there? Answer: Because this *is* one of the primary causes of the obesity and disease epidemics in our country! Let me explain: Just because fat on your body is bad does not mean that fat in your mouth is bad. Fat is needed for a number of physiological processes, including fat burning. We will cover more about this later, but for now it suffices to say that fat is not bad. I was once in an argument with a registered dietician (one of many), and we were arguing over the Atkins style of eating. While I am only a proponent of Atkins' style as a short–term diet option and not a lifestyle, I am in the same ballpark when it comes to a lot of the complex (I call them active carbohydrates, as you will see below) carbohydrates causing a number of problems. The registered dietician's argument was, "You cannot remove an entire food group from someone's diet and lose weight or be healthy." My response was simple in turn: "What have you and the whole American Dietetics Association done with fat? You have removed an entire food group." All of these low–fat foods have one thing in common: high sugar. Diet foods cut the fat and add sugar in its place, thereby reducing calories but exposing the body to more harmful substances. Not all calories are created equal! I will elucidate this more in future writings, but for now please know that diet foods and low fat foods are a problem, not a solution to our overweight epidemic.

Here comes another paradigm revolution: Food is a drug! By every term and definition of a drug, food fits. My definition of a drug is any substance that affects the structure or functioning of a living organism.

In my experience, once my patients have come to this realization, once their paradigm has shifted, a few key events take place: They realize that food (like drugs) has specific effects, interactions, and side effects. They understand that food has consequences. They understand that like most prescription drugs, you occasionally need *another* drug to combat the side effects of the first (and it can occasionally become exponential in process). They realize that food is very powerful and cannot only affect them *while they eat*, in terms of cravings, fat storage, etc., but sometimes *up to seventy–two hours later*. Francis Bacon said, "Knowledge and human power are synonymous," and "Knowledge itself is power." Believe me, gaining a firm understanding that food is a drug is one of the most powerful things you can do for your health, your body, and your longevity.

"Knowledge Itself is Power."

-Francis Bacon

One shining example of this comes in the form of some of the most developed and meticulous bodies around: bodybuilders and physique artists (such as models and fitness stars). These dedicated individuals can tell you precisely the five W's (Who, What, Where, When, and Why) of food intake and how it affects their bodies. For them to, as we call it in the sport, "dial in" just right for that very short period of time of perfection (when their bodies are at the lowest imaginable body fat, lean mass is at its current peak, hydration status is perfected, etc.) takes the most painstaking and all–inclusive familiarity with the way food interacts with the system (please see Table 13–1). Bodies and, therefore, contests can be flawless, or failed, simply on the basis of the type and amount of food taken in the night before. It is that powerful. But that knowledge is not privy; the fine details are obviously individualized, but the process is right here in this book!

Another fact I tell all my clients that seems to take them off guard: There is no such thing as a bad food. I am convinced that there are foods that are better than others and some that can be utilized at more optimum times, but overall no food is or should be completely avoided because it is "bad." This is where food timing comes in. Food, which you now recognize as a drug, has all sorts of metabolic, hormonal, and chemical responses that follow its intake. When you time the type of food you eat with other daily events, you optimize that food. More importantly, *you optimize the effect that food has on you.* This is a vital part of understanding optimal health. By following the recommended eating schedule, you will gain an understanding of *how* to eat; you will start to see the dramatic effects of food timing. This is part of the real–life properties of this program. Knowledge of the type of food and the timing involved allows you to eat the foods you enjoy without the dreaded diet connotation. Before we get deeper in that subject, we need to review some food basics. These are what I call the Fundamental Facts of Food.

There is no such thing as a bad food!

Table 13-1:

> Speaking of power, marketing has some unique tricks it pulls on the American public, especially in the area of weight loss, muscular development, etc. The "look" we have all become accustomed to and desire: that lean, muscular, well-developed look without blemish, infraction, or scar is a product of time, computer enhancing, and makeup. Makeup and computer enhancing are self-explanatory; time, on the other hand, is something less well known. You see, photo shoots are not randomly done. The model or physique artist has plenty of time to utilize food and exercise programs to "dial in" to the preferred look the camera is after. Those people do not look like that all the time! I have been there, and though I am able to maintain a degree of accomplishment, that perfected, onstage look is not possible to maintain *all the time*. Do not fall for false goals! And above all, avoid setting expectations that cannot be obtained. You, too, with the proper knowledge and training, may have the potential to be there one day, but do not expect it without first obtaining the knowledge it takes to do so.

The Fundamental Facts of Food

There are a number of resources out there to help you learn as much (and occasionally more) as you will ever need. The knowledge of food, types of food, and other basic facts is, in my opinion, essential for day–to–day living. This information should not be avoided. It should not be saved for the dietitians or other nutritional specialists. This is just good, clean information for every person who engages in the practice of eating. As with the rest of this book, we will disregard the esoteric and cut to the information you need to be successful in your own age–management program.

The Basic Food Types

Carbohydrates

Contrary to (current) popular belief, carbohydrates are not bad. Remember, there is no such thing as a bad food, only bad choices and bad timing. Carbohydrates are essential for energy, especially the energy needed for sports, exercise, etc. They play a vital role in the body's ability to increase lean mass, a primary objective of this book. Carbohydrates' most essential role is that of fuel for the ole noggin (i.e., the brain). For purposes of this book and the accompanying eating program, we will define carbohydrates as two primary types: active and free.

Active Carbohydrates

Active Carbohydrates are also called, depending on whom you read, starchy carbohydrates, white carbohydrates, high–glycemic carbohydrates, etc. These foods have a powerful effect on the hormonal and biochemical system of the body; hence *active carbohydrates*. Now it goes without saying that all foods have some influence; however, we are looking at food in the big picture as it relates to your optimum health and body. Active carbohydrates cause a rise in blood sugar. The rate is dependent on the glycemic index of the food (continue reading and see Appendix III) and a resulting rise in insulin, the hormone responsible for getting sugar out of the blood and into tissues, including muscles and fat. We consider these active because they have a direct influence on your energy, thought processes, cravings, emotions, and body in terms of lean and fat mass. These carbohydrates, as I stated earlier, are not bad, nor should they be avoided.

They just need to be regulated. As a matter of fact, these foods are very powerful and can be essential in helping you reach any fitness or body goal you may have when used correctly. Food is a drug, and this type of food exemplifies the true power of this little–known paradigm. Reviewing the drug effects of food involves understanding that the timing of specific foods is also essential in overall health and in the attainment of body–oriented goals, something we covered earlier. An example/partial list of active carbohydrates has been provided in Table 13–2.

TABLE 13-2: Partial List of Active Carbohydrates

Barley	Sweet potatoes
Yams	Long-grain rice
Oatmeal	Potatoes
Red beans	Popcorn
Tomatoes	Lentils
Blackeyed peas	Pasta
Corn	Peas

An analogy I use with my clients when it comes to active carbohydrates involves a cup. Get a cup and place it right in front of you. Imagine that cup as your ability to handle active carbohydrates. When that cup is half full, your body will utilize the energy from the carbohydrates and the energy from fat. As that cup approaches fullness, however, the body is more inclined to utilize the energy from the active carbohydrates and leave the fat alone (survivalist response). When you eat too many active carbohydrates, "the cup runneth over" and that excess is (gulp) stored as fat! On the opposite extreme, when that cup is empty, your body has little energy to perform activities of daily living and exercise (See Table 13–3).

Table 13-3:

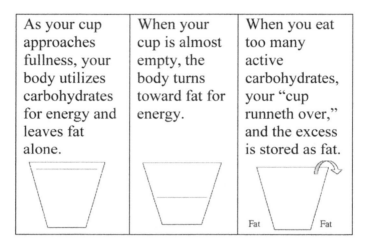

As your cup approaches fullness, your body utilizes carbohydrates for energy and leaves fat alone.	When your cup is almost empty, the body turns toward fat for energy.	When you eat too many active carbohydrates, your "cup runneth over," and the excess is stored as fat.

This analogy is also applicable to utilizing the free window (Chapter 15). Though not essential all the time, one method of using the free window is to purposely drain the cup by eating a lower active–carbohydrate plan for a few days prior to your free window and fill the cup up with your free window.

This acts as a virtual carbohydrate load, such as the ones athletes do prior to competition. This, in turn, helps the lean mass maintain/gain, while you are utilizing a lower active carbohydrate–eating plan. But remember, do not let the cup flow over...

Free Carbohydrates

Free carbohydrates are also called fibrous carbohydrates, non–active carbohydrates, low glycemic carbohydrates, etc. These are the carbohydrates that do not have the dramatic effect on blood sugar and insulin that active carbohydrates do. Free carbohydrates can be utilized whenever and as often as you need them. They are great fillers, adding bulk to your diet, as well as satisfying that strong oral fixation we all have. I have had a number of clients complain that diets do not let them have enough food, not in the hunger sense, but the "sit down and take your time eating" sense. Free carbohydrates fill this void and should be utilized as needed. Free carbohydrates are also good for you. They are fibrous and (besides a few of them) vitamin packed. They provide a variety of tastes, textures, and colors that we need when following an eating program. Free carbohydrates have been the lifesaver of a number of dieters. I highly encourage them and would suggest they become a mainstay in your optimal health lifestyle program.

TABLE 13-4: Partial List of Free Carbohydrates

Zucchini	Mushrooms
Green beans	Cauliflower
Squash	Lettuce (of all kinds)
Broccoli	Cucumber
Spinach	Pickles
Red peppers	Green peppers
Celery	

For now, and for the rest of your healthy life, understand carbohydrates as active and free. Apply appropriate timing for both in the discussed time frames (hours, days, weeks), and always be vigilant in your determination to make the right decision!

Proteins

Proteins are, in my opinion, one of the most vital nutrient/food types there are. The word "protein" is derived from the Greek word meaning *of prime importance*. They are comprised of building blocks called amino acids. There are approximately twenty amino acids available that combine to form a large number of different proteins. Out of the amino acids, we have subdivided groups called essential, nonessential, and semi–essential. Essential amino acids means the body needs you to take them in, as it cannot make them on its own. Nonessential amino acids (the word does not indicate that they are less important) means the body can synthesize them from compounds ordinarily found in the body at a rate needed to maintain function. Many purists may argue against the final subclassification of amino acids, but I believe it is important with what we are doing here. Semi–essential amino acids are amino acids that the body can make, but extra may be needed from the outside, depending on the activities and needs of the individual.

Amino acids provide the major substrate for synthesis of cellular components and tissue. Proteins are essential and present in all cells of the body and make up important structures, such as the cell membrane and intracellular material. They are essential for muscle contraction and movement and are vital in the formation of regulatory hormones and the activation of selected vitamins. They are also deeply involved in the regulatory, metabolic, and physiologic actions the body performs on a daily basis.

Protein tends to be filling, give your metabolism a boost, and, when consumed with carbohydrates helps keep blood sugar swings in check. Protein also has the highest thermic effect of the foods. This means that it takes more energy, or calories, to digest proteins than it does fats or carbohydrates. Some studies have shown that up to thirty percent of the calories in protein are lost as heat in the digestion process. This may be one of the most powerful determining factors of success in high protein, low carb diets!

Protein sources include all animal products, including meat and dairy and a variety of vegetable sources. I use the word "variety" in the sense that a complete protein regimen intake in those who do not eat animal products (i.e., vegans) needs to come from a combination of plant sources. It is beyond the scope of this book to delve into vegetarian eating habits, so I will leave it at that. A list of some of my favorite protein sources is provided in the table below:

TABLE 13-5: Lean Protein Sources

Eggs	Lean beef (10-15% fat)
Low fat/fat free cottage cheese	Chicken
Low fat/fat free cheese	Shrimp, crab, and lobster
Tofu	Whey protein powder
Fish	Tuna, can

Fats

The word "fat" has a bad connotation. It has been unfairly deemed the bad guy and the cause of obesity both in America and around the world. First, you must change your paradigm and become convinced of the fact that fat is not bad! It is absolutely essential for optimum function and daily living on all levels! A few of the noteworthy functions of fat include:

• Protection and insulation of vital organs and the central nervous system

- Providing the body with large amounts of stored and potential energy
- Acting as a carrier for the fat–soluble vitamins including D, E, A, and K

Fat is also essential in its function of controlling hunger pangs and giving the feeling of fullness (satiety). This is one reason all these low– to no–fat diets fail everyone who attempts them. If you are always hungry and craving food, you cannot expect to live a normal, productive life!

Fat is vital in body function on a cellular and full–scale level, from the central nervous system (the brain and spinal cord) to the production of red blood cells, hormones, etc.

Fat is not your enemy. Fat is an essential part of your diet, an absolute must in any eating program, and an indispensable ingredient in the quest for optimum health.

In the average American diet, visible fat constitutes about thirty percent of the total fat intake. This includes butter, lard, cooking oils, mayonnaise, etc. The remaining seventy percent comes from invisible fat found in meats, dairy products, vegetables, nuts, and seeds.

Both plants and animals synthesize fats. Fats can be classified into three groups: simple fats, compound fats (made up of a simple fat with another chemical attached such as protein), and derived fats, such as cholesterol, which is a combination of simple and compound fats. In the media's current anti–fat propaganda, I must give them credit for distinguishing saturated from unsaturated fats. Saturated fats can be, even in my opinion, the bad fats. These guys are typically more prominent in animal products, such as meat and dairy. They are the ones linked to elevated blood cholesterol and the associated cardiac risk factors. A general rule of thumb (obviously not all–inclusive) for you optimum health seekers out there is saturated fats are hard at room temperature. Moderate to controlled intake of these guys is important. Unsaturated fats have been associated with improved cardiac profiles and can be found predominantly in uncooked nuts, seeds, and plant sources.

As we hope to utilize our storage fat (see Chapter 9, The Fallacy of Scale Weight), it is important to understand food timing as described below. During light to moderate exercise, fat contributes to about fifty percent of the energy requirements. As exercise continues and food timing is taken into consideration, the role of stored fat increases and may provide eighty percent of needed energy requirements. That is a lot of fat burning! Sound good? If so, let's continue on with *food timing*, one of the most important topics.

Chapter Fourteen

Food Timing

No other fact should be more fundamentally understood than the following: There is no such thing as a bad food. What is important to know is *when* to utilize the foods we like to eat. The timing of food intake in relation to our sleep/wake cycle, exercise, work, playtime, and all other activities of daily living is what needs to be understood. Once this has been embedded, you will begin to see results of your quest for optimal health on a new level. You will actually learn to *benefit* from pizza and other indulges of the taste buds. No, that is not a typing error. I said *benefit* from what most diets would consider horrific foods. Food timing is elementary in your quest for optimal health. Your understanding of the fundamental facts about foods (see above) and the difference between active carbohydrates, free carbohydrates, proteins, and fats will allow you to place foods strategically in your day according to your activities and plans. The following will provide instructions for utilizing foods and the reasons why I suggest certain things and at specific times.

Before I delve into it, however, I would like to clarify something. The basis for my reasoning is very scientific and well researched both in the lab (from which the articles I read were written) and also in my clinical experience. I will not bore you with the detailed physiology behind my reasons. Rather, I will illustrate the reasons with a few simplistic cartoons and graphs. The numbers I will use are to exemplify a point, and they are not intended to be taken at face value. I will not use proper units of measure, nor will I try to provide you with the exactness necessary in some more technical writings. I am trying to help you understand *why* food timing is important. Forget the esoteric. As we have already discussed, there are a number of variables involved with everything we see and can demonstrate in life and the lab. I want to provide you with one of the reasons food timing is so important. The other reasons? Give me a call, buy me lunch, and I'll tell you.

Insulin

This is the mother of all hormones for this particular discussion. We learned in Chapter 6 that hormones are powerhouses in the body, responsible for all sorts of different functions, including growth, feelings, etc. Insulin is one of these powerhouses. Insulin is released by the pancreas, a fish–shaped organ (or at least that's what I think it looks like) in the belly directly under the rib cage and slightly left of midline. This hormone is constantly released into the body but increases in response to sugar in the blood, and, some would argue, even thoughts of sugar in the blood. It rapidly responds according to the glycemic index of the food you just started chewing (see above and Appendix III). One of its actions is to transport sugar in the blood into cells, including muscle, liver, and fat cells. Insulin is not the only hormone that deals with blood sugar. Glucagon, epinephrine (adrenaline) and cortisol also play a role in the fine balancing act of blood sugar control, but again we will limit our discussion to insulin, as it will serve to demonstrate the importance of food timing.

Of note, insulin also increases protein synthesis, increases transport of amino acids into muscle cells, and reduces protein degradation (break down), all essential in our quest to increase lean mass, one of the primary goals of this book.

Insulin can be your best friend or worst enemy. You have most likely heard about it in negative connotations in the media (a spin they are infamous for), and I would like to elucidate a bit in this area, as I feel it is important.

Insulin resistance is a condition where the body has trouble utilizing blood sugar because it is resistant to the effect of insulin. This condition is a *lifestyle–related* condition! It is caused by poor diet, obesity, and lack of exercise. It greatly increases one's cardiovascular risk for such things as heart attack and stroke, as well as the risk for diabetes. However, diabetes does not have to be the end result of insulin resistance. Studies have show diabetes can be avoided (even in the face of insulin resistance) with exercise and a good eating program. Diabetes is a disorder of blood sugar usage/metabolism. People with type 1 diabetes do not produce enough insulin and need to inject it so they can get some control over their blood sugar. In type 2 diabetes, insulin is present, but unable to take sugar into the cells, as the cells are resistant to its actions.

So why are we focusing on insulin in our quest for optimal health? Well, for one thing, problems with insulin and blood sugar are a setup for a variety of potentially serious or even life–threatening obstacles, including kidney disease, stroke, eye damage, and heart attacks. These are not things we want in our pursuit of optimal health.

More relative to our discussion is insulin's involvement in building tissue, particularly lean tissue and fat tissue. Insulin is responsible for the storage of energy (in the form of sugars) in both fat and muscle. It deposits this energy into either fat or muscle based on food timing, activity level, when we ate last, the last time insulin was raised (in response to blood sugar), and a variety of other factors. Again, avoiding the esoteric, using insulin's response to food, we will develop a timing system to optimize lean mass gain (while minimizing fat gain) and maximize fat loss (while maintaining lean mass). So how does this work? Generally speaking, the body will not utilize fat when sugar is present to burn and use for energy. As you will recall, we are survivalistic, and our bodies will do anything to protect fat for what is believed to be the up–and–coming starvation that is required to endure. If we repeatedly feed it active carbohydrates throughout the day, we cause insulin to continually spike, thereby setting up the environment for fat storage (see Table 14–1). Energy in the form of active carbohydrates is present to feed the brain, and the body is as happy as can be. It is never required to turn to fat stores for energy.

> Lean mass gain and fat loss are based on food *timing*, not the *type* of food you choose.

Now what we want to do is trick the system into thinking it needs to burn fat for energy. How? Decrease the amount of sugar present, thereby decreasing the insulin and forcing the body to turn to fat stores. This is, of course, a gross oversimplification, but it makes the point. Make your body burn fat by decreasing the active carbohydrates throughout the day.

In an ideal situation, we utilize active carbohydrates at two times during the day: first thing in the morning upon waking from our overnight "fast," and then immediately after a workout. This is because exercise utilizes the storage form of sugars in the muscles and sets up the environment for needing to replenish energy. This causes insulin to rise and deposit the energy into our hungry muscles. Optimally, one would get up and exercise, *then* eat active carbohydrates, as this would combine the best of both worlds in the quest for maximum fat loss and muscle gain. The rest of the day, we slowly decrease our active carbohydrates, allowing a drop in sugar and resulting in a drop in insulin. Our body is then forced into fat–burning mode, because insulin is no longer depositing sugar.

Sound complicated? It is actually quite simple. This may sound obvious, but your eating habits influence fat gain or loss and/or muscle gain or loss. More importantly, the *timing* of the food you eat has a direct influence on this process. Let's review what a typical, overweight, out–of–shape person does: Our example wakes up in the morning, may, on occasion, eat something, and throughout the day snacks on all sorts of simple sugars and processed foods, such as crackers, potato chips, candy, etc. As you recall from above, these are all active carbohydrates, and they directly affect insulin by causing it to rise and, being ever so dutiful, deposit the energy (calories) into the most reasonable receptacle, in this case, fat. Though this person claims to have "just nibbled" all day, the hormonal response was rapid, repeated spikes in the insulin causing deposition of calories into fat. Then, to top it off, he sits down to a large active carbohy-drate and fat–filled dinner, allowing the perfect setup for fat gain. This is illustrated in the following chart:

Table 14-1:

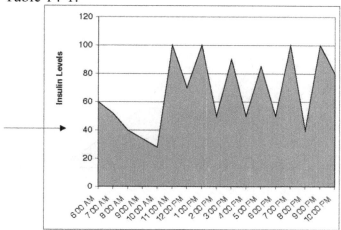

Back to ideal: What should happen is, we wake up in the morning after our over nightly "fast," blood sugar and insulin at their lowest. We exercise, burning more fat and muscle sugar stores, setting our muscles up for "eating" and growing. Following exercise, we have our biggest active carbohydrate meal of the day, spike insulin, and store that energy in the muscles for growth and maintenance of our lean mass tissue. The rest of the day we slowly decrease our active carbohydrate intake, allowing a steady drop in insulin, causing the body to return to fat stores for energy while we are carrying out our daily activities. We fast once again all night, burning fat for fuel, and wake up and repeat the process. This is illustrated pictorially in the following graph (Table 14–2):

Table 14-2:

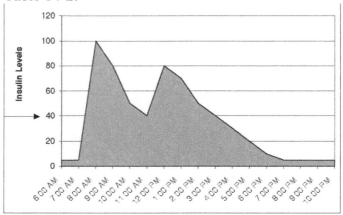

This is one of the foundations of this program. *Lean mass gain and fat loss are based on food timing, not the type of food you choose.*

You will also notice the arrow on both graphs pointing to the forty number/line. Using another simplistic illustration, let's say this is the "magic line of fat loss." Any time insulin falls below this line, the body starts resorting to fats for energy. If, as in Table 14–1, the insulin levels never fall below that line, fat loss does not occur because there is plenty of sugar to be utilized for energy. The body will not burn the fat if it does not have to; it protects it when sugar and, therefore, insulin are available. Now look at the "magic line of fat loss" in Table 14–2. The insulin level falls below it for the majority of the day, causing you to become a fat–burning machine!

So let's review an ideal day in a stepwise fashion: Wake up in the morning in a fasting state when the blood sugar and insulin are at they're lowest. Exercise right away, before eating, to burn fat and utilize muscle glycogen, preparing the muscles for growth because, again, sugar is not present and sets us up for number three. Eat or drink a high glycemic load or meal to cause insulin to spike and distribute the energy to the ready muscles to cause them to grow.

Gradually decrease your active carbohydrates throughout the day to get your insulin below that "magic line of fat loss." Wake up in the morning and start over.

One option for getting into the habit of proper food timing is to utilize Appendix III, The Glycemic Index, as it has been categorized by the time of day foods are most advantageous. Simply use the list as a guide as to when to eat certain foods. You could try this before utilizing the accompanying eating plans, but obviously, your best results will come about by following the eating plans as they are laid out.

I hope this chapter has helped you understand the basics of optimal eating. What follows are some tools you can incorporate into your newfound understanding of food and food timing, such as The Free Window, Holiday and Vacation Eating, and actual diet examples for you to follow and design yourself.

Chapter Fifteen

The Free Window

The free window is also an indispensable part of the optimal eating program described in this book. The free window is essential not only psychologically, but also physiologically. You can actually benefit from eating whatever you want and as much as you want with the free window. How's that for another paradigm shift? I mentioned this in my client interview in How This Book Came About, but now let's discuss how to plan a free window and why and how a free window can benefit you.

Psychologically, the free window gives your mind and emotions a break from the daily routine of eating correctly. You will eventually get to a point where you know only a healthy eating style, and the free window will be there as a matter of convenience and to aid in your deliberate efforts to build muscle mass. Convenient, as the free window will allow you to indulge in foods that are not necessarily bad (remember, there is no such thing as a bad food) but, more importantly, in uninhibited amounts and at a less–than–ideal time.

This can be utilized to your advantage in a number of situations, from a dinner party with friends to an important business lunch with your company's executives. The free window allows you more autonomy in your optimal eating system. How can eating to your heart's content assist in your goal for optimal health? To understand this, we must first review a few simple facts about the eating style this book describes.

The pattern of eating, as presented in Chapter 16, allows for maximization of metabolic hormones such as insulin, growth hormone, and testosterone. It also increases the body's sensitivity to those hormones. In other words, those hormones have a greater effect on the body with the style of eating described. The gradual decrease in active carbohydrates throughout the day causes a hormone called glucagon to increase and thereby burn more fat while at the same time causing a decrease and stabilization of insulin for efficient metabolism of carbohydrates and fats. The body responds to this style of eating by increasing the amount of enzymes available for essential metabolic processes, including muscle growth and repair, fat burning and utilization, and, as some research has shown, an anti–aging mechanism by the control of dangerous free radicals. This eating style also acts to detoxify the body by neutralizing, breaking down, and eliminating wastes.

The Free Window fits right into the scheme of things. Let me summarize a few of the key facts behind the occasional episode of overeating:

1. Increase Your Metabolism

The free window allows your body to literally "turn up the heat" when it is exposed to a large amount of food. Your body turns into a thermogenic machine and your metabolism skyrockets in response. Thyroid hormones, adrenal hormones, and sex hormones such as testosterone all increase, bringing about this metabolic surge. A phenomenon called diet–induced thermogenesis, or the ability of food to increase energy expenditure, also increases by forty percent following carbohydrate overfeeding.[1] This occurs not only during your food frenzy, but also for some time following (see Table 15–1).

2. Increase the Anabolic (Growth) Process

With this sudden increase in food and the resultant increase in metabolism, the food you have eaten is assimilated more quickly, and tissue repair and muscle growth occur. This is due to the increase in growth–promoting hormones and number three described below.

3. Replenish the Glycogen Stores

As you recall from the portion on food timing and eating a high–glycemic load following your early morning exercise, the free window acts even more powerfully and really fills the glycogen stores in the muscles, what some have termed *supercompensation.* This process in and of itself is a muscle–promoting activity!

4. Refuel the Mind

An essential role of the free window is to allow the emotional, mental, and psychological aspects of food to be enjoyed to their fullest.

Table 15-1: Free Window/Overeating Experiences

I love to talk to clients after a free window, especially following the first time they experience it. They give a classic description of heat radiating from their bodies to the point of having to undress or go outside to cool off and of feeling full only and, to their surprise, hungry again a very short time later. They then tell of waking up the next morning and feeling all their muscles are "full," as if they had just completed a full body workout. They describe energy and a sense of actually being *leaner* the following day. To their amazement, they are *still hungry* the following day due to the metabolism boost. Those who are willing to take the time to measure their body composition find a substantial increase in lean mass with very little, if any increase in fat mass. The free window has been a powerful tool in the quest for optimal health and the desired increase in lean mass and decrease in fat mass.

There are a few other physiologic and psychological health benefits to the free window, but the above information is what is most essential.

There are two types of free windows I like to utilize. The first one is the three–hour time block. The second is the full–day window.

The Three–Hour Window

The three–hour window is a three–hour time block in which you can eat as much as you want, when you want for a three–hour time period. The three–hour window is advantageous in the sense that you can have more than one a week. Dinner parties or engagements such as a date with your spouse can be planned using the three–hour window. It can be used at any time during the day, a free breakfast, lunch, or dinner, on any day of the week. I encourage people not to use more than two three–hour windows a week, as the habit of nightly free windows sneaks up on us. The biggest advantage is you can plan your weekly eating around your three–hour free window, which can be very valuable for people with busy schedules.

The Full–Day Window

The full–day window is basically a free eating time from sunup to bedtime. It can be utilized for those hard–to–control days like a family picnic at the zoo. It can also be used when you just need a full day to relax and let life and eating happen. This window can be utilized around your weekly schedule as well. I have found that a very successful technique for the busy working participant is to eat well controlled and scheduled meals during the week (when everything else in our lives is being dictated) and then use the full–day window on one of the weekend days. One other option is to start your full–day free window one evening and end it with a large, free breakfast the following morning. In general, and as you start down the road to optimal health, I would suggest one three–hour free window each week, or one full–day window every two weeks. Once you become accustomed to the optimal eating you have learned in this book and when you see that lean mass climbing and the fat falling off, you can slowly increase your windows to fit your needs. I would encourage you to be a high self–monitor however. If you feel you are not gaining as you think you should, evaluate your free windows to see if they are being open too often or possibly not often enough.

There are also some basic rules to follow during your free window utilization. This may sound contradicting, as rules remove the freedom of the window, so let me rephrase it by saying there are some general *guidelines* that should be applied in the ideal situation. This is not set in stone, as I would rather you enjoy your free window in whatever form it may take, but the following seems to be most effective for maximizing your free window.

1. Start your free window with fibrous carbs, such as a salad, mixed vegetables, etc.

2. Following the fibrous carbs, move to proteins and fats, such as a large steak with sautéed mushrooms and onions.

3. Then move to your active carbohydrates, such as rice or potatoes.

4. Eat as many different textures and tastes as you can come up with.

5. Add jalapeños, habanero, and cayenne peppers to your meal. These all contain capsaicin (gives peppers their "kick"), a chemical shown to help increase metabolism.

6. Listen to your body. If you are full to the point of bursting, do not push it. One other method that seems to work well is eating to the point of excessive thirst. This may be the signal that you are done, but if you are still hungry after a few minutes, go back to it.

7. Try to keep a few hours between your feeding and bedtime.

8. The day after a free window, get up really early and exercise like crazy! Do a lot of cardio and possibly work your weakest body part (like legs), as the higher glycogen stored in the muscles will allow some intense training and optimal results. It will also help start the glycogen depletion so the body quickly returns to fat burning.

Be a high self—monitor!
Utilize the free windows with a lot of thought!

Free windows can be a lot of fun. I always open my window in the company of good friends, most of who are doing one of my eating plans anyway. We all do them together, as this support and accountability are powerful tools in your quest for optimal health. The free window is a powerful tool in your quest. The benefits far exceed those described in this book. You literally have to see it to believe it. Go for it!

Chapter Sixteen

Eating Plans

This chapter will provide you with an actual eating plan to follow in your quest for optimal health, fat loss, and muscle gain. The style is simple and follows all the rules and guidelines set up in the previous chapters. The actual plans are found in Appendix I, with an example and explanation below. The sample foods with amounts based on total daily caloric needs are found in Appendix I as well.

Prior to beginning your optimal health eating program, you need to determine your total caloric needs. I have taken the liberty of determining amounts of protein, carbohydrates, and fat proportions you will consume, but the total calories are something you will need to determine and change on an ongoing basis. I have provided a very simple equation for you to use in this caloric determination (see Table 16–1).

The foods listed in Appendix I are broken down according to the way foods were described in Chapter 13. For each caloric amount, there is an active carbohydrate list and a protein list with appropriate amounts so you can stay within your caloric determinant. Free carbohydrates can be found in Appendix I alongside the Protein Sources. The calculation you will be utilizing is a simple conversion of your scale weight in pounds to your scale weight in kilograms. After this has been found, you will multiply your scale weight in kilograms by the eating variable. The eating variable is a number I have established to help you find your average daily caloric needs. This eating variable will differ based on your amount of exercise and your progress. For example: As shown in Table 16–1, a person who exercises at least three times a week for thirty or more minutes will use the eating variable of 24. A nonexerciser will use the eating variable of 22 and so forth. By changing this number, as directed below and based on your objective and subjective changes, you will be able to determine your daily caloric needs, meet your body goals, and obtain and maintain optimal health!

Table 16-1: Determining Daily Caloric Needs

If you exercise at least three times a week for thirty minutes a session, use the following equation:

Take your scale weight in pounds and divide by 2.2 to get your scale weight in kilograms. Then multiply your scale weight in kilograms by the Eating Variable 24. This will give you your suggested daily caloric need. Find the corresponding food list in Appendix I.

Example: Scale Weight = 175 pounds
Divide 175 pounds by 2.2 = weight in kilograms
175 / 2.2 = 79.5

Multiply your weight in kilograms by 24
79.5 x 24 = 1908 calories a day
Rounding off to the nearest calorie amount:
Your total caloric needs will be 1900 calories a day.

> If you *do not* exercise at least three times a week
> for thirty minutes a session, use the following
> equation:
>
> Take your scale weight in pounds and divide by
> 2.2 to get your scale weight in kilograms.
> Multiply your scale weight in kilograms by the
> Eating Variable 22. This will give you your
> suggested daily caloric need. Find the
> corresponding food list in Appendix I.
>
> Example: Scale Weight = 175 pounds
> Divide 175 pounds by 2.2 = weight in kilograms
> 175 / 2.2 = 79.5
>
> Multiply your weight in kilograms by 22
> 79.5 x 22 = 1749 calories a day
> Rounding off to the nearest calorie amount:
> Your total caloric needs will be 1700 calories a
> day.

Once you have established your daily caloric need, find the matching calorie food list in Appendix I. Round your value to the closest caloric number provided (in increments of 100). For example, if you determine that your total caloric need is 1,635 calories a day, utilize the 1,600–calorie–a–day eating plan. If you find your caloric need to be 1,472 calories a day, round your calories to 1,500.

This eating plan will work well for any person, no matter what size or shape. However, I would suggest that people who weigh more than 280 pounds (scale weight) get their body composition determined and use their lean mass in the caloric calculations. For example, if you weighed 325 pounds scale weight and determined your lean mass to weigh 210 pounds, divide 210 pounds by 2.2, then multiply that number by your eating variable.

$$210/2.2 = 95.5 \text{ x eating variable (24)} = 2{,}290$$

Round your calories to the nearest 100 and use the 2,300–calorie eating plan.

If you have no way of determining your lean mass, please use Appendix IX to order a skin caliper and how–to book. If you cannot do this either, use the following sliding scale in your calculations.

To use the sliding scale, determine your scale weight and subtract that number from the number in the right column. For example, if you weighed 325 pounds scale weight, subtract 85 from 325 (off the chart below) to get 240. Then divide 240 by 2.2, and then multiply that number by your eating variable.

$$240/2.2 = 109 \text{ x eating variable (24)} = 2{,}618$$

Round your calories to the nearest 100 and use the 2,600–calorie eating plan.

Obviously, determining your lean mass will be most accurate, but the sliding scale shown below works very well.

If your scale weight is:	Subtract the following number (in the column below) from your scale weight and use that number in your determination of caloric amounts.
280 - 350	85
351 - 380	115
381 - 400	135
401 - 425	160
426 - 450	185
451 - 500	235
501 +	300

Now that you have determined your daily caloric need, we will review the actual menu plan. Below is an example of a menu plan with an explanation where I felt it was appropriate.

1000 Calories		
Suggested amounts and types of foods. Keep track of what you are eating		

Name: _____

Date: _____

Exercise: 30 – 40 min in AM Before Food		Write what you eat here:
Meal 1 **Time:** _____	**1 Protein Source** **2 Active Carbohydrates**	
Meal 2 **Time:** _____	1 oz Raw Almonds	
Meal 3 **Time:** _____	**1 Protein Source** **1 Active Carbohydrates** **Free Carbohydrates** (as much as you want)	
Meal 4 **Time:** _____	1/2 LOW CARB protein bar (OR) 1 scoop Whey Protein Powder in water	
Meal 5 **Time:** _____	**1 Protein Source** **0 Active Carbohydrates** **Free Carbohydrates** (as much as you want)	
Bed Time Meal **(Optional)**	**Sugar Free Jell-O 1 cup**	
Add fiber supplement in evening such as Metamucil or other (sugar FREE). Add spices, pepper, etc. as needed. Try to eat every two to three hours Drink ¾ of a gallon of water EVERY DAY! May have up to 2 diet pops **(or)** 2 cups a coffee a day		

Suggestions for added flavor, fluid intake, etc.

The following is an example of the food list with the recommended amount next to it.

The way to utilize the eating plan is to do the following in this order:

- Determine your current daily caloric needs.
- Find the closest matching caloric diet example in Appendix I.
- Each item listed with its amounts is *one serving*. For example, on the 2,000–calorie–a day menu, breakfast could be as follows:

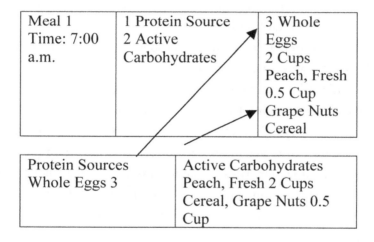

Meal 1 Time: 7:00 a.m.	1 Protein Source 2 Active Carbohydrates	3 Whole Eggs 2 Cups Peach, Fresh 0.5 Cup Grape Nuts Cereal

Protein Sources Whole Eggs 3	Active Carbohydrates Peach, Fresh 2 Cups Cereal, Grape Nuts 0.5 Cup

It is that simple! Determine your numbers, pick the eating program, choose the foods on your eating program list (or similar foods and amounts), and eat!

The suggested serving size is based on your total caloric needs (by your calculation). As I said before, I have determined the amounts of carbohydrates, proteins, and fats for each eating plan based on my experience and success with my clients. Try to stay as close to your portions as you can, as this will allow you to track your total calories very well. At first, it will take some extra time to measure foods, but after one or two practice runs, you will be able to visualize the portion sizes, enabling you to toss the scale or other measuring device.

This menu plan follows the suggested guidelines we reviewed earlier. The majority of your active carbohydrates are in the morning, with a small amount at lunch and none in the evening. Protein sources are basically steady all day long, and free carbohydrates come in at lunch and dinner. I have provided two between meal snacks, nuts in the morning, and a low–carbohydrate protein bar in the afternoon. Nuts provide the good fats you need for energy throughout the day, not to mention their cardiovascular protection and benefits to total health and fat loss. The low–carbohydrate bar offers a good protein source without too many active carbohydrates and a soothing for that common late afternoon sweet tooth. I have not mentioned brand names of bars, as no one pays me enough for endorsements; however, I will say there are a number out there that are very good. Try to find a low–carbohydrate protein bar with fewer than seven grams of active carbohydrates in it. I also have included an optional late night snack in the form of Sugar–free Jell–O. This can be mixed with your sugar–free fiber replacement for a different texture and also has the advantage of helping with the late night sweet tooth.

How to Make Dietary Changes
via the Tracking System

Dietary changes are a very important part of your eating program. Change offers a break in possible perceived monotony, it interferes with your body's tendency to adapt then stagnate to what you are doing, and it encourages continual, positive change. Before I get into the discussion of changing your eating plan based on your results, I feel it is important to review a few facts. You will hear arguments contending that *weight loss* is nothing more than calories in (how much you eat) to calories out (how much activity you are involved with). While I agree with this, let's examine the statement. Weight loss indicates scale weight, which, as you are being repeatedly reminded in this book, does not differentiate fat mass from lean mass. You will lose scale weight by cutting your calories or cutting off your leg. You will also lose scale weight by increasing your exercise or cardiovascular activity. Both things, increasing exercise and decreasing calories, will cause you to utilize more than you take in, causing scale weight loss. In the sport of bodybuilding we often balance calories to cardio (cardio is short for cardiovascular training) to help us make a weight class or lean up a little more. It is a never–ending game of exercising more so we can eat more or vice versa. This is not an uncommon practice outside the sport of bodybuilding either.

As I have been adamant about describing the difference between lean and fat mass, I feel it is also important to stress to you that calories in to calories out is only part of the picture. On multiple occasions, with a large number of people, I have kept calories and cardio constant, yet they have still made changes in their fat–to–lean mass by changing the amounts of carbohydrates, fats, and proteins they utilized. This statement is bound to get some arguments from the mainstream dietary world. Fine. "Bring them on." I have data to prove it. I do it to myself all the time, and I will elucidate it in great detail in my next book. For now, it suffices to say that changing the amount of exercise you are doing and/or changing the number of calories you are taking in is just one part of the picture. We will, however, use these two variables in our tracking and change system, as described below. I brought the other up so you would be aware of it and so you would have a better understanding of why I chose to design the diets the way I did. The calculated amounts for each diet plan are designed to help you acquire and then maintain lean mass. Therefore, sticking to the program as outlined, utilizing the calories to cardio changes that we are about to cover will do wonders for your ability to continually make positive changes! The other diet programs out there do not do that. If you hit a wall and stop progressing, use the suggestions in Chapter 19, Progression Through Roadblocks, Walls, and Plateaus. I have taken the time to calculate each and every food and caloric amount, so you progress in the direction you want.

Now, back to the tracking system. The tracking system reviewed in Chapter 10 will allow you to continually monitor and make appropriate changes to your optimal health program. To quickly review, the tracking system follows objective and subjective changes that you will experience during your efforts. If, at weekly intervals and reviews, you have two of the four objective changes and four of the eight subjective changes, you will need to advance your diet. What I mean by advance is this (hold on to your seat): You, on occasion, are going to increase your calories. Though it may appear to be yet another perceived typing error, it is not. If you are progressing, you need to change your eating. This is done by utilizing the calculations in Table 16–2.

Let me delve a little deeper with this concept. Contrary to popular belief, heavier people have *faster* metabolisms. As they drop scale weight, their caloric needs also drop. However, when scale weight is ignored and lean mass versus fat mass (as well as the other objective and subjective measures) is followed, we occasionally need to increase our caloric intake to keep up with the metabolic changes. Now this is not progressive to the point of eventually needing/getting to 10,000 calories a day! This occurs for a short time until you accomplish two things: 1) You reach your goals, and 2) you are able to maintain your goals. Remember, life is dynamic, always changing, always needing to be changed. That's why I have set up this system with the eating variable. You will not always *need* to change your calories. Following objective and subjective events allows you to see *when* you may need a change, as this will shock the system *into* change. Again, this is done by utilizing the calculations in Table 16–2.

Table 16-2: Dietary Changes for those who are answering fifty percent of the Objective and Subjective questions with YES answers.

If you exercise at least three times a week for thirty minutes a session, use the following equation:

Take your scale weight in pounds and divide by 2.2 to get your scale weight in kilograms. Multiply your scale weight in kilograms by the Eating Variable 25. This will give you your *new* suggested daily caloric need. Find the corresponding food list in Appendix I.

Example: Scale Weight = 175 pounds
Divide 175 pounds by 2.2 = weight in kilograms
175 / 2.2 = 79.5

Multiply your weight in kilograms by 25
79.5 x 25 = 1988 calories a day.

Rounding off to the nearest calorie amount, your total caloric needs will be 2000 calories a day.

If you *do not* exercise at least three times a week for thirty minutes a session, use the following equation:

Take your scale weight in pounds and divide by 2.2 to get your scale weight in kilograms. Multiply your scale weight in kilograms by the Eating Variable 23. This will give you your suggested daily caloric need. Find the corresponding food list in Appendix I.

Example: Scale Weight = 175 pounds
Divide 175 pounds by 2.2 = weight in kilograms
175 / 2.2 = 79.5
Multiply your weight in kilograms by 23
79.5 x 23 = 1829 calories a day

Rounding off to the nearest calorie amount, your total caloric needs will be 1800 calories a day.

Table 16-3: Dietary Changes for those who are *not* answering fifty percent of the Objective and Subjective questions with a *yes* answer.

If you exercise at least three times a week for thirty minutes a session, use the following equation:

Take your scale weight in pounds and divide by 2.2 to get your scale weight in kilograms. Multiply your scale weight in kilograms by the Eating Variable 23. This will give you your *new* suggested daily caloric need. Find the corresponding food list in Appendix I.

Example: Scale Weight = 175 pounds
Divide 175 pounds by 2.2 = weight in kilograms
175 / 2.2 = 79.5

Multiply your weight in kilograms by 23
79.5 x 23 = 1829 calories a day.
Rounding off to the nearest calorie amount, your total caloric needs will be 1800 calories a day.

If you *do not* exercise at least three times a week for thirty minutes a session, use the following equation:

Take your scale weight in pounds and divide by 2.2 to get your scale weight in kilograms. Multiply your scale weight in kilograms by the Eating Variable 21. This will give you your suggested daily caloric need. Find the corresponding food list in Appendix I.

Example:
Scale Weight = 175 pounds
Divide 175 pounds by 2.2 = weight in kilograms
175 / 2.2 = 79.5

Multiply your weight in kilograms by 21
79.5 x 21 = 1670 calories a day

Rounding off to the nearest calorie amount, your total caloric needs will be 1700 calories a day.

If you have not answered at least fifty percent of the objective and subjective questions with *yes* answers, answer the questions on the back of the form. They include: Did I follow the eating plan at least eighty percent of the time? Did I exercise to the best of my abilities and according to the schedule? Did I schedule my food intake according to my schedule every day? Were there any confounding variables that I did not account for (stress, illness, etc.)? Answer these questions honestly and make adjustments where you can. After that, recalculate your daily caloric need using the equations in table 16–3.

I have purposely given the above example for the nonexerciser to show that occasionally with the calculations, your dietary caloric value will not change. This is purposeful, a part of the eating variables benefits. In this situation I want you to go back and *truly* review the questions on the back of the form and continue with the current dietary recommendations. If you go two weeks without change, drop the eating variable by 1 (one) and go for it again with your new numbers.

One other effective method in "getting things moving" is to increase your cardiovascular training and/or exercise in general. I encourage weightlifting, as the more lean mass you have, the more you burn, as we have already discussed. Increasing exercise is effective if you like your caloric amount where it is. I, however, am more apt to change the food intake, as this is a much more powerful tool in your quest. I tell people all the time, "Anyone can exercise, but the ones who know how to eat are the ones who really make a difference in their bodies." This entire eating system is very effective in the way it can reward you for positive results with more foods. In turn, it also ensures that your lean mass will be protected.

Description of the Food List

The foods listed in all the different caloric plans are foods that I use most commonly and my clients have requested most often. Obviously, this list is not all–inclusive. I would encourage you to use the foods on the list, and as you develop the habit of eating correctly, substitute foods that are similar, utilizing similar amounts. I did not include recipes with this book because in my experience, the simpler, the better, and a lot of people do not cook. The basics foods are there. If you have the ability, talent, and time to prepare dishes, I highly encourage it. The way it is written, all can benefit if you cook or not.

When I developed this eating plan, I took into account the amount of protein, carbohydrates, and fats. Using some math, I determined what the probability was that you would follow the eating plan exactly and averaged the caloric intake to span a seven–day course. This includes the use of condiments (see below).

As you review the different food lists, you will see some unusual amounts, such as 0.88 of a cup. This is not an exact measurement, as far as you needing to measure that exact amount. If you can exactly measure 0.88 of a cup, great! I do not expect you to. What I would like is for you to find a midway point between 0.75 and 1 cup. Follow a similar pattern for other odd amounts. You will also note that some of the foods and their amounts are the same for a few of the caloric amounts. This is due to the fact that other foods have been changed to compensate and/or I may have increased the amount of your mid–morning or mid–afternoon snack. Again, I have utilized some math and statistical reasoning, and this has been incorporated into the eating program as well.

I did not include a separate section on fats, as I felt that would be too burdensome for you to keep track of. I have accounted for the amount of fat you will be ingesting in the eating program within the amounts of proteins and, in some cases, carbohydrates. For you vegetarians out there, this plan is limited. It will work well for the ovo–laco vegetarians, but obviously limiting for true vegans. I have had the privilege of working with a number of vegetarians who all did very well in obtaining their goals, and I do not want to leave this population out. Currently, I am working on a food plan for vegetarians that fits my schematic here. Please refer to Appendix IX to contact me, and I will be sure to get you a copy of that food list when it is complete.

A Quick Word on Fast Foods

I have no problem with fast foods. There is no such thing as a bad food, remember? I understand some people's schedules and need for quickness and availability as well. Fast foods fill that void. Fast foods, though not the *best choice* in foods, as they are expensive and out of your control in preparation, do work. I have included a short list of fast foods here, but it would be preferable if you used whole foods. These foods are cheaper (see Table 16–4) and better accounted for. Fast foods can be substituted in place of the foods listed with relatively little thought. Stick to your food timing and the amounts provided and you can substitute as needed. For example, substitute a protein source and an active carbohydrate source from your list with a chicken sandwich from Burger King. Then add free carbohydrates on top with your condiment selection and voila! You are still following the eating plan! One simple suggestion: When I mention a sandwich in the menu items, such as a Subway 6–inch cold turkey breast, eat one–half of the bread/bun to cut back on some calories.

Table 16-4: The "Cost" of This Eating Plan

I have been told more times than I can recall how inexpensive this program is. People have noted a large decrease in their grocery bills and overall food budgets while following this plan. This is due to the fact that we utilize mostly whole foods, minimal processed foods, and, hopefully, limits the amount of restaurant foods you consume. That, in my opinion, is part of optimal health: protecting your wallet!

Dividing Portions

As you get higher in the caloric amounts, you will note that some of the foods have extreme amounts in the serving size. This is from my serving–size calculations for each diet, for each food listed. I would encourage you to divide the serving size in half when this occurs and substitute it for half of another food listed. For example: On the 2,000–calorie–a–day food list, you will find, under active carbohydrates, 13.5 ounces of canned corn, no sodium, from Del Monte. Instead of eating all 13.5 ounces, unless you want to, eat 7 ounces and then take half of another food off the list for the remainder. This little trick will allow you a large number of options for your lifestyle–eating program!

Condiments

I have added a page at the end of the food list section (Appendix I) that contains a list of the most commonly asked for condiments in my practice. I have divided this list into active condiments and free condiments. No matter what diet plan you are on, you may have two active condiments a day before 3:00 p.m. and unlimited free condiments.

Feel free to use two active condiments each day before 3:00 pm. Use free condiments as needed.

Active Condiments		Free Condiments	
Food Type	Serving Size	Food Type	Serving Size
Butter, unsalted	1 Tspn	Apple Cider Vinegar	1 Tblsp
Dressing, Kraft Fat Free Ranch	1 Tblsp	Chicken broth, Sfwy, FF/low sodium	1 Cup
Hidden Bal. Orig. FF Ranch w/bacon	1 Tblsp	Dressing, Kraft Free Italian	1 Tblsp
Dressing, Kraft Free Blue Cheese	1 Tblsp	Dressing Kraft Free Red Wine Vinegar	1 Tblsp
Kraft Lite Done Right Roka Blue Cheese	1 Tblsp	Bernstein's FF Parmes. Cheese Dressing	1 Tblsp
Wishbone Just 2 Good Blue Cheese	1 Tblsp	Kraft Fat Free Mayo	1 Tblsp
Knorr Spring Veggy Soup/Dip Mix	1 Tblsp	Mustard	1 Tblsp
Jam, Smuckers Reduced Sugar	1 Tblsp	Cinnamon, ground	1 Tspn
Heinz Ketchup	1 Tblsp	Pace Picante Sauce	1 Tblsp
Hunts Ketchup	1 Tblsp	La Victoria Salsa Supreme	1 Tblsp
Del Monte Ketchup	1 Tblsp	Tostitos Salsa	1 Tblsp

Mayonnaise Best Foods Low Fat	1 Tblsp	Rotel Extra Hot Tomatoes	1 Oz
Pasta sauce, Hunt's Homestyle	0.5 Cup	Rotel Mild Tomatoes	1 Oz
Pasta sauce, SW Verdi Sel. mush/onion	0.5 Cup		
Peter Pan Creamy Peanut Butter	1 Tspn		
Soynut Butter	1 Tspn		
Tartar sauce, Best Foods Low Fat	1 Tblsp		
Kraft Cocktail Sauce	0.25 Cup		
Heinz Cocktail Sauce	0.25 Cup		
Kraft Fat Free Parmesan	1 Tspn		

Supplements

I have added some vitamin and supplement recommendations in Appendix VI. These are only a universal suggestion. Obviously, we all have different needs and indications for supplements. I have added a suggested list that can be used as a reference, but before taking any supplement, discuss it with your doctor to ensure that you have no contraindications or potential interactions with other medications or supplements. The ones I have suggested have worked very well with almost all of my clients and are an excellent part of an optimal health plan.

This eating plan should be your daily guide. If you follow it as directed, with the occasional free window (see Chapter 15), you will be well on your way to optimal health and the ideal body. This program has proved itself over and over again. I would encourage you to first understand the previous chapters as to *why* this program works and then give it a full scale, all–out effort to make the most of it. I will be reviewing holiday and vacation eating in the next chapter, as these are the only two events I can think of where you may diverge from the lifestyle program presented here. The style of eating, the use of free windows, drinking the suggested amount of water, and utilizing the recommended supplements (after your doctor's approval) will allow you to reach your goals.

As one more aid in your quest, I have summarized the style of eating presented in Appendix VII. These twelve rules will assist you in your quest. This is a lifestyle, not a diet. Focus on gain, not loss! You can do it!

Chapter Seventeen

Holiday and Vacation Meal Planning and Eating

I get questions all the time about how to eat during vacations and holidays. Clients who are doing very well with their newfound lifestyle and eating habits are frightened to death to go on vacation or "make it through" a holiday and blow all of their progress. This is a very valid fear, as we all have experienced the scale skyrocketing following Thanksgiving or other noted holidays, such as birthdays.

Let me help you with that fear by pointing out a few facts. As we discussed in Chapter 9, The Fallacy of Scale Weight, post–holiday scale weight gain needs to be recognized as either fat gain or lean mass gain. You can gain good weight, i.e. lean mass, during holiday eating. That's right! You can actually *benefit* from your holiday pig–out. This was reviewed in Chapter 15, The Free Window, and is applicable for holiday/vacation eating as well. We will get into more detail below, but first, let's continue with resolving our fears. Prior to this chapter, you entered the holidays with a "full cup" (see cup analogy in Chapter 13, Developing an Understanding of Food (Table 13–3)). Your extra eating had no place to go but your hips, stomach, and backside. After you read below, you will enter the holidays with your cup empty, ready to be filled with all the delectable treats you would like! Another fear alleviator is the fact that you now have an understanding of food timing and can apply it to your pig–out sessions, thereby limiting possible detrimental effects from said feasting.

Holiday Eating

That sets us up for a discussion on preparing your body for holiday eating. Holidays provide every taste and texture imaginable. I encourage everyone to enjoy all of them if possible, but obviously, that can be a lot of food! So how do we survive holiday eating? Consider a holiday a free window with one difference: your body needs a little more prep. We need to be sure our "cup" is as empty as possible for a few days leading into the holiday. This is done by limiting the *active carbohydrates* to the best of your ability for two or three days before the holiday. To make up for calories and help satisfy the hunger that will occur, add some extra protein to your day, specifically to meals one and three. This will allow your cup to be filled first and will limit the "spill over" into fat that has likely occurred in the past. Following the holiday, it is a good idea to allow your body to recover from your eating frenzy. You can do this by allowing the cup to get low again by limiting the *active carbohydrates* to the best of your ability for two or three days following the holiday before returning to your normal eating program. As stated above, make up for calories by adding a protein source to meals one and three. This is a very effective way to maximize lean mass gains, prevent the addition of body fat, and still enjoy the heck out of the holiday foods! I have summarized the above in the following steps:

1. Two or three days prior to the holiday, cut your active carbohydrates out of your diet. To make up for calories, add 1 protein source to meals one and three.

2. Eat like crazy on the holiday.

3. The day after the holiday, cut the active carbohydrates out of your diet for another two or three days. To make up for calories, add 1 protein source to meals one and three.

4. Exercise vigorously the morning following the feast.

5. Resume your regular eating program following a few days without active carbohydrates.

Vacation Eating

Holiday and vacation eating should, first and foremost, be fun! You are, after all, on vacation and/or it is a holiday! I have provided some general rules/guidelines to follow for prepping your body for vacation eating below. These rules can be applied to any situation that requires travel or time away from your normal daily activities.

1. *Remember, you are on vacation!* First rule to remember: Have fun! A lifestyle program like this one is just as the words imply: *Life*, because that's how long it will last, and *style*, "a way of doing something." You have the style, now live life!

2. The portion size of a protein choice is equivalent to the size and shape of your palm.

3. Active carbohydrates portion sizes are also equivalent to the size and shape of your palm.

4. Free carbohydrates are still free carbohydrates even on vacation. Eat away!

5. Drink *as much water as you can* and as bathrooms/rest stops allow!

6. In restaurants, specify your food and how it is to be cooked. Some general guidelines are as follows: try to avoid complex/ processed (active) carbohydrates such as pasta and breads. One

way to determine if it is an active carbohydrate is to think of the process that it went through to get to your plate. If it required too many human interventions, avoid it.

7. If you go overboard with eating, try to eat more vegetables and salads (free carbs)!

8. Always have your nuts and protein bar available in case you can't get to food (carry extra in case that's all you get…). In other words, do not let your hunger get to the point where you settle for anything you see. If you fail to plan, you plan to fail!

9. If you drink alcohol, avoid beers, malts, and ales and only have non–sweetened mixed drinks (i.e. rum in a Diet Coke). See the list below for the "better to worst" suggestions.

10. Continue a.m. exercise whenever possible!

Travel eating, with the program given in this book, is actually very easy. Your style of eating can remain the same no matter where you are. I realize the difficulty in some situations, so I have provided a sample travel menu that I have used with my clients before they venture on a vacation. One of my clients cut out the boxes and laminated them, placed them on a key ring, and traveled all over the place with an eating plan similar to that below. She did very well while on vacation and actually made some notable progress! The foods and drinks are listed best to worst according to the glycemic index (see Appendix III). The meal plan should be the one you are currently using. As I have mentioned before, this is just a guideline and sample travel–eating plan, so you get the idea reiterated in a different format.

TABLE 17-1

Alcohol choices:	Fruit (best to worst):	Meal Plan:
For straight alcohol, the lower the "proof," the lower the calories.	Apple	Utilize the designated meal plan and style you have determined from the book.
	Cherries	P = Protein
	Grapefruit	C = Carbohydrate
	Apricot	M = Mixed
	Pears	Protein/Carbohydrate
	Coconut	(equal to ½ protein
Pick "light" beers over dark.	Plums	and ½ carb)
	Peach	
	Orange	
Mixed Drinks (best to worst)	Pear	
	Grapes	
Bloody Mary	Banana	
Bourbon and soda	Mango	
Tom Collins	Pineapple	
Tequila Sunrise	Dates	
Martini	Watermelon	
Gin and Tonic		
Manhattan		
Screwdriver		
Margarita		
"Fruit" Daiquiri		
Piña Colada		

Travel Foods (best to worst):	General "Rules" of travel dieting:
(P) All meats/cheeses (V) Vegetables (C) Protein-enriched Spaghetti (M) Beans (M) Whole Milk (C) Fettuccine (C) Mixed grain breads (C) Cereal (C) Muffins/pastries (C) Rice (C) Taco shells (C) Potatoes (C) White/wheat bread (C) Pretzels (C) Mashed Potatoes	1. *Remember, you are on vacation!* 2. Protein sources are equal to one palm-sized portion. 3. Active carbohydrates portion sizes are also equivalent to the size and shape of your palm. 4. Free carbohydrates are still free carbohydrates, even on vacation! Eat away! 5. In restaurants, specify your food and how it is to be cooked. 6. If you go overboard with eating, try to eat more vegetables and salads (free carbs)! 7. Always have your nuts and protein bar available in case you can't get to food. 8. If you drink alcohol, avoid beers, malts, and ales and only have *unsweetened* mixed drinks (i.e. rum in a Diet Coke) 9. Continue a.m. exercise.

Chapter Eighteen

The Importance of Exercise, or Developing an Exercise Routine

There are a number of exercise programs, books, videos, and self-help guides available. In writing this book, I felt it important to encourage and help you understand the importance of movement in your quest for ultimate health. Initially, I was planning to add a full exercise program with descriptions and accompanying pictures. However, I found it to be burdensome, not for me, but for you, the reader. My goal of keeping this book concise was defeated by the length of the exercise routine. In Appendix IV, I have provided a basic structure and style of walking program that can be used by anyone in a quest for ultimate health. Feel free to take the program and make it a bike riding or running program, or any type of movement you desire. The style (timed intervals of slow– and fast–paced movement) has been shown to be very effective in cardiovascular health and fat loss. In Appendix V, I have provided a basic resistance–training program that can be done at home using common, household items. Those of you with access to a health facility, let me encourage you to find a well–rounded personal trainer to help you develop your own program. The following is some reasoning behind why I preach exercise like I do medicine—to me, they are one in the same.

Every one of us has had one experience or another with medicine. The word "medicine" brings many things to mind, such as white coats, stethoscopes, the smell of rubbing alcohol, the occasional shot, and medication. Some of us can add surgery to that list. *Webster's* defines medicine as "the science and art of diagnosing, treating, curing, and preventing disease, diminishing pain, and improving and preserving health." As we reviewed in Chapter 4, Understanding the Process of Health, almost everything in this definition involves us. Leaving the diagnosing to health care providers, we need to be an integral part of treating and curing ourselves, preventing disease, relieving pain, and improving and preserving health. One way this can be done is with exercise. Taking this responsibility does not require a medical degree; it does, however, require some information.

What exactly does exercise do for you? We have all been lectured on the benefits of exercise, but can exercise be included under the definition of medicine? If we were to change our paradigm and include exercise in our definition of medicine, would that also allow us to accept it on the same scale of importance? When we get sick, we think of getting better. We think of doctors and medication to help us reach that objective. If we grasp the concept that exercise is medicine, wouldn't the thought prevail that if you want to avoid (or treat) disease, stay healthy, and enjoy life, you had better exercise?

Exercise, like medication and surgery, is at the crux of disease treatment and prevention, fat loss and lean mass gain. If we arm ourselves with the knowledge of what exercise can do, I believe we will be more apt to partake in it. I hope to demonstrate that just like medication and surgery, exercise can be used to treat and, in many cases, cure a lot of disease states we all fear. Exercise also has the distinct advantage of preventing disease, whereas only a few medications and a few surgeries are actually preventative. The rest are needed after the fact.

Research has demonstrated protective effects between physical activity and risk for several chronic diseases. Regular physical activity also contributes to better balance, coordination, and agility that, in turn, may help prevent falls.[43]

In the following paragraphs, I will briefly summarize how exercise is medicine. Recall our definition of medicine as you read the following. I will focus on a few of the more common disease states and provide references that can be utilized if more information about a particular subject or disease is needed.

General Health

A large number of scientific studies[1,2] and controlled experimental investigation[3] have demonstrated that adults engaged in physical activity or exercise, in contrast to their sedentary counterparts, tend to develop and maintain higher levels of physical fitness. Not only has being involved with exercise demonstrated benefits, *lack* of exercise has shown actual detriments! Studies have shown that habitually low levels of physical activity and of physical fitness are associated with markedly increased all–cause mortality (death) rates.[4,22] Even if one were to start an exercise program at mid–life, there would be a decreased mortality risk.[23] It has been estimated that as many as 250,000 deaths per year in the United States (approximately 12% of the total) are attributable to a lack of regular physical activity.[24,25,45]

Cardiovascular Disease

Cardiovascular disease is one of the leading killers in our society. Exercise has been shown not only to prevent the occurrence of cardiovascular disease, but also to modify its course once it is present.[4-8,40-42,44] Experimental studies indicate that exercise training improves all aspects of cardiovascular risk factors, including blood lipid profile (cholesterol level),[26] resting blood pressure,[9,27-29] body composition,[30-32] glucose (sugar) tolerance and insulin sensitivity having to do with the onset and control of diabetes (another major risk factor in heart disease).[33,34]

High Blood Pressure

High blood pressure, or hypertension, is a leading risk factor in heart disease, strokes, kidney disease, eye problems, etc. Exercise has been shown not only to help prevent the onset of hypertension, but also to help modify the treatment of it.[9,10-12] I have had the opportunity in my practice of lowering or even eliminating blood pressure medications for some patients because they began and maintained an exercise and eating program.

Type 2 Diabetes Mellitus

Diabetes is a major cause of health problems ranging from heart disease, kidney disease, blindness, vascular complications, and neuropathy, or loss of sensation and/or increased pain in extremities. Exercise has been shown not only to help prevent this form of diabetes, but to help control it and thereby increase life vitality and expectancy.[13-15]

Osteoporosis

Osteoporosis is a degenerative disease of the bones, which causes increased risk for fracture, disability, and chronic pain syndromes. It affects activities of daily living and can be related to increased mortality due to associated fractures and further complications. Exercise has been shown to slow down the occurrence of osteoporosis and to increase the density of bone, thereby reducing the risk of fractures and associated complications.[16-18,35] Of note, exercise benefits are site specific. A walking program, though beneficial for the hips, will do nothing for your wrists. A well–rounded weightlifting program, on the other hand, benefits the whole body and prevents osteoporosis at all sites involved!

Colon Cancer

Even cancer is affected by exercise. Exercise has actually been shown to decrease the risk of colon cancer.[19]

Psychiatric Conditions

Psychological function and exercise have shown an emphatic relationship. Exercise not only makes you feel good in the short run, but also has been shown to positively influence anxiety and depression.[20,21,38] Exercise is also beneficial, as it allows interaction with others. This increases social opportunities, which have also been shown to decrease depression.

Immune Function

The function of your immune system, or internal disease–fighting complex, can be improved by utilizing exercise.[36,37] This has a profound impact not only on major diseases such as cancer, but also on everyday cold and viral syndromes.

Most of the studies cited above have been utilizing cardiovascular exercise such as running or biking in preventing chronic diseases. However, one cannot overlook the importance of flexibility and strength training in viewing the importance of exercise. Clinical experience and studies suggest that people who maintain or improve their strength and flexibility may be better able to perform daily activities, may be less likely to develop back pain, and may be better able to avoid disability, especially as they advance into older age.

As I am personally biased toward strength training (weightlifting), I want to spend some time acquainting you with the importance of a strength–training program in the quest for optimal health.

As you learned in How This Book came About and 13, it is essential that we focus on *lean mass gain,* not necessarily fat loss. Fat loss is the side effect of muscle gain! Admittedly, I have clients who do not use resistance training on a regular basis. They did and do well even so, as their eating was fine–tuned to near perfection. In my experience, however, those who take the time to do a strength–training program within the confines of the suggestions below reap the benefits of their lifestyle quicker and easier.

I will briefly review the basics of strength training. It is my hope that you will take the information and begin to develop your own program. I will start with some terminology that you will see and use as you explore strength–training literature:

Cardiovascular endurance–the ability of the respiratory system and the circulatory system to supply oxygen and nutrients to the muscle cells so an activity can continue for a long period of time.
Muscular endurance–the ability of a muscle to produce force repeatedly over a period of time. *Intensity* is the difficulty of training (time or speed of movement, pounds lifted).

Power–strength in addition to speed.

A *repetition* (abbreviated as "rep") is one movement of that exercise.

A *set* is a series of counted repetitions, or repetitions over a specified time period.

A *spotter* is another person who can assist you in exercises that are very difficult to manage alone.

Strength–the ability of a muscle to produce force.

Volume is the total amount of training (reps, sets).

I will now cover some basic rules that need to be applied to any strength–training program, be it at your house or in the gym:

- *Commit to your program and be consistent!* If you want to improve, you've got to put forth your best effort. Avoid getting distracted or disheartened. Results come with effort. A big barrier to continual progress is missing a workout or wasting time and effort during workouts. I cannot tell you the number of times I have witnessed my clients justifying missing one workout, thinking it's a well–deserved break, or that "missing just one won't hurt." The problem with a neglected workout is that it makes it that much easier to miss another, and before you know it, you are not exercising at all!

- *Limit your strength–training workout time to 40–60 minutes.* The body's natural hormonal response is maximized during this time frame. Working out wisely will ensure maximum results in the shortest time possible. If you are taking the time to do it, do it right!

- *Practice good exercise form and speed.* Your exercise movements should be done in a smooth and deliberate fashion. Injuries can result from improper form, speed, or overexertion. Take about 3 to 6 seconds for each repetition, unless otherwise specified. Deliberately pause at both the top and bottom of each repetition. Do not hold your breath at any point while exercising. Breathe with slow, deliberate breaths by inhaling as you lower the weight and exhaling as you raise or exert effort against the weight.

- *Warm up before exercise.* This can be a brisk five–minute jog or bike ride. This gets the blood flowing and prepares the body for the up–and–coming exercises. After your warm–up, briefly stretch in accordance to a good stretching routine. Stretching is a form of exercise and is essential in preparing the muscles, ligaments, and tendons for resistance training.

- *Listen to your body.* If something does not feel right or becomes painful, stop the exercise. I would suggest that you feel the muscles working to the point of a slight burning sensation, but do not go to the point of pain. Always be aware of what you are doing and be sure to concentrate while performing the movements.

- *Start easy and work your way up.* I would start by using lighter weights and high repetitions for each set and exercise. Gradually increase your intensity in the form of heavier weights, more repetitions, and/or sets, or for longer time periods.

Appendix V gives a basic strength–training program with pictures to help you decipher the movement. Both novice and more advanced weightlifters can use the program I have included in this book. Regardless of the modalities used (soup cans, dumbbells, etc.), the style is very effective. It is a variation of a weightlifting technique called *Timed Sets/Reps* or *Time Under Tension.* Following the exercise instructions, you will perform 2 sets of each exercise for 40 seconds each, followed by 60 seconds of rest. We are not counting repetitions with this particular technique; we are just doing the repetitions in a slow and controlled fashion for a total of 40 seconds a set. To advance your program, I would suggest one of two things: Increase the amount of resistance for the same time period, or keep the resistance the same and increase the time. This should be done when the set becomes too easy and you no longer feel you are putting forth much effort.

I would highly encourage the use of resistance training in your quest for optimal health. The benefits to your lean mass for fat burning, balance, coordination, strength in activities of daily living, and changing your body shape cannot be repeated enough. If you have some fears or trepidations about a resistance–training program, I would encourage you to attempt it for a month and see if you notice a difference. I would lay my last dollar on a bet that you will.

Chapter Nineteen

Progression Through Roadblocks, Walls, and Plateaus

Any attempt at health maximization includes confrontation with the dreaded wall. This plateau not only affects your quest, but can have detrimental effects on your psyche as well. I have added this brief chapter to help you through this commonly met roadblock. First, I will let you in on a little secret: You are going to hit a wall! Everyone does, has, and will, including me, and it is not just one wall either. It is wall after wall after wall. I must say, however, that this is a good thing. I have made most of my personal progress as well as helped clients' progress when this occurs. Breaking through walls allows us to understand what our body is doing in relation to the situation we are placing it in. It also prevents monotony, the deadly killer of all eating and exercise programs.

The human body is the most amazingly adaptive system on the planet. Given enough time, we can acclimatize to any condition, internal (such as diet), or external (such as the weather). One very obvious example is that of someone who engages in drinking alcohol on a regular basis. When they first started, it only took a beer or two to obtain their desired effect. After a while, however, it takes multiple beers and hard drinks to get that same effect.

The lifestyle changes that initially have such a profound and dramatic outcome will eventually slow down. This does not mean it stopped working or will not work again in the future. The body just gets used to what we are doing until we tell it differently. That is one of the keys to understanding how to break past these common endpoints.

> The body just gets used to what we are doing until we tell it differently.

Once you notice that your objective and subjective changes are slowing down or have halted, it is time to shock the system. As I have said above, our bodies adapt to everything we do to them, so we need to jumpstart them so progress will continue. Remember our definition of health: "a continuing process of *transformation*, both physical and mental, that allows your body and mind to take the next step into maximal living." It is a process, and part of that process involves not allowing our bodies to get used to our techniques.

The following is a list of ten tried and true techniques to help you break past plateaus:

1. Take a break. Nothing can be more effective both physiologically and psychologically than just taking a week off. Eat what you want, avoid the gym, and forget it. Just be sure to get back to your program within a week!

2. Alternate your caloric intake. After calculating your daily energy requirements (see Chapter 16), change your eating variable by 2 or 3 every other day for a while and see how you do. This provides the metabolism enough confusion that it will help break up and prevent that evil wall.

3. Alternate your free window. If you have been using a free day, change to a free evening twice a week and vice versa. Change your free window to the morning. Utilize it at lunchtime. Change it

up according to your schedule, needs, or wants. Monitor it as well. Are you *over*utilizing or *under*utilizing the free window? (See Table 19–1)

4. Eat your day's calories in fewer or more meals. For example: If you calculated your energy requirements to be 2,000 calories a day and you have been following the five–meal–a–day plan provided, eat the same diet over three meals or eat it over ten meals.

5. Take a supplement holiday. When you meet a wall, try cutting all supplements out for one week. This has been very successful in my practice, and it is a good and easy technique to apply.

6. Try a new form of exercise. If you are a walker, try riding a bike. If you are a weightlifter, change your sets and reps. For example, if you have been doing 3 sets of 10 reps per exercise, change it to 2 sets of 30 reps per exercise.

7. Cut out all of your active carbohydrates for a few days. I will cover different diets and dietary techniques in my next book, but for now it suffices to say that cutting out active carbohydrates completely for a few days is a good shock to the system. Just remember to continue your daily fiber, as this technique has a tendency to cause constipation.

8. Do a short fast. Pick one day and just drink water, lots of it. Avoid all foods and the act of chewing (as this will make you hungry) for a twenty–four–hour period.

9. Change your foods. This may sound obvious, but we are creatures of habit. Review your eating plan and make drastic changes everywhere you can with the type of food eaten. Maintain your food timing, however.

10. Add more unsaturated fat to your diet. As you have likely added more protein to your eating program following this plan, and, therefore, an increase in saturated fat, take a few days and add fish oils and vegetable oils in place of the protein. Watch your calories, as fat packs a lot of them (9 kcals/g).

Table 19-1: Not Using the Free Window *Enough*!

A very common erroneous belief is that the free window can hamper or even harm your progress. It is such a paradigm shift that a lot of people have a hard time accepting the fact that they can do it. A familiar roadblock I often see in clients is the fact that they *do not* use their free window as often as they should. Their lean mass does not get the benefit of a free window, and it starts to decline, slowing the fat loss, and a vicious cycle begins. Make sure you are using your free windows! They are part of your optimal health and eating plan!

Epilogue

The question posed at the beginning of this book was intended to make you think about optimal health, the multiple factors and variables involved, how it can be obtained, and who is responsible for it. The direct question is applicable: Does your health care provider practice what he preaches? What does he look like under that lab coat or suit? How does he eat, and does he exercise regularly? More importantly, however, is the indirect meaning of the question. To understand this we must first pose a question in its place: *Who* really is your health care provider? Is it your medical doctor? Is it your chiropractor or massage therapist? When I present the question, "What does your doctor look like naked?" what I really want to know is, "Do you know *who your* health care provider is?"

I hope the answer has become clear throughout the book. The answer can be found in front of your bedroom mirror. In reality, neither you nor I should care what we look like, but we do. Part of optimal health is obtaining the preferred look and physical characteristics we admire. More important, however, is that we take the responsibility for our health, longevity, and happiness. Utilizing the instruments and knowledge provided in this book will allow you to further delve into optimal health attainment. I tell my clients on a regular basis: My job is to give you the tools. *Your* job is to use them. If I were to give you a handsaw and nail and ask you to hang a picture, it might be done, but not without some difficulty. What I have provided you with are a hammer and a nail, with instructions, so you can properly and easily hang that picture. My job is done. Now it is up to you to utilize the tools provided.

This book and all of the information in it can be summed up as follows:

- Understand health and disease as processes that you have control over.
- Have knowledge of and apply the five basics of Age–management Medicine.
  - Nutrition.
    - Use the eating program in this book for optimal intake, lean mass gain, and fat loss.
  - Supplementation.
    - Use the suggested supplements (after discussing them with your doctor) to maximize your quest for optimal health.
  - Exercise.
    - Move daily! Develop an exercise routine that will capitalize on your lean mass gain.
  - Stress Reduction.
    - Review and practice the ten proposals on stress reduction every day!
  - Preventative Screening.
    - Utilize suggested preventative screening to ensure health maximization. Be on your guard for problems with screening exams. Every test is a setup for another test.
- Be familiar with hormone replacement therapy and its implications in your optimal health.
- Avoid the scale as an independent measuring device! Use objective and subjective data to track and then make changes to your lifestyle program.

- Develop an understanding of food and its power by concentrating on the following:
  - Food is a drug!
  - It is based on food *timing*, not the *type* of food you choose.
    - There is no such thing as a bad food.
  - Use the Eating Variable to adjust your caloric intake and capitalize on lean mass gain and fat loss.
  - Make use of the free window to take full advantage of your eating program.
  - Know you can eat to your benefit even on holidays and vacations.
- Appreciate the importance of exercise in your daily routine!
- Use the suggested techniques to break through roadblocks, walls, and plateaus.
  - Use the same techniques to *shock the system* from time to time.

As I mentioned earlier, this book's approach is clear and simple: Commit to a healthy lifestyle and stick with it. Evaluate your progress regularly and make adjustments based on your needs and results. Expect to make consistent and measurable improvements by utilizing the techniques described above.

In the very near future I will publish what I consider to be the end–all diet book. It will contain the details of the programs others and I have had so much success with. A basic understanding is still needed before utilizing that tool. That is why this book came first.

I hope you have enjoyed getting a basic and necessary understanding of optimal health. If you are currently attempting or are willing to attempt the eating program or exercise program, or have questions about preventative screening or hormone replacement, or if you just hit the wall we spoke of and cannot get around it, please feel free to contact me (see Appendix IX). It is my passion to see you succeed. Let me help if I can.

Until next time: Focus on gaining, not losing. Remember, there is no such thing as a bad food. It's all about the food timing, not the food type, and always train with your brain!

J. Warren Willey

Appendix I

Food Lists

Description of the Food List

Each caloric total (from 1,000 to 3,500 in increments of 100) consists of a Menu Plan, Active Carbohydrate List, Protein Source List, and Free Carbohydrate List (on the Protein Source page). Once you have calculated your caloric needs (Chapter 16), find the Menu Plan, Active Carbohydrate List, Protein Source List, and Free Carbohydrate List (on the Protein Source page) for that caloric total.

The foods listed in all the different caloric plans are foods that I use most commonly and my clients have requested most often. Obviously, this list is not all–inclusive. I would encourage you to use the foods on the list, and as you develop the habit of eating correctly, substitute foods that are similar, utilizing similar amounts. The amount of protein, carbohydrates, and fats has been accounted for with each eating plan and at each caloric level. The design is a simple "cut and paste" format. If your menu plan suggests one protein source, go to the Protein Source page and pick one item at the suggested amount, and so forth. It is that simple!

As you review the different food lists, you will see some unusual amounts, such as 0.88 of a cup. This is not an exact measurement as far as you needing to measure that exact amount. If you can exactly measure 0.88 of a cup, great! I do not expect you to. What I would like is for you to find a midway point between 0.75 and 1 cup. Follow a similar pattern for other odd amounts. You will also note that some of the foods and their amounts are the same for a few of the caloric amounts. This is due to the fact that other foods have been changed to compensate and/or I may have increased the amount of your mid–morning or mid–afternoon snack

1000 Calories/Day Eating Plan		
What Does Your Doctor Look Like Naked?		
Name: _____		
Date: _____		
Exercise: 30-40 min. in a.m. before food		Write what you eat here:
Meal 1 Time: _____	1 Protein Source 2 Active Carbohydrates	
Meal 2 Time: _____	1 oz Raw Almonds	
Meal 3 Time: _____	1 Protein Source 1 Active Carbohydrates Free Carbohydrates (as much as you want)	
Meal 4 Time: _____	½ LOW CARB protein bar (OR) 1 scoop Whey Protein Powder in water	
Meal 5 Time: _____	1 Protein Source 0 Active Carbohydrates Free Carbohydrates (as much as you want)	
Bedtime Meal (Optional)	Sugar Free Jell-O 1 cup	

Add fiber supplement in evening, such as Metamucil or other (sugar FREE).
Add spices, pepper, etc. as needed.
Try to eat every two to three hours.
Drink ¾ of a gallon of water EVERY DAY!
May have up to 2 diet pops (or) 2 cups a coffee a day.

Active Carbohydrates 1000 Calories

Fruit and Vegetables

APPLE	1.45	3 INCH
APPLESAUCE, MOTT'S	0.54	CUP
APRICOTS (CAN/DEL MONTE LITE)	1	CUP
APRICOTS (DRIED)	1.7	OZ
APRICOTS (FRESH 12/LB)	6.9	MEDIUM
ASPARAGUS	32	OZ
BANANA	1.13	MEDIUM
BLUEBERRIES (FRESH)	1.44	CUP
BRUSSELS SPROUTS, BOILED	1.97	CUP
CABBAGE, SHREDDED	6.6	CUP
CANTALOUPE	0.63	5 INCH
CARROT (FRESH)	10.7	OZ
CAULIFLOWER	4.5	CUP
CELERY	29.5	OZ
CHERRIES, FRESH, SWEET W/PIT	1.135	CUP
CHERRIES, DARK (CAN/DEL MONTE)	0.59	CUP
COLLARD GREENS (CAN)	1.968	CUP
COLLARD GREENS (FRESH)	9.84	CUP
CORN CAKE	3.374	CAKE
CORN (CAN/DEL MONTE NO SODIUM)	8.62	OZ
CUCUMBER, SLICED	8.43	CUP
EGGPLANT	5.37	CUP
FRUIT, MIXED FROZEN	1.312	CUP
GARLIC, 1 CLOVE	29.5	CLOVE
GARLIC, TRIMMED	2.81	OZ
GRAPES	1.035	CUP
GRAPEJIUCE/VERYFINE	6.3	OZ
GRAPEFRUIT	1.283	4 INCH
GREEN BEANS (CAN/DEL MONTE NO SALT)	2.95	CUP
GREEN PEPPER	5.9	MEDIUM
KIWI	7.95	OZ
MUSHROOMS, FRESH	6.56	CUP
ONION, FRESH/CHOPPED	1.968	CUP
ORANGE, NAVAL	1.816	3 INCH

ORANGE, JUICE	8.59	OZ
PAPAYA	1.01	LB.
PAPAYA, PEELED/CUBED	2.19	CUP
PEACH, FRESH, SLICED	1.6	CUP
PEACH (CAN/DEL MONTE EXTRA LITE)	0.985	CUP
PEARS (CAN)	3.94	HALF
PEAS, BLACKEYED (CAN)	0.656	CUP
PEAS (CAN/DEL MONTE NO SODIUM)	8.6	OZ
PEAS, GREEN GIANT FROZEN, SWEET	1.12	CUP
PEAS, EDIBLE-PODDED	1.97	CUP
PINEAPPLE, FRESH/DICED	1.515	CUP
PINEAPPLE, DEL MONTE SNACK CAN (LITE)	1.688	3.5 OZ
PINEAPPLE, (CAN/DOLE LITE SYRUP)	6.95	SLICE
PRUNES, DOLE, DRIED	1.69	OZ
PUMPKIN (CAN)	2.36	CUP
RAISENS	0.246	CUP
RED PEPPER	5.9	MEDIUM
STRAWBERRIES (FRESH)	1.22	PINT
STRAWBERRIES (FROZEN)	1.575	CUP
SQUASH, CAN, STOKLEY	1.18	CUP
SQUASH, FRESH BAKED	1.038	CUP
TANGERINE	3.2	2.5 INCH
TOMATO, CANNED	11.03	OZ
TOMATO, FRESH	4.55	3 INCH
TOMATO, JUICE	18.9	OZ
VEGETABLES, MIXED (FROZEN)	1.311	CUP
WATERMELLON	0.78	1X10 INCH
ZUCCHINI, FRESH, SLICED	6.56	CUP

Yogurts and Desserts

DING DONG	0.738	DING
DREYERS FROZEN FAT FREE YOGURT	0.656	CUP
FRUIT ROLL-UP	1.686	ROLL UP
POPCORN, WHITE	2.36	TBLSP
TCBY, SOFT SERVE (NON FAT/NO SUGAR)	0.74	CUP
YOGURT, FAT FREE, MOUNTAIN HIGH	8	OZ
YOGURT, FAT FREE, DANNON	8	OZ
LUCERN, YOGURT (NONFAT, LITE)	8	OZ

YOGURT, YOPLAIT (FAT FREE, LITE)	6	OZ
YOGURT,YOPLAIT ORIGINAL/99% FAT FREE	6	OZ
YOGURT, HORIZON, FF/BLUEBERRY	5	OZ
PLANTER DRIED WALNUT PIECES	0.15	CUP
RAW ALMONDS, TOASTED	0.7	OZ
PECANS, DRIED	0.6	OZ
PEANUTS, DRY ROASTED	0.14	CUP
HOT CHOCOLATE	1	ENVEL.
ALMONDS, SHELLED	0.7	OZ

Cereals

CEREAL, CHEERIOS	1.08	CUP
CEREAL, COCOA KRISPIES	0.74	CUP
CEREAL, GRAPENUTS	0.296	CUP
CEREAL, HONEY NUT TOASTY O'S	1.07	CUP
CEREAL, WHEATIES	1.07	CUP
CEREAL, KELLOGG'S ALL BRAN	0.74	CUP
CEREAL, KELLOGG'S CORN FLAKES	1.07	CUP
CEREAL, KELLOGG'S RAISIN BRAN	0.69	CUP
CEREAL, KELLOGG'S CRACKLIN' OAT BRAN	0.45	CUP
CEREAL, NABISCO SHREDDED WHEAT	1.48	PIECE
CEREAL, NAB. SHREDDED WHEAT (SPOON)	0.69	CUP
CEREAL, RICE KRISPIES	1.35	CUP
CEREAL, BENEFIT NUTRITION, PROTEIN+	0.565	CUP
CREAM OF WHEAT	2.95	TBL/DRY
GRANOLA, CW POST HEARTY	0.281	CUP
GRANOLA, KELLOGG'S LOW FAT	3	CUP
OATMEAL (PRE-COOK MEASUREMENT)	0.422	CUP

Breads

BREAD, OROWHEAT LITE	2.95	SLICE
BREAD, SUSAN'S HOMEMADE/18 SLICES	1.31	SLICE
BREAD, SUSAN'S HOMEMADE	0.072	LOAF
BUN, WONDER REDUCED CALORIE LITE	1.48	BUN
CRACKER, ZESTA SALTINES	9.84	CRACKER
TORTILLA (CAROLYN)	0.695	TORT
TORTILLA, TORTILLA'S MEXICO, FLOUR	1.074	TORT

TORTILLA, TORTILLA'S MEXICO, CORN	1.31	TORT
TRISCUITS	0.844	OZ
WAFFLE, EGGO, HOMESTYLE	1.074	WAFFLE
WHOLE GRAIN/WHOLE WHEAT FLOUR	0.29	CUP

Rice/Potatoes/Beans

BLACK BEANS (BOILED)	0.52	CUP
BLACK BEANS (DRY)	0.42	CUP
CHICKPEAS/GARBANZO BEANS	0.17	CUP
KIDNEY BEANS (BOILED)	0.18	CUP
LIMA BEANS (BOILED)	0.568	CUP
NAVY BEANS (BOILED)	0.4574	CUP
NAVY BEANS (CAN)	0.492	CUP
PINTO BEANS (BOILED)	0.505	CUP
PINTO BEANS (CAN)	0.622	CUP
PINTO BEANS (DRY)	0.197	CUP
PORK & BEANS/VAN CAMPS	0.537	CUP
POTATO, SWEET	1	5"X2"
POTATO	7	OZ
RICE CAKE	2.36	CAKE
RICE, WHITE, BASMATI	0.492	CUP (C)
RICE, BROWN LONG GRAIN	0.59	CUP (C)
RICE, INSTANT, MINUTE BRAND	0.369	CUP(UC)
RICE, WHITE, LONG GRAIN	0.185	CUP(UC)
SOYBEANS (BOILED)	0.45	CUP
YAM, BOILED OR BAKED	0.747	CUP

Pasta

MACARONI, DAVINI TWIST	0.449	CUP/DRY
MACARONI, HOSPITALITY ELBOW	0.246	CUP/DRY
MACARONI, AM. BEAUTY ELBOW	0.281	CUP/DRY
PASTA, CREAMETTE PLAIN	1.124	OZ
SPAGHETTI, EDEN WHOLE WHEAT	1.125	OZ/UC

Protein Sources 1000 Calories

White Meat

CHICKEN BREAST (HORMEL/CAN)	0.787	CAN
CHICKEN BREAST (SKINLESS)	3.94	OZ
CHICKEN (LEG W/SKIN & BONE)	0.447	
CHICKEN (THIGH W/SKIN & BONE)	0.775	
CHICKEN (LEG & THIGH W/SKIN & BONE)	0.283	
HAM, BAR S, XTRA LEAN, 96% FAT FREE	3.38	OZ
HAM, DAK CANNED	3.94	OZ
PORK, SIRLOIN, LEAN W/FAT	1.18	OZ
TURKEY BREAST (SKINLESS)	2.21	OZ
TURKEY BREAST (HORMEL/CAN)	0.676	CAN
TURKEY BRST/OVEN ROAST/SFWY/89% FF	4.7	OZ
VENISON/ANTELOPE	2.65	OZ

Red Meat

HAMBURGER (10% FAT)	2.1	OZ
HAMBURGER (15% FAT)	1.74	OZ
HAMBURGER (20% FAT)	1.69	OZ
HAMBURGER (27% FAT)	1.43	OZ
LAMB, SHOULDER	1.35	OZ
STEAK, BOTTOM ROUND	2	OZ
STEAK, BRISKET (FLAT HALF)	1.88	OZ
STEAK, CHUCK, ARM	1.94	OZ
STEAK, CHUCK, BLADE	1.67	OZ
STEAK, EYE ROUND	2.48	OZ
STEAK, FLANK	2.02	OZ
STEAK, NEW YORK STRIP	2.36	OZ
STEAK, PORTERHOUSE	1.92	OZ
STEAK, RIBEYE	1.86	OZ
STEAK, ROUND TIP	2.26	OZ
STEAK, SHANK (CROSSCUTS)	2.08	OZ
STEAK, T-BONE	1.95	OZ
STEAK, TENDERLOIN	1.99	OZ
STEAK, TOP LOIN	2.02	OZ
STEAK, TOP ROUND	2.3	OZ

STEAK, TOP SIRLOIN	2.15	OZ
STEAK, TYSON SEASONED BEEF STRIPS	2.53	OZ
TACO/BURRITO MEAT/SMART GROUND	0.615	CUP
OSCAR MAYER BACON	3.94	SLICE
LITTLE SIZZLER BROWN/SERVE SAUSAGE	1.54	LINK

Sea Food

BASS, FRESHWATER, DRY HEAT	2.86	OZ
BASS, STRIPED, DRY HEAT	3.38	OZ
COD, ATLANTIC, DRY HEAT	4	OZ
CRAB, ALASKA KING, MOIST HEAT	4.33	OZ
CRAB, BLUE, MOIST HEAT	4.1	OZ
FLOUNDER, DRY HEAT	3.6	OZ
HADDOCK, DRY HEAT	3.75	OZ
HALIBUT, DRY HEAT	2.98	OZ
LOBSTER, NORTHERN, MOIST HEAT	4.3	OZ
MAHI MAHI	4.9	OZ
ORANGE ROUGHY, DRY HEAT	4.68	OZ
PERCH, DRY HEAT	3.6	OZ
PERCH, OCEAN/ATLANTIC, DRY HEAT	3.45	OZ
SALMON, ATLANTIC, DRY HEAT	2.27	OZ
SHRIMP, MOIST HEAT	4.22	OZ
TROUT, DRY HEAT	2.2	OZ
TUNA BURGER, AHI/OMEGA FOODS	4.22	OZ
TUNA, LOW SODIUM, CANNED	0.675	CAN
TUNA, WATER, CANNED	0.6	CAN
TUNA, WHITE/LOW SALT, CAN (1 CAN/5 OZ)	0.676	CAN
TUNA, WHITE, CAN (1 CAN/5 OZ)	0.676	CAN
TUNA, FILLET/STEAK	2.7	OZ
WALLEYE, BAKED/BROILED/MICRO	3.5	OZ

Vegetarian

IVES VEG. COUSINE VEGGY DOG	1.96	DOG
SOY MILK (TRIS)	1.25	CUP
SOY MILK (SYLVIA)	1.15	CUP

Eggs/Dairy

1% COTTAGE CHEESE, NORDICA	0.74	CUP
2% COTTAGE CHEESE (LOW FAT)	0.59	CUP
COTTAGE CHEESE (LUCERNE FAT FREE)	0.74	CUP
COTT CHEESE MARIGOLD/DRY CURD	1.13	CUP
COTT CHEESE MARIGOLD/DRY CURD	18	TBLSP
COTT CHEESE BREAKSTONES FAT FREE	0.74	CUP
CHEDDER, SHREDDED, FAT FREE, KHF	0.66	CUP
CHEDDER, SHREDDED, 94% FAT FREE, HC	0.59	CUP
CHEESE, COLBY/MOZZARELLA	1.08	OZ
EGG WHITE	6.95	
EGG, WHOLE	1.58	
EGG BEATERS	0.98	CUP
MOZZARELLA SHREDDED, FAT FREE, KHF	0.59	CUP
SKIM MOZZARELLA STRING CHEESE	1.48	OZ

Free Carbs, Supplements, Fast Foods
1000 calories

Free Carbs

ASPARAGUS
BROCCOLI
CABBAGE
CAULIFLOWER
CELERY
CUCUMBER
GREEN BEANS
GREEN PEPPERS
GREEN SQUASH
LETTUCE, ICEBERG
LETTUCE, LEAF/SHREDDED
MUSHROOMS
ONION
PICKLES (DILL)
RADISH

RED PEPPERS
SPINACH (CAN/NO SALT)
SPINACH (FRESH)
TOMATO (EXCLUDING JUICE)
ZUCCHINI

Supplements/Fast Foods

ATKINS BAR	0.5	BAR
EAS ADVANTEDGE, C&C/LEM/BLUE	0.5	BAR
BAR, ZONE	0.5	BAR
BAR, PURE PROTEIN, 50 G.	0.5	BAR
BAR, W.W. PURE PROTEIN, 78 G.	0.33	BAR
BAR, PROTEIN REVOLUTION, PBJ	0.5	BAR
BAR, FIBAR, PEANUT BUTTER, 1.2 OZ	0.75	BAR
BAR, PREMIER 1, PROTEIN 8, CHOC/COCO	0.33	BAR
BAR, PREFERRED BAR, CHOC./FUDG/RAS	0.5	BAR
BAR, PREFERRED BAR, CHOC./FUDG/BROW	0.5	BAR
ALIVE, HI CARB POWDER	3	TBLSP
POWERADE	1.5	SERVING
PROTEIN,GNC P.P. EGG/WHEY	1	SERVING
PROTEIN. GNC P.PERF. WHEY	2.75	SCOOP
OPTIMUM NUTRITION WHEY	1	SCOOP
SYNTRAX WHEY PROTEIN	1	SCOOP
TRI PROTEIN PLUS POWDER	0.75	SERVING
HW STRAWBERRY PROT. POWD.	1.25	SCOOP
BIOCHEM WHEY PRO 290	1.25	SCOOP
HUMAN DEV. TECH. WHEY	0.75	SCOOP
NATURADE 100% SOY PROTEIN	0.33	CUP
SUPER GREEN PRO 96 - SOY	0.33	CUP
100% PURE WHEY, PROLAB	0.75	SCOOP
ECLIPSE BULK UP WHEY	1.25	SCOOP
VITAMIN WORLD WHEY 100%	1	SCOOP
ULT. NUT. PROSTAR WHEY	1	SCOOP
RED WINE	4	OZ
MET RX CH.RST.PNT.PRO + BAR	0.33	BAR
MET RX BAV. MINT. PRO + BAR	0.33	BAR
MET AFTER FX BAR	0.33	BAR
MET RX CH. CH. CHIP PRO + BAR	0.33	BAR

MET RX SOURCE ONE BAR	0.5	BAR
MET RX CHOC. GRAHCRK CHIP BAR	0.33	BAR
MET RX PEANUT BUTTER BAR	0.33	BAR
MET RX DRINK MIX, MRP	0.33	SERVING
MET RX PRO 50, ANABOLIC DRIVE	0.33	SERVING
MET RX PRO 60, ANABOLIC DRIVE	0.33	SERVING
MET RX PROTEIN PLUS	1.7	SCOOP
MET RX KETO PRO	1.5	SCOOP
NUTRI FORCE DRINK MIX, MRP	0.33	SERVING
EAS MYO. DEL. CH/PB BAR	0.33	BAR
EAS MYOPLEX + DELUXE	0.33	SERVING
EAS MYOPLEX LITE	0.5	SERVING
ADVANT EDGE QUICK STIR PROTEIN DRINK	0.5	SERVING
EAS NEUROGAIN	2.5	SCOOP
EAS PHOSPHAGEN HP	0.75	SCOOP
EAS PRECISION PROTEIN	1	SCOOP
EAS SIMPLY PROTEIN	2	SCOOP
EAS WHEY PROTEIN	1	SCOOP
EAS SUPPER SHAKE	0.25	SHAKE
VITAMIN WORLD DAILY RX, MRP	0.45	SHAKE
VITAMIN WORLD PROTOPLEX DELUXE, MRP	0.35	SHAKE
VITAMIN WORLD PRE. ENG. WHEY PROT.	1.25	SCOOP
PERFECT RX, MRP, CHOCOLATE	0.5	SHAKE
OPTI PRO	0.35	SHAKE
ARBY'S CHICK. SAND. R.DELX.LITE	0.33	BURGER
ARBY'S SIDE SALAD	1	SALAD
ARBY'S GARDEN SALAD	1	SALAD
ARBY'S RST. CHCK. SALAD	0.75	SALAD
ARBY'S RED. CAL. ITAL. DRESSING	1	PACKET
ARBY'S RED RANCH DRESSING	1	PACKET
MCD'S VINAG. LITE SALAD DR.	1	PACKET
MCD'S GARDEN SALAD	1	SALAD
MCD'S VINAG. LITE SALAD DR.	1	PACKET
P.HUT. HAND-TOSS CHEESE	0.5	SLICE
P.HUT. HAND-TOSS HAM	0.5	SLICE
P.HUT. HAND-TOSS VEG. LUV.	0.5	SLICE
P.HUT. HAND-TOSS PEPPERON	0.5	SLICE
P.HUT. THIN/CRISP CHEESE	0.5	SLICE

P.HUT. THIN/CRISP HAM	0.5	SLICE
P.HUT. THIN/CRISP VEG. LUV.	0.5	SLICE
P.HUT. THIN/CRISP PEPPERON	0.5	SLICE
SW 6" COLD SUB/VEGG. DELIT	1	SUB
SW 6" COLD SUB/TURK. BRST.	1	SUB
SW 6" COLD SUB/TURK.B/HAM	1	SUB
SW 6" COLD SUB/HAM	1	SUB
SW 6" COLD SUB/ROAST BEEF	1	SUB
SW 6" COLD SUB/SFOOD,CRAB	1	SUB
SW 6" COLD SUB/COLD CUT 3	1	SUB
SW 6" COLD SUB/TUNA	1	SUB
SW 6" HOT SUB/RST.CHICK.BR.	1	SUB
SW 6" HOT SUB/STAK/CHEESE	1	SUB
SW 6" HOT SUB/SUB MELT	1	SUB
SW VEGGIE DELITE SALAD	1	SALAD
SW TURKEY BREAST SALAD	1	SALAD
SW ROAST BEEF SALAD	1	SALAD
SW TURK. BRST/HAM SALAD	1	SALAD
SW RST. CHICK. BR. SALAD	0.75	SALAD
SW SEAFOOD/CRAB SALAD	0.75	SALAD
SW STEAK/CHEESE SALAD	0.5	SALAD
SW SUBWAY MELT SALAD	0.5	SALAD
SW COLD CUT 3 SALAD	0.5	SALAD
SW FAT FREE ITALIAN DRESS	1	OZ
SW FAT FREE FRENCH DRESS	1	OZ
SW FAT FREE RANCH DRESS	1	OZ
SW DELI STYLE TURKEY BR.	0.5	SNDWCH
SW DELI STYLE HAM	0.5	SNDWCH
SW DELI STYLE ROAST BEEF	0.5	SNDWCH
TB GRILLED STEAK SOFT TACO	0.5	TACO
WAHOO'S CHBROIL FISH TACO	0.5	TACO
WENDI'S SIDE SALAD	1	SALAD
WENDI'S FF FRENCH DRESSING	1	OZ
WENDI'S ITALIAN RED. F/C DRESS	1	OZ
WENDI'S SMALL CHILI	0.5	BOWL
WENDI'S GRILLED CHICK. FILLET	1	MEAT

1100 Calories/Day Eating Plan		
What Does Your Doctor Look Like Naked?		

Name: _____

Date: _____

Exercise: 30-40 min in a.m. before food		Write what you eat here:
Meal 1 Time: _____	1 Protein Source 2 Active Carbohydrates	
Meal 2 Time: _____	1 oz Raw Almonds	
Meal 3 Time: _____	1 Protein Source 1 Active Carbohydrates Free Carbohydrates (as much as you want)	
Meal 4 Time: _____	½ LOW CARB protein bar (OR) 1 scoop Whey Protein Powder in water	
Meal 5 Time: _____	1 Protein Source 0 Active Carbohydrates Free Carbohydrates (as much as you want)	
Bedtime Meal (Optional)	Sugar Free Jell-O 1 cup	

Add fiber supplement in evening such as Metamucil or other (sugar FREE).
Add spices, pepper, etc. as needed.
Try to eat every two to three hours.
Drink ¾ of a gallon of water EVERY DAY!
May have up to 2 diet pops (or) 2 cups a coffee a day.

Active Carbohydrates 1100 Calories

Fruit and Vegetables

APPLE	1.67	3 INCH
APPLESAUCE, MOTT'S	0.614	CUP
APRICOTS (CAN/DEL MONTE LITE)	1.125	CUP
APRICOTS (DRIED)	1.93	OZ
APRICOTS (FRESH 12/LB)	7.95	MEDIUM
ASPARAGUS	36.5	OZ
BANANA	1.29	MEDIUM
BLUEBERRIES (FRESH)	1.65	CUP
BRUSSELS SPROUTS, BOILED	2.25	CUP
CABBAGE, SHREDDED	7.5	CUP
CANTALOUPE	0.63	5 INCH
CARROT (FRESH)	0.72	OZ
CAULIFLOWER	12.17	CUP
CELERY	5.2	OZ
CHERRIES, FRESH, SWEET W/PIT	1.3	CUP
CHERRIES, DARK (CAN/DEL MONTE)	0.68	CUP
COLLARD GREENS (CAN)	2.25	CUP
COLLARD GREENS (FRESH)	11.3	CUP
CORN CAKE	3.85	CAKE
CORN (CAN/DEL MONTE NO SODIUM)	9.9	OZ
CUCUMBER, SLICED	9.7	CUP
EGGPLANT	6.1	CUP
FRUIT, MIXED FROZEN	1.5	CUP
GARLIC, 1 CLOVE	34	CLOVE
GARLIC, TRIMMED	3.23	OZ
GRAPES	1.19	CUP
GRAPE JUICE/VERYFINE	7.2	OZ
GRAPEFRUIT	1.47	4 INCH
GREEN BEANS (CAN/DEL MONTE NO SALT)	3.38	CUP
GREEN PEPPER	6.7	MEDIUM
KIWI	9.1	OZ
MUSHROOMS, FRESH	7.5	CUP
ONION, FRESH/CHOPPED	2.25	CUP
ORANGE, NAVAL	2.1	3 INCH

ORANGE, JUICE	9.8	OZ
PAPAYA	1.16	LB.
PAPAYA, PEELED/CUBED	2.5	CUP
PEACH, FRESH, SLICED	1.83	CUP
PEACH (CAN/DEL MONTE EXTRA LITE)	1.12	CUP
PEARS (CAN)	4.5	HALF
PEAS, BLACKEYED (CAN)	0.75	CUP
PEAS (CAN/DEL MONTE NO SODIUM)	9.9	OZ
PEAS, GREEN GIANT FROZEN, SWEET	1.29	CUP
PEAS, EDIBLE-PODDED	2.25	CUP
PINEAPPLE, FRESH/DICED	1.73	CUP
PINEAPPLE, DEL MONTE SNACK CAN (LITE)	1.94	3.5 OZ
PINEAPPLE, DOLE CAN (LITE SYRUP)	8	SLICE
PRUNES, DOLE, DRIED	1.93	OZ
PUMPKIN (CAN)	2.7	CUP
RAISINS	0.283	CUP
RED PEPPER	6.75	MEDIUM
STRAWBERRIES (FRESH)	1.4	PINT
STRAWBERRIES (FROZEN)	1.8	CUP
SQUASH, CAN, STOKLEY	1.35	CUP
SQUASH, FRESH BAKED	1.19	CUP
TANGERINE	3.65	2.5 INCH
TOMATO, CAN	12.7	OZ
TOMATO, FRESH	5.2	3 INCH
TOMATO, JUICE	21.5	OZ
VEGETABLES, MIXED (FROZEN)	1.5	CUP
WATERMELLON	0.09	1X10 INCH
ZUCCHINI, FRESH, SLICED	7.5	CUP

Yogurts and Desserts

DING DONG	0.84	DING
DREYERS FROZEN FAT FREE YOGURT	0.75	CUP
FRUIT ROLL-UP	1.94	ROLL UP
POPCORN, WHITE	2.7	TBLSP
TCBY, SOFT SERVE, NON FAT/NO SUGAR	0.84	CUP
YOGURT, FAT FREE, MOUNTAIN HIGH	8	OZ
YOGURT, FAT FREE, DANNON	8	OZ
LUCERN, YOGURT, NONFAT, LITE	8	OZ

YOGURT, YOPLAIT, FAT FREE, LITE	6	OZ
YOGURT,YOPLAIT ORIGINAL/99% FAT FREE	6	OZ
YOGURT, HORIZON, FF / BLUEBERRY	6	OZ
PLANTER DRIED WALNUT PIECES	0.18	CUP
RAW ALMONDS, TOASTED	0.8	OZ
PECANS, DRIED	0.7	OZ
PEANUTS, DRY ROASTED	0.16	CUP
HOT CHOCOLATE	2	ENVEL.
ALMONDS, SHELLED	0.8	OZ

Cereals

CEREAL, CHEERIOS	1.23	CUP
CEREAL, COCOA KRISPIES	0.845	CUP
CEREAL, GRAPENUTS	0.338	CUP
CEREAL, HONEY NUT TOASTY O'S	1.23	CUP
CEREAL, WHEATIES	1.23	CUP
CEREAL, KELLOGG'S ALL BRAN	0.845	CUP
CEREAL, KELLOGG'S CORN FLAKES	1.23	CUP
CEREAL, KELLOGG'S RAISIN BRAN	0.7955	CUP
CEREAL, KELLOGG'S CRACKLIN' OAT BRAN	0.515	CUP
CEREAL, NABISCO SHREDDED WHEAT	1.69	PIECE
CEREAL, NAB. SHREDDED WHEAT (SPOON)	0.7955	CUP
CEREAL, RICE KRISPIES	1.543	CUP
CEREAL, BENEFIT NUTRITION, PROTEIN +	0.64	CUP
CREAM OF WHEAT	3.38	TBL/DRY
GRANOLA, CW POST HEARTY	0.32	CUP
GRANOLA, KELLOGG'S LOW FAT	12	CUP
OATMEAL (PRE-COOK MEASUREMENT)	0.48	CUP

Breads

BREAD, OROWHEAT LITE	3.38	SLICE
BREAD, SUSAN'S HOMEMADE/18 SLICES	1.489	SLICE
BREAD, SUSAN'S HOMEMADE	0.083	LOAF
BUN, WONDER REDUCED CALORIE LITE	1.69	BUN
CRACKER, ZESTA SALTINES	11.3	CRACKER
TORTILLA (CAROLYN)	0.79	TORT
TORTILLA, TORTILLA'S MEXICO, FLOUR	1.23	TORT

TORTILLA, TORTILLA'S MEXICO, CORN	1.5	TORT
TRISCUITS	0.96	OZ
WAFFLE, EGGO, HOMESTYLE	1.23	WAFFLE
WHOLE GRAIN/WHOLE WHEAT FLOUR	0.33	CUP

Rice/Potatoes/Beans

BLACK BEANS (BOILED)	0.598	CUP
BLACK BEANS (DRY)	0.483	CUP
CHICKPEAS/GARBANZO BEANS	0.2	CUP
KIDNEY BEANS (BOILED)	0.21	CUP
LIMA BEANS (BOILED)	0.65	CUP
NAVY BEANS (BOILED)	0.52	CUP
NAVY BEANS (CAN)	0.56	CUP
PINTO BEANS (BOILED)	0.575	CUP
PINTO BEANS (CAN)	0.71	CUP
PINTO BEANS (DRY)	0.225	CUP
PORK & BEANS/VAN CAMPS	0.61	CUP
POTATO, SWEET	1.15	5"X2"
POTATOE	8	OZ
RICE CAKE	2.7	CAKE
RICE, WHITE, BASMATI	0.565	CUP (C)
RICE, BROWN LONG GRAIN	0.68	CUP (C)
RICE, INSTANT, MINUTE BRAND	0.42	CUP(UC)
RICE, WHITE, LONG GRAIN	0.21	CUP(UC)
SOYBEANS (BOILED)	0.5	CUP
YAM, BOILED OR BAKED	0.85	CUP

Pasta

MACARONI, DAVINI TWIST	0.515	CUP/DRY
MACARONI, HOSPITALITY ELBOW	0.28	CUP/DRY
MACARONI, AM. BEAUTY ELBOW	0.32	CUP/DRY
PASTA, CREAMETTE PLAIN	1.29	OZ
SPAGHETTI, EDEN WHOLE WHEAT	1.29	OZ/UC

Protein Sources 1100 Calories

White Meat

CHICKEN BREAST (HORMEL/CAN)	0.9	CAN
CHICKEN BREAST (SKINLESS)	4.5	OZ
CHICKEN (LEG W/ SKIN & BONE)	0.51	
CHICKEN (THIGH W/SKIN & BONE)	0.883	
CHICKEN (LEG & THIGH W/SKIN & BONE)	0.323	
HAM, BAR S, XTRA LEAN, 96% FAT FREE	3.86	OZ
HAM, DAK CAN	4.5	OZ
PORK, SIRLOIN, LEAN W/ FAT	1.35	OZ
TURKEY BREAST (SKINLESS)	2.53	OZ
TURKEY BREAST (HORMEL/CAN)	0.772	CAN
TURKEY BRST/OVEN ROAST/SFWY/89% FF	5.4	OZ
VENISON / ANTELOPE	3.033	OZ

Red Meat

HAMBURGER (10% FAT)	2.4	OZ
HAMBURGER (15% FAT)	1.99	OZ
HAMBURGER (20% FAT)	1.93	OZ
HAMBURGER (27% FAT)	1.63445	OZ
LAMB, SHOULDER	1.535	OZ
STEAK, BOTTOM ROUND	2.28	OZ
STEAK, BRISKET (FLAT HALF)	2.15	OZ
STEAK, CHUCK, ARM	2.22	OZ
STEAK, CHUCK, BLADE	1.9	OZ
STEAK, EYE ROUND	2.832	OZ
STEAK, FLANK	2.31	OZ
STEAK, NEW YORK STRIP	2.7	OZ
STEAK, PORTERHOUSE	2.19	OZ
STEAK, RIBEYE	2.121	OZ
STEAK, ROUND TIP	2.58	OZ
STEAK, SHANK (CROSSCUTS)	2.37	OZ
STEAK, T-BONE	2.23	OZ
STEAK, TENDERLOIN	2.265	OZ
STEAK, TOP LOIN	2.302	OZ
STEAK, TOP ROUND	2.65	OZ

STEAK, TOP SIRLOIN	2.46	OZ
STEAK, TYSON SEASONED BEEF STRIPS	2.9	OZ
TACO/BURRITO MEAT/SMART GROUND	0.704	CUP
OSCAR MAYER BACON	4.5	SLICE
LITTLE SIZZLER BROWN/SERVE SAUSAGE	1.755	LINK

Sea Food

BASS, FRESHWATER, DRY HEAT	3.25	OZ
BASS, STRIPED, DRY HEAT	3.86	OZ
COD, ATLANTIC, DRY HEAT (DRY HEAT)	4.551	OZ
CRAB, ALASKA KING, MOIST HEAT	5	OZ
CRAB, BLUE, MOIST HEAT	4.66	OZ
FLOUNDER, DRY HEAT	4.09	OZ
HADDOCK, DRY HEAT	4.3	OZ
HALIBUT, DRY HEAT	3.4	OZ
LOBSTER, NORTHERN, MOIST HEAT	4.885	OZ
MAHI MAHI	5.58	OZ
ORANGE ROUGHY, DRY HEAT	5.33	OZ
PERCH, DRY HEAT	4.09	OZ
PERCH, OCEAN/ATLANTIC, DRY HEAT	3.94	OZ
SALMON, ATLANTIC, DRY HEAT	2.6	OZ
SHRIMP, MOIST HEAT	4.83	OZ
TROUT, DRY HEAT	2.2	OZ
TUNA BURGER, AHI / OMEGA FOODS	4.83	OZ
TUNA, LOW SODIUM, CAN	0.772	CAN
TUNA, WATER, CAN	0.9001	CAN
TUNA, WHITE / LO SALT, CAN (1 CAN / 5 OZ)	0.774	CAN
TUNA, WHITE, CAN (1 CAN / 5 OZ)	0.774	CAN
TUNA, FILLET/STEAK	3.07	OZ
WALLEYE, BAKED/BROILED/MICRO	4	OZ

Vegetarian

IVES VEG. COUSINE VEGGY DOG	2.25	DOG
SOY MILK (TRIS)	1.5	CUP
SOY MILK (SYLVIA)	1.25	CUP

Eggs/Dairy

1% COTTAGE CHEESE, NORDICA	0.845	CUP
2% COTTAGE CHEESE (LOW FAT)	0.675	CUP
COTTAGE CHEESE (LUCERNE FAT FREE)	0.845	CUP
COTT CHEESE MARIGOLD/DRY CURD	1.29	CUP
COTT CHEESE MARIGOLD/DRY CURD	20.6	TBLSP
COTT CHEESE BREAKSTONES FAT FREE	0.845	CUP
CHEDDER, SHREDDED, FAT FREE, KHF	0.75	CUP
CHEDDER, SHREDDED, 94% FAT FREE, HC	0.675	CUP
CHEESE, COLBY/MOZZARELLA	1.23	OZ
EGG WHITE	7.95	
EGG, WHOLE	1.8	
EGG BEATERS	1.125	CUP
MOZZARELLA SHREDDED, FAT FREE, KHF	0.675	CUP
SKIM MOZZARELLA STRING CHEESE	1.69	OZ

Free Carbs, Supplements, Fast Foods
1100 calories

Free Carbs

ASPARAGUS
BROCCOLI
CABBAGE
CAULIFLOWER
CELERY
CUCUMBER
GREEN BEANS
GREEN PEPPERS
GREEN SQUASH
LETTUCE, ICEBERG
LETTUCE, LEAF/SHREDDED
MUSHROOMS
ONION
PICKLES (DILL)
RADISH

RED PEPPERS
SPINACH (CAN/NO SALT)
SPINACH (FRESH)
TOMATO (EXCLUDING JUICE)
ZUCCHINI

Supplements/Fast Foods

ATKINS BAR	0.5	BAR
EAS ADVANTEDGE, C&C/LEM/BLUE	0.5	BAR
BAR, ZONE	0.5	BAR
BAR, PURE PROTEIN, 50 G.	0.5	BAR
BAR, W.W. PURE PROTEIN, 78 G.	0.33	BAR
BAR, PROTEIN REVOLUTION, PBJ	0.5	BAR
BAR, FIBAR, PEANUT BUTTER, 1.2 OZ	0.75	BAR
BAR, PREMIER 1, PROTEIN 8, CHOC/COCO	0.33	BAR
BAR, PREFERRED BAR, CHOC./FUDG/RAS	0.5	BAR
BAR, PREFERRED BAR, CHOC./FUDG/BROW	0.5	BAR
ALIVE, HI CARB POWDER	3	TBLSP
POWERADE	1.75	SERVING
PROTEIN,GNC P.P. EGG/WHEY	1	SERVING
PROTEIN. GNC P.PERF. WHEY	2.75	SCOOP
OPTIMUM NUTRITION WHEY	1	SCOOP
SYNTRAX WHEY PROTEIN	1.5	SCOOP
TRI PROTEIN PLUS POWDER	1	SERVING
HW STRAWBERRY PROT. POWD.	1.33	SCOOP
BIOCHEM WHEY PRO 290	1.25	SCOOP
HUMAN DEV. TECH. WHEY	1	SCOOP
NATURADE 100% SOY PROTEIN	0.33	CUP
SUPER GREEN PRO 96-SOY	0.33	CUP
100% PURE WHEY, PROLAB	0.75	SCOOP
ECLIPSE BULK UP WHEY	1.5	SCOOP
VITAMIN WORLD WHEY 100%	1	SCOOP
ULT. NUT. PROSTAR WHEY	1	SCOOP
RED WINE	5	OZ
MET RX CH.RST.PNT.PRO + BAR	0.33	BAR
MET RX BAV. MINT. PRO + BAR	0.5	BAR
MET AFTER FX BAR	0.5	BAR
MET RX CH. CH. CHIP PRO + BAR	0.5	BAR

MET RX SOURCE ONE BAR	0.55	BAR
MET RX CHOC. GRAHCRK CHIP BAR	0.33	BAR
MET RX PEANUT BUTTER BAR	0.33	BAR
MET RX DRINK MIX, MRP	0.5	SERVING
MET RX PRO 50, ANABOLIC DRIVE	0.5	SERVING
MET RX PRO 60, ANABOLIC DRIVE	0.33	SERVING
MET RX PROTEIN PLUS	1.9	SCOOP
MET RX KETO PRO	1.7	SCOOP
NUTRI FORCE DRINK MIX, MRP	0.5	SERVING
EAS MYO. DEL. CH/PB BAR	0.33	BAR
EAS MYOPLEX + DELUXE	0.33	SERVING
EAS MYOPLEX LITE	0.68	SERVING
ADVANT EDGE QUICK STIR PROTEIN DRINK	0.5	SERVING
EAS NEUROGAIN	2.5	SCOOP
EAS PHOSPHAGEN HP	0.88	SCOOP
EAS PRECISION PROTEIN	1.25	SCOOP
EAS SIMPLY PROTEIN	2.25	SCOOP
EAS WHEY PROTEIN	1.2	SCOOP
EAS SUPPER SHAKE	0.25	SHAKE
VITAMIN WORLD DAILY RX, MRP	0.45	SHAKE
VITAMIN WORLD PROTOPLEX DELUXE, MRP	0.35	SHAKE
VITAMIN WORLD PRE. ENG. WHEY PROT.	1.25	SCOOP
PERFECT RX, MRP, CHOCOLATE	0.5	SHAKE
OPTI PRO	0.5	SHAKE
ARBY'S CHICK. SAND. R.DELX.LITE	0.5	BURGER
ARBY'S SIDE SALAD	1	SALAD
ARBY'S GARDEN SALAD	1	SALAD
ARBY'S RST. CHCK. SALAD	0.75	SALAD
ARBY'S RED. CAL. ITAL. DRESSING	1	PACKET
ARBY'S RED RANCH DRESSING	1	PACKET
MCD'S VINAG. LITE SALAD DR.	1	PACKET
MCD'S GARDEN SALAD	1	SALAD
MCD'S VINAG. LITE SALAD DR.	1	PACKET
P.HUT. HAND-TOSS CHEESE	0.5	SLICE
P.HUT. HAND-TOSS HAM	0.5	SLICE
P.HUT. HAND-TOSS VEG. LUV.	0.5	SLICE
P.HUT. HAND-TOSS PEPPERON	0.5	SLICE
P.HUT. THIN/CRISP CHEESE	0.5	SLICE

P.HUT. THIN/CRISP HAM	0.5	SLICE
P.HUT. THIN/CRISP VEG. LUV.	0.5	SLICE
P.HUT. THIN/CRISP PEPPERON	0.5	SLICE
SW 6" COLD SUB/VEGG. DELIT	1	SUB
SW 6" COLD SUB/TURK. BRST.	1	SUB
SW 6" COLD SUB/TURK.B/HAM	1	SUB
SW 6" COLD SUB/HAM	1	SUB
SW 6" COLD SUB/ROAST BEEF	1	SUB
SW 6" COLD SUB/SFOOD,CRAB	1	SUB
SW 6" COLD SUB/COLD CUT 3	1	SUB
SW 6" COLD SUB/TUNA	1	SUB
SW 6" HOT SUB/RST.CHICK.BR.	1	SUB
SW 6" HOT SUB/STAK/CHEESE	1	SUB
SW 6" HOT SUB/SUB MELT	1	SUB
SW VEGGIE DELITE SALAD	1	SALAD
SW TURKEY BREAST SALAD	1	SALAD
SW ROAST BEEF SALAD	1	SALAD
SW TURK. BRST/HAM SALAD	1	SALAD
SW RST. CHICK. BR. SALAD	0.75	SALAD
SW SEAFOOD/CRAB SALAD	0.75	SALAD
SW STEAK/CHEESE SALAD	0.5	SALAD
SW SUBWAY MELT SALAD	0.5	SALAD
SW COLD CUT 3 SALAD	0.5	SALAD
SW FAT FREE ITALIAN DRESS	1	OZ
SW FAT FREE FRENCH DRESS	1	OZ
SW FAT FREE RANCH DRESS	1	OZ
SW DELI STYLE TURKEY BR.	0.5	SNDWCH
SW DELI STYLE HAM	0.5	SNDWCH
SW DELI STYLE ROAST BEEF	0.5	SNDWCH
TB GRILLED STEAK SOFT TACO	0.5	TACO
WAHOO'S CHBROIL FISH TACO	0.75	TACO
WENDI'S SIDE SALAD	1	SALAD
WENDI'S FF FRENCH DRESSING	1	OZ
WENDI'S ITALIAN RED. F/C DRESS	1	OZ
WENDI'S SMALL CHILI	0.5	BOWL
WENDI'S GRILLED CHICK. FILLET	1	MEAT

1200 Calories/Day Eating Plan		
What Does Your Doctor Look Like Naked?		
Name: _____ Date: _____		
Exercise: 30-40 min in a.m. before food		Write what you eat here:
Meal 1 Time: _____	1 Protein Source 2 Active Carbohydrates	
Meal 2 Time: _____	1 oz Raw Almonds	
Meal 3 Time: _____	1 Protein Source 1 Active Carbohydrates Free Carbohydrates (as much as you want)	
Meal 4 Time: _____	½ LOW CARB protein bar (OR) 1 scoop Whey Protein Powder in water	
Meal 5 Time: _____	1 Protein Source 0 Active Carbohydrates Free Carbohydrates (as much as you want)	
Bedtime Meal (Optional)	Sugar Free Jell-O 1 cup	

Add fiber supplement in evening, such as Metamucil or other (sugar FREE).
Add spices, pepper, etc. as needed.
Try to eat every two to three hours.
Drink ¾ of a gallon of water EVERY DAY!
May have up to 2 diet pops (or) 2 cups a coffee a day.

Active Carbohydrates 1200 Calories

Fruit and Vegetables

APPLE	1.87	3 INCH
APPLESAUCE, MOTT'S	0.69	CUP
APPLESAUCE, MUSSELMAN'S	7.5	OZ
APRICOTS (CAN/DEL MONTE LITE)	1.26	CUP
APRICOTS (DRIED)	2.17	OZ
APRICOTS (FRESH 12/LB)	8.9	MEDIUM
ASPARAGUS	41	OZ
BANANA	1.44	MEDIUM
BLUEBERRIES (FRESH)	1.85	CUP
BRUSSELS SPROUTS, BOILED	2.5	CUP
CABBAGE, SHREDDED	8.4	CUP
CANTALOUPE	0.8	5 INCH
CARROT (FRESH)	13.6	OZ
CAULIFLOWER	5.8	CUP
CELERY	37.9	OZ
CHERRIES, FRESH, SWEET W/PIT	1.45	CUP
CHERRIES, DARK (CAN/DEL MONTE)	0.75	CUP
COLLARD GREENS (CAN)	2.5	CUP
COLLARD GREENS (FRESH)	12.6	CUP
CORN CAKE	4.3	CAKE
CORN (CAN/DEL MONTE NO SODIUM)	11	OZ
CUCUMBER, SLICED	10.8	CUP
EGGPLANT	6.9	CUP
FRUIT, MIXED FROZEN	1.68	CUP
GARLIC, 1 CLOVE	38	CLOVE
GARLIC, TRIMMED	3.6	OZ
GRAPES	1.33	CUP
GRAPE JUICE/VERYFINE	8	OZ
GRAPEFRUIT	1.65	4 INCH
GREEN BEANS (CAN/DEL MONTE NO SALT)	3.8	CUP
GREEN PEPPER	7.6	MEDIUM
KIDNEY BEANS (BOILED)	0.675	
KIWI	10.2	OZ
LETTUCE, ICEBURG	2.15	

LETTUCH, LEAF/SHREDDED	15	
MUSHROOMS, FRESH	8.4	CUP
ONION, FRESH/CHOPPED	2.5	CUP
ORANGE, NAVAL	2.33	3 INCH
ORANGE, JUICE	11	OZ
PAPAYA	1.3	LB.
PAPAYA, PEELED/CUBED	2.8	CUP
PEACH, FRESH, SLICED	2.05	CUP
PEACH (CAN/DEL MONTE EXTRA LITE)	1.25	CUP
PEARS (CAN)	5	HALF
PEAS, BLACKEYED (CAN)	0.84	CUP
PEAS, (CAN/DEL MONTE NO SODIUM)	11	OZ
PEAS, GREEN GIANT FROZEN, SWEET	1.44	CUP
PEAS, EDIBLE-PODDED	2.5	CUP
PINEAPPLE, FRESH/DICED	1.94	CUP
PINEAPPLE, DEL MONTE SNACK CAN (LITE)	2.15	3.5 OZ
PINEAPPLE (CAN/DOLE LITE SYRUP)	8.9	SLICE
PRUNES, DOLE, DRIED	2.15	OZ
PUMPKIN (CAN)	3	CUP
RAISINS	0.315	CUP
RED PEPPER	7.5	MEDIUM
STRAWBERRIES (FRESH)	1.55	PINT
STRAWBERRIES (FROZEN)	2	CUP
SQUASH, CAN, STOKLEY	1.5	CUP
SQUASH, FRESH BAKED	1.33	CUP
TANGERINE	4.1	2.5 INCH
TOMATO, CAN	14.2	OZ
TOMATO, FRESH	5.8	3 INCH
TOMATO, JUICE	24	OZ
VEGETABLES, MIXED (FROZEN)	1.68	CUP
WATERMELLON	1	1X10 INCH
ZUCCHINI, FRESH, SLICED	8.4	CUP

Yogurts and Desserts

DING DONG	0.94	DING
DREYERS FROZEN FAT FREE YOGURT	0.84	CUP
FRUIT ROLL-UP	2.17	ROLL-UP
POPCORN, WHITE	3	TBLSP

TCBY, SOFT SERVE/NON FAT/NO SUGAR	0.95	CUP
YOGURT, FAT FREE, MOUNTAIN HIGH	8	OZ
YOGURT, FAT FREE, DANNON	8	OZ
LUCERN, YOGURT, NONFAT, LITE	8	OZ
YOGURT, YOPLAIT, FAT FREE, LITE	6	OZ
YOGURT, YOPLAIT ORIGINAL/99% FAT FREE	6	OZ
YOGURT, HORIZON, FF / BLUEBERRY	6	OZ
PLANTER DRIED WALNUT PIECES	0.2	CUP
RAW ALMONDS, TOASTED	0.88	OZ
PECANS, DRIED	0.8	OZ
PEANUTS, DRY ROASTED	0.17	CUP
HOT CHOCOLATE	2.5	ENVEL.
ALMONDS, SHELLED	0.9	OZ

Cereals

CEREAL, CHEERIOS	1.38	CUP
CEREAL, COCOA KRISPIES	0.94	CUP
CEREAL, GRAPENUTS	0.38	CUP
CEREAL, HONEY NUT TOASTY O'S	1.38	CUP
CEREAL, WHEATIES	1.38	CUP
CEREAL, KELLOGG'S ALL BRAN	0.94	CUP
CEREAL, KELLOGG'S CORN FLAKES	1.38	CUP
CEREAL, KELLOGG'S RAISIN BRAN	0.89	CUP
CEREAL, KELLOGG'S CRACKLIN' OAT BRAN	0.575	CUP
CEREAL, NABISCO SHREDDED WHEAT	1.9	PIECE
CEREAL, NAB. SHREDDED WHEAT (SPOON)	0.89	CUP
CEREAL, RICE KRISPIES	1.71	CUP
CEREAL, BENEFIT NUTRITION, PROTEIN +	0.72	CUP
CREAM OF WHEAT	3.75	TBL/DRY
GRANOLA, CW POST HEARTY	0.36	CUP
GRANOLA, KELLOGG'S LOW FAT	1	CUP
OATMEAL (PRE-COOK MEASUREMENT)	0.54	CUP

Breads

BREAD, OROWHEAT LITE	3.8	SLICE
BREAD, SUSAN'S HOMEMADE/18 SLICES	1.67	SLICE
BREAD, SUSAN'S HOMEMADE	0.093	LOAF

BUN, WONDER REDUCED CALORIE LITE	1.9	BUN
CRACKER, ZESTA SALTINES	12.9	CRACKER
TORTILLA (CAROLYN)	0.89	TORT
TORTILLA, TORTILLA'S MEXICO, FLOUR	1.38	TORT
TORTILLA, TORTILLA'S MEXICO, CORN	1.68	TORT
TRISCUITS	1.08	OZ
WAFFLE, EGGO, HOMESTYLE	1.38	WAFFLE
WHOLE GRAIN/WHOLE WHEAT FLOUR	0.37	CUP

Rice/Potatoes/Beans

BLACK BEANS (BOILED)	0.67	CUP
BLACK BEANS (DRY)	0.54	CUP
CHICKPEAS/GARBANZO BEANS	0.22	CUP
KIDNEY BEANS (BOILED)	0.675	CUP
LIMA BEANS (BOILED)	0.73	CUP
NAVY BEANS (BOILED)	0.59	CUP
NAVY BEANS (CAN)	0.63	CUP
PINTO BEANS (BOILED)	0.645	CUP
PINTO BEANS (CAN)	0.8	CUP
PINTO BEANS (DRY)	0.25	CUP
PORK & BEANS / VAN CAMPS	0.69	CUP
POTATO, SWEET	1.28	5"X2"
POTATOE	9	OZ
RICE CAKE	3	CAKE
RICE, WHITE, BASMATI	0.63	CUP (C)
RICE, BROWN LONG GRAIN	0.75	CUP (C)
RICE, INSTANT, MINUTE BRAND	0.47	CUP(UC)
RICE, WHITE, LONG GRAIN	0.235	CUP(UC)
SOYBEANS (BOILED)	0.45	CUP
YAM, BOILED OR BAKED	0.96	CUP

Pasta

MACARONI, DAVINI TWIST	0.575	CUP/DRY
MACARONI, HOSPITALITY ELBOW	0.315	CUP/DRY
MACARONI, AM. BEAUTY ELBOW	0.36	CUP/DRY
PASTA, CREAMETTE PLAIN	1.44	OZ
SPAGHETTI, EDEN WHOLE WHEAT	1.44	OZ/UC

Protein Sources 1200 Calories

White Meat

CHICKEN BREAST (HORMEL/CAN)	1	CAN
CHICKEN BREAST (SKINLESS)	5	OZ
CHICKEN (LEG W/SKIN & BONE)	0.57	
CHICKEN (THIGH W/SKIN & BONE)	0.99	
CHICKEN (LEG & THIGH W/SKIN & BONE)	0.36	
HAM, BAR S, XTRA LEAN, 96% FAT FREE	4.3	OZ
HAM, DAK CAN	5	OZ
PORK, SIRLOIN, LEAN W/FAT	1.5	OZ
TURKEY BREAST (SKINLESS)	2.83	OZ
TURKEY BREAST (HORMEL/CAN)	0.86	CAN
TURKEY BRST/OVEN ROAST/SFWY/89% FF	6	OZ
VENISON/ANTELOPE	3.38	OZ

Red Meat

HAMBURGER (10% FAT)	2.7	OZ
HAMBURGER (15% FAT)	2.23	OZ
HAMBURGER (20% FAT)	2.15	OZ
HAMBURGER (27% FAT)	1.83	OZ
LAMB, SHOULDER	1.72	OZ
STEAK, BOTTOM ROUND	2.55	OZ
STEAK, BRISKET (FLAT HALF)	2.4	OZ
STEAK, CHUCK, ARM	2.5	OZ
STEAK, CHUCK, BLADE	2.1	OZ
STEAK, EYE ROUND	3.2	OZ
STEAK, FLANK	2.58	OZ
STEAK, NEW YORK STRIP	3	OZ
STEAK, PORTERHOUSE	2.45	OZ
STEAK, RIBEYE	2.38	OZ
STEAK, ROUND TIP	2.9	OZ
STEAK, SHANK (CROSSCUTS)	2.65	OZ
STEAK, T-BONE	2.5	OZ
STEAK, TENDERLOIN	2.53	OZ
STEAK, TOP LOIN	2.58	OZ
STEAK, TOP ROUND	3	OZ

STEAK, TOP SIRLOIN	2.75	OZ
STEAK, TYSON SEASONED BEEF STRIPS	3.25	OZ
TACO/BURRITO MEAT/SMART GROUND	0.79	CUP
OSCAR MAYER BACON	5	SLICE
LITTLE SIZZLER BROWN/SERVE SAUSAGE	1.95	LINK

Sea Food

BASS, FRESHWATER, DRY HEAT	3.65	OZ
BASS, STRIPED, DRY HEAT	4.3	OZ
COD, ATLANTIC, DRY HEAT	5.1	OZ
CRAB, ALASKA KING, MOIST HEAT	5.5	OZ
CRAB, BLUE, MOIST HEAT	5.2	OZ
FLOUNDER, DRY HEAT	4.6	OZ
HADDOCK, DRY HEAT	4.75	OZ
HALIBUT, DRY HEAT	3.8	OZ
LOBSTER, NORTHERN, MOIST HEAT	5.5	OZ
MAHI MAHI	6.2	OZ
ORANGE ROUGHY, DRY HEAT	6	OZ
PERCH, DRY HEAT	4.6	OZ
PERCH, OCEAN/ATLANTIC, DRY HEAT	4.4	OZ
SALMON, ATLANTIC, DRY HEAT	2.9	OZ
SHRIMP, MOIST HEAT	5.4	OZ
TROUT, DRY HEAT	2.8	OZ
TUNA BURGER, AHI/OMEGA FOODS	5.4	OZ
TUNA, LOW SODIUM, CAN	0.87	CAN
TUNA, WATER, CAN	1	CAN
TUNA, WHITE/LOW SALT, CAN (5 OZ)	0.86	CAN
TUNA, WHITE, CAN (5 OZ)	0.86	CAN
TUNA, FILLET/STEAK	3.45	OZ
WALLEYE, BAKED/BROILED/MICRO	4.5	OZ

Vegetarian

IVES VEG. COUSINE VEGGY DOG	2.5	DOG
SOY MILK (TRIS)	1.25	CUP
SOY MILK (SYLVIA)	1.15	CUP

Eggs/Dairy

1% COTTAGE CHEESE, NORDICA	0.945	CUP
2% COTTAGE CHEESE (LOW FAT)	0.755	CUP
COTTAGE CHEESE (LUCERNE FAT FREE)	0.945	CUP
COTT CHEESE MARIGOLD/DRY CURD	1.44	CUP
COTT CHEESE MARIGOLD/DRY CURD	23	TBLSP
COTT CHEESE BREAKSTONES FAT FREE	0.945	CUP
CHEDDER, SHREDDED, FAT FREE, KHF	0.84	CUP
CHEDDER, SHREDDED, 94% FAT FREE, HC	0.75	CUP
CHEESE, COLBY/MOZZARELLA	1.38	OZ
EGG WHITE	8.9	
EGG, WHOLE	8.2	
EGG BEATERS	1.26	CUP
MOZZARELLA SHREDDED, FAT FREE, KHF	0.75	CUP
SKIM MOZZARELLA STRING CHEESE	1.9	OZ

Free Carbs, Supplements, Fast Foods
1200 calories

Free Carbs

ASPARAGUS
BROCCOLI
CABBAGE
CAULIFLOWER
CELERY
CUCUMBER
GREEN BEANS
GREEN PEPPERS
GREEN SQUASH
LETTUCE, ICEBERG
LETTUCE, LEAF/SHREDDED
MUSHROOMS
ONION
PICKLES (DILL)
RADISH
RED PEPPERS

SPINACH (CAN) NO SALT
SPINACH (FRESH)
TOMATO (EXCLUDING JUICE)
ZUCCHINI

Supplements/Fast Foods

ATKINS BAR	0.5	BAR
EAS ADVANTEDGE, C&C/LEM/BLUE	0.5	BAR
BAR, ZONE	0.5	BAR
BAR, PURE PROTEIN, 50 G.	0.5	BAR
BAR, W.W. PURE PROTEIN, 78 G.	0.33	BAR
BAR, PROTEIN REVOLUTION, PBJ	0.5	BAR
BAR, FIBAR, PEANUT BUTTER, 1.2 OZ	0.75	BAR
BAR, PREMIER 1, PROTEIN 8, CHOC/COCO	0.5	BAR
BAR, PREFERRED BAR, CHOC./FUDG/RAS	0.5	BAR
BAR, PREFERRED BAR, CHOC./FUDG/BROW	0.5	BAR
ALIVE, HI CARB POWDER	3	TBLSP
POWERADE	2	SERVING
PROTEIN,GNC P.P. EGG/WHEY	1.25	SERVING
PROTEIN. GNC P.PERF. WHEY	3	SCOOP
OPTIMUM NUTRITION WHEY	1.25	SCOOP
SYNTRAX WHEY PROTEIN	1.59	SCOOP
TRI PROTEIN PLUS POWDER	1	SERVING
HW STRAWBERRY PROT. POWD.	1.33	SCOOP
BIOCHEM WHEY PRO 290	1.75	SCOOP
HUMAN DEV. TECH. WHEY	1	SCOOP
NATURADE 100% SOY PROTEIN	0.33	CUP
SUPER GREEN PRO 96-SOY	0.33	CUP
100% PURE WHEY, PROLAB	1	SCOOP
ECLIPSE BULK UP WHEY	1.5	SCOOP
VITAMIN WORLD WHEY 100%	1	SCOOP
ULT. NUT. PROSTAR WHEY	1	SCOOP
RED WINE	6	OZ
MET RX CH.RST.PNT.PRO + BAR	0.5	BAR
MET RX BAV. MINT. PRO + BAR	0.5	BAR
MET AFTER FX BAR	0.5	BAR
MET RX CH. CH. CHIP PRO + BAR	0.5	BAR
MET RX SOURCE ONE BAR	0.55	BAR

MET RX CHOC. GRAHCRK CHIP BAR	0.33	BAR
MET RX PEANUT BUTTER BAR	0.33	BAR
MET RX DRINK MIX, MRP	0.5	SERVING
MET RX PRO 50, ANABOLIC DRIVE	0.5	SERVING
MET RX PRO 60, ANABOLIC DRIVE	0.5	SERVING
MET RX PROTEIN PLUS	1.9	SCOOP
MET RX KETO PRO	1.7	SCOOP
NUTRI FORCE DRINK MIX, MRP	0.5	SERVING
EAS MYO. DEL. CH/PB BAR	0.33	BAR
EAS MYOPLEX + DELUXE	0.5	SERVING
EAS MYOPLEX LITE	0.75	SERVING
ADVANT EDGE QUICK STIR PROTEIN DRINK	0.5	SERVING
EAS NEUROGAIN	3	SCOOP
EAS PHOSPHAGEN HP	1	SCOOP
EAS PRECISION PROTEIN	1.25	SCOOP
EAS SIMPLY PROTEIN	2.5	SCOOP
EAS WHEY PROTEIN	1.33	SCOOP
EAS SUPPER SHAKE	0.33	SHAKE
VITAMIN WORLD DAILY RX, MRP	0.5	SHAKE
VITAMIN WORLD PROTOPLEX DELUXE, MRP	0.55	SHAKE
VITAMIN WORLD PRE. ENG. WHEY PROT.	1.75	SCOOP
PERFECT RX, MRP, CHOCOLATE	0.5	SHAKE
OPTI PRO	0.5	SHAKE
ARBY'S CHICK. SAND. R.DELX.LITE	0.5	BURGER
ARBY'S SIDE SALAD	1	SALAD
ARBY'S GARDEN SALAD	1	SALAD
ARBY'S RST. CHCK. SALAD	1	SALAD
ARBY'S RED. CAL. ITAL. DRESSING	1	PACKET
ARBY'S RED RANCH DRESSING	1	PACKET
MCD'S VINAG. LITE SALAD DR.	1	PACKET
MCD'S GARDEN SALAD	1	SALAD
MCD'S VINAG. LITE SALAD DR.	1	PACKET
P.HUT. HAND-TOSS CHEESE	0.5	SLICE
P.HUT. HAND-TOSS HAM	0.5	SLICE
P.HUT. HAND-TOSS VEG. LUV.	0.5	SLICE
P.HUT. HAND-TOSS PEPPERON	0.5	SLICE
P.HUT. THIN/CRISP CHEESE	0.5	SLICE
P.HUT. THIN/CRISP HAM	0.75	SLICE

1300 Calories/Day Eating Plan		
What Does Your Doctor Look Like Naked?		

Name: _____

Date: _____

Exercise: 30-40 min in a.m. before food		
		Write what you eat here:
Meal 1 Time: _____	1 Protein Source 2 Active Carbohydrates	
Meal 2 Time: _____	1 oz Raw Almonds	
Meal 3 Time: _____	1 Protein Source 1 Active Carbohydrates Free Carbohydrates (as much as you want)	
Meal 4 Time: _____	½ LOW CARB protein bar (OR) 1 scoop Whey Protein Powder in water	
Meal 5 Time: _____	1 Protein Source 0 Active Carbohydrates Free Carbohydrates (as much as you want)	
Bedtime Meal (Optional)	Sugar Free Jell-O 1 cup	

Add fiber supplement in evening such as Metamucil or other (sugar FREE).
Add spices, pepper, etc. as needed.
Try to eat every two to three hours.
Drink ¾ of a gallon of water EVERY DAY!
May have up to 2 diet pops (or) 2 cups a coffee a day.

Active Carbohydrates 1300 Calories

Fruit and Vegetables

APPLE	2.08	3 INCH
APPLESAUCE, MOTT'S	0.76	CUP
APRICOTS (CAN/DEL MONTE LITE)	1.4	CUP
APRICOTS (DRIED)	2.4	OZ
APRICOTS (FRESH 12/LB)	9.9	MEDIUM
ASPARAGUS	45.5	OZ
BANANA	1.6	MEDIUM
BLUEBERRIES (FRESH)	2.05	CUP
BRUSSELS SPROUTS, BOILED	2.8	CUP
CABBAGE, SHREDDED	9.3	CUP
CANTALOUPE	0.9	5 INCH
CARROT (FRESH)	15.2	OZ
CAULIFLOWER	6.5	CUP
CELERY	42	OZ
CHERRIES, FRESH, SWEET W/PIT	1.62	CUP
CHERRIES, DARK (CAN, DEL MONTE)	0.84	CUP
COLLARD GREENS (CAN)	2.8	CUP
COLLARD GREENS (FRESH)	14	CUP
CORN CAKE	4.8	CAKE
CORN (CAN/DEL MONTE NO SODIUM)	12.3	OZ
CUCUMBER, SLICED	12	CUP
EGGPLANT	7.6	CUP
FRUIT, MIXED FROZEN	1.86	CUP
GARLIC, 1 CLOVE	42	CLOVE
GARLIC, TRIMMED	4	OZ
GRAPES	1.48	CUP
GRAPE JUICE/VERYFINE	9	OZ
GRAPEFRUIT	1.83	4 INCH
GREEN BEANS (CAN/DEL MONTE NO SALT)	4.2	CUP
GREEN PEPPER	8.4	MEDIUM
KIWI	11.4	OZ
MUSHROOMS, FRESH	2.81	CUP
ONION, FRESH/CHOPPED	1.968	CUP
ORANGE, NAVAL	2.6	3 INCH

ORANGE, JUICE	12.2	OZ
PAPAYA	1.44	LB.
PAPAYA, PEELED/CUBED	3.1	CUP
PEACH, FRESH, SLICED	2.28	CUP
PEACH (CAN/DEL MONTE EXTRA LITE)	1.4	CUP
PEARS (CAN)	5.6	HALF
PEAS, BLACKEYED (CAN)	0.93	CUP
PEAS (CAN/DEL MONTE NO SODIUM)	12.3	OZ
PEAS, GREEN GIANT FROZEN, SWEET	1.6	CUP
PEAS, EDIBLE-PODDED	2.8	CUP
PINEAPPLE, FRESH/DICED	2.15	CUP
PINEAPPLE, DEL MONTE SNACK CAN (LITE)	2.4	3.5 OZ
PINEAPPLE (CAN/DOLE LITE SYRUP)	9.9	SLICE
PRUNES, DOLE, DRIED	2.4	OZ
PUMPKIN (CAN)	3.35	CUP
RAISINS	0.35	CUP
RED PEPPER	8.4	MEDIUM
STRAWBERRIES (FRESH)	1.75	PINT
STRAWBERRIES (FROZEN)	2.25	CUP
SQUASH, CAN, STOKLEY	1.68	CUP
SQUASH, FRESH BAKED	1.48	CUP
TANGERINE	4.55	2.5 INCH
TOMATO, CAN	15.7	OZ
TOMATO, FRESH	6.45	3 INCH
TOMATO, JUICE	27	OZ
VEGETABLES, MIXED (FROZEN)	1.87	CUP
WATERMELLON	1.1	1X10 INCH
ZUCCHINI, FRESH, SLICED	9.3	CUP

Yogurts and Desserts

DING DONG	1.05	DING
DREYERS FROZEN FAT FREE YOGURT	0.9	CUP
FRUIT ROLL-UP	2.4	ROLL-UP
POPCORN, WHITE	3.35	TBLSP
TCBY, SOFT SERVE/NONFAT/NO SUGAR	1.05	CUP
YOGURT, FAT FREE, MOUNTAIN HIGH	8	OZ
YOGURT, FAT FREE, DANNON	8	OZ
LUCERN, YOGURT, NONFAT, LITE	8	OZ

YOGURT, YOPLAIT, FAT FREE, LITE	6	OZ
YOGURT, YOPLAIT ORIGINAL/99% FAT FREE	6	OZ
YOGURT, HORIZON, FF/BLUEBERRY	6	OZ
PLANTER DRIED WALNUT PIECES	0.2	CUP
RAW ALMONDS, TOASTED	1	OZ
PECANS, DRIED	0.88	OZ
PEANUTS, DRY ROASTED	0.2	CUP
HOT CHOCOLATE	3	ENVEL.
ALMONDS, SHELLED	1	OZ

Cereals

CEREAL, CHEERIOS	1.53	CUP
CEREAL, COCOA KRISPIES	1.05	CUP
CEREAL, GRAPENUTS	0.42	CUP
CEREAL, HONEY NUT TOASTY O'S	1.53	CUP
CEREAL, WHEATIES	1.53	CUP
CEREAL, KELLOGG'S ALL BRAN	1.05	CUP
CEREAL, KELLOGG'S CORN FLAKES	1.53	CUP
CEREAL, KELLOGG'S RAISIN BRAN	1	CUP
CEREAL, KELLOGG'S CRACKLIN' OAT BRAN	0.64	CUP
CEREAL, NABISCO SHREDDED WHEAT	2.1	PIECE
CEREAL, NAB. SHREDDED WHEAT (SPOON)	0.99	CUP
CEREAL, RICE KRISPIES	1.9	CUP
CEREAL, BENEFIT NUTRITION, PROTEIN+	0.8	CUP
CREAM OF WHEAT	4.2	TBL/DRY
GRANOLA, CW POST HEARTY	0.4	CUP
GRANOLA, KELLOGG'S LOW FAT	2	CUP
OATMEAL (PRE-COOK MEASUREMENT)	0.6	CUP

Breads

BREAD, OROWHEAT LITE	4.2	SLICE
BREAD, SUSAN'S HOMEMADE/18 SLICES	1.86	SLICE
BREAD, SUSAN'S HOMEMADE	0.103	LOAF
BUN, WONDER REDUCED CALORIE LITE	2.1	BUN
CRACKER, ZESTA SALTINES	14	CRACKER
TORTILLA (CAROLYN)	0.99	TORT
TORTILLA, TORTILLA'S MEXICO, FLOUR	1.53	TORT

TORTILLA, TORTILLA'S MEXICO, CORN	1.87	TORT
TRISCUITS	1.2	OZ
WAFFLE, EGGO, HOMESTYLE	1.53	WAFFLE
WHOLE GRAIN/WHOLE WHEAT FLOUR	0.412	CUP

Rice/Potatoes/Beans

BLACK BEANS (BOILED)	0.74	CUP
BLACK BEANS (DRY)	0.6	CUP
CHICKPEAS/GARBANZO BEANS	0.2	CUP
KIDNEY BEANS (BOILED)	0.25	CUP
LIMA BEANS (BOILED)	0.81	CUP
NAVY BEANS (BOILED)	0.65	CUP
NAVY BEANS (CAN)	0.7	CUP
PINTO BEANS (BOILED)	0.72	CUP
PINTO BEANS (CAN)	0.88	CUP
PINTO BEANS (DRY)	0.28	CUP
PORK & BEANS/VAN CAMPS	0.76	CUP
POTATO, SWEET	1.43	5"X2"
POTATO	10	OZ
RICE CAKE	3.35	CAKE
RICE, WHITE, BASMATI	0.7	CUP (C)
RICE, BROWN LONG GRAIN	0.84	CUP (C)
RICE, INSTANT, MINUTE BRAND	0.525	CUP(UC)
RICE, WHITE, LONG GRAIN	0.263	CUP(UC)
SOYBEANS (BOILED)	0.66	CUP
YAM, BOILED OR BAKED	1.06	CUP

Pasta

MACARONI, DAVINI TWIST	0.64	CUP/DRY
MACARONI, HOSPITALITY ELBOW	0.35	CUP/DRY
MACARONI, AM. BEAUTY ELBOW	0.4	CUP/DRY
PASTA, CREAMETTE PLAIN	1.6	OZ
SPAGHETTI, EDEN WHOLE WHEAT	1.6	OZ/UC

Protein Sources 1300 Calories

White Meat

CHICKEN BREAST (HORMEL/CAN)	1.12	CAN
CHICKEN BREAST (SKINLESS)	5.6	OZ
CHICKEN (LEG W/ SKIN & BONE)	0.64	
CHICKEN (THIGH W/ SKIN & BONE)	1.1	
CHICKEN (LEG & THIGH W/ SKIN & BONE)	0.4	
HAM, BAR S, XTRA LEAN, 96% FAT FREE	4.25	OZ
HAM, DAK CAN	5.6	OZ
PORK, SIRLOIN, LEAN W/ FAT	1.68	OZ
TURKEY BREAST (SKINLESS)	3.14	OZ
TURKEY BREAST (HORMEL/CAN)	0.96	CAN
TURKEY BRST/OVEN ROAST/SFWY/89% FF	6.7	OZ
VENISON/ANTELOPE	3.75	OZ

Red Meat

HAMBURGER (10% FAT)	3	OZ
HAMBURGER (15% FAT)	2.48	OZ
HAMBURGER (20% FAT)	2.4	OZ
HAMBURGER (27% FAT)	2.04	OZ
LAMB, SHOULDER	1.92	OZ
STEAK, BOTTOM ROUND	2.84	OZ
STEAK, BRISKET (FLAT HALF)	2.68	OZ
STEAK, CHUCK, ARM	2.77	OZ
STEAK, CHUCK, BLADE	2.38	OZ
STEAK, EYE ROUND	3.53	OZ
STEAK, FLANK	2.87	OZ
STEAK, NEW YORK STRIP	3.35	OZ
STEAK, PORTERHOUSE	2.74	OZ
STEAK, RIBEYE	2.65	OZ
STEAK, ROUND TIP	3.22	OZ
STEAK, SHANK (CROSSCUTS)	2.95	OZ
STEAK, T-BONE	2.8	OZ
STEAK, TENDERLOIN	2.83	OZ
STEAK, TOP LOIN	2.88	OZ
STEAK, TOP ROUND	3.3	OZ

STEAK, TOP SIRLOIN	3.06	OZ
STEAK, TYSON SEASONED BEEF STRIPS	3.6	OZ
TACO/BURRITO MEAT/SMART GROUND	0.88	CUP
OSCAR MAYER BACON	5.6	SLICE
LITTLE SIZZLER BROWN/SERVE SAUSAGE	2.2	LINK

Sea Food

BASS, FRESHWATER, DRY HEAT	4.08	OZ
BASS, STRIPED, DRY HEAT	4.8	OZ
COD, ATLANTIC, DRY HEAT	5.65	OZ
CRAB, ALASKA KING, MOIST HEAT	6.15	OZ
CRAB, BLUE, MOIST HEAT	5.8	OZ
FLOUNDER, DRY HEAT	5.1	OZ
HADDOCK, DRY HEAT	5.3	OZ
HALIBUT, DRY HEAT	4.25	OZ
LOBSTER, NORTHERN, MOIST HEAT	6.1	OZ
MAHI MAHI	6.9	OZ
ORANGE ROUGHY, DRY HEAT	6.6	OZ
PERCH, DRY HEAT	5.1	OZ
PERCH, OCEAN/ATLANTIC, DRY HEAT	4.9	OZ
SALMON, ATLANTIC, DRY HEAT	1.68	OZ
SHRIMP, MOIST HEAT	3.25	OZ
TROUT, DRY HEAT	3.1	OZ
TUNA BURGER, AHI/OMEGA FOODS	6	OZ
TUNA, LOW SODIUM, CAN	0.96	CAN
TUNA, WATER, CAN	1.12	CAN
TUNA, WHITE/LOW SALT, CAN (5 OZ)	0.96	CAN
TUNA, WHITE, CAN (5 OZ)	0.96	CAN
TUNA, FILLET/STEAK	3.8	OZ
WALLEYE, BAKED/BROILED/MICRO	5	OZ

Vegetarian

IVES VEG. COUSINE VEGGY DOG	2.8	DOG
SOY MILK (TRIS)	1.87	CUP
SOY MILK (SYLVIA)	1.5	CUP

Eggs/Dairy

1% COTTAGE CHEESE, NORDICA	1.05	CUP
2% COTTAGE CHEESE (LOW FAT)	0.84	CUP
COTTAGE CHEESE (LUCERNE FAT FREE)	1.05	CUP
COTT CHEESE MARIGOLD/DRY CURD	1.6	CUP
COTT CHEESE MARIGOLD/DRY CURD	25.7	TBLSP
COTT CHEESE BREAKSTONES FAT FREE	1.05	CUP
CHEDDER, SHREDDED, FAT FREE, KHF	0.93	CUP
CHEDDER, SHREDDED, 94% FAT FREE, HC	0.84	CUP
CHEESE, COLBY/MOZZARELLA	1.53	OZ
EGG WHITE	9.9	
EGG, WHOLE	2.25	
EGG BEATERS	1.4	CUP
MOZZARELLA SHREDDED, FAT FREE, KHF	0.84	CUP
SKIM MOZZARELLA STRING CHEESE	2.1	OZ

Free Carbs, Supplements, Fast Foods
1300 calories

Free Carbs

ASPARAGUS
BROCCOLI
CABBAGE
CAULIFLOWER
CELERY
CUCUMBER
GREEN BEANS
GREEN PEPPERS
GREEN SQUASH
LETTUCE, ICEBERG
LETTUCE, LEAF/SHREDDED
MUSHROOMS
ONION
PICKLES (DILL)
RADISH
RED PEPPERS
SPINACH (CAN) NO SALT

SPINACH (FRESH)
TOMATO (EXCLUDING JUICE)
ZUCCHINI

Supplements/Fast Foods

ATKINS BAR	0.75	BAR
EAS ADVANTEDGE, C&C/LEM/BLUE	0.75	BAR
BAR, ZONE	0.75	BAR
BAR, PURE PROTEIN, 50 G.	0.75	BAR
BAR, W.W. PURE PROTEIN, 78 G.	0.5	BAR
BAR, PROTEIN REVOLUTION, PBJ	0.5	BAR
BAR, FIBAR, PEANUT BUTTER, 1.2 OZ	1	BAR
BAR, PREMIER 1, PROTEIN 8, CHOC/COCO	0.5	BAR
BAR, PREFERRED BAR, CHOC./FUDG/RAS	0.5	BAR
BAR, PREFERRED BAR, CHOC./FUDG/BROW	0.5	BAR
ALIVE, HI CARB POWDER	3	TBLSP
POWERADE	2	SERVING
PROTEIN,GNC P.P. EGG/WHEY	1.25	SERVING
PROTEIN. GNC P.PERF. WHEY	4	SCOOP
OPTIMUM NUTRITION WHEY	1.5	SCOOP
SYNTRAX WHEY PROTEIN	1.75	SCOOP
TRI PROTEIN PLUS POWDER	1	SERVING
HW STRAWBERRY PROT. POWD.	1.5	SCOOP
BIOCHEM WHEY PRO 290	2	SCOOP
HUMAN DEV. TECH. WHEY	1.25	SCOOP
NATURADE 100% SOY PROTEIN	0.5	CUP
SUPER GREEN PRO 96-SOY	0.5	CUP
100% PURE WHEY, PROLAB	1.25	SCOOP
ECLIPSE BULK UP WHEY	1.25	SCOOP
VITAMIN WORLD WHEY 100%	1.25	SCOOP
ULT. NUT. PROSTAR WHEY	1.25	SCOOP
RED WINE	4	OZ
MET RX CH.RST.PNT.PRO + BAR	0.5	BAR
MET RX BAV. MINT. PRO + BAR	0.5	BAR
MET AFTER FX BAR	0.5	BAR
MET RX CH. CH. CHIP PRO + BAR	0.5	BAR
MET RX SOURCE ONE BAR	0.55	BAR
MET RX CHOC. GRAHCRK CHIP BAR	0.5	BAR

MET RX PEANUT BUTTER BAR	0.5	BAR
MET RX DRINK MIX, MRP	0.5	SERVING
MET RX PRO 50, ANABOLIC DRIVE	0.5	SERVING
MET RX PRO 60, ANABOLIC DRIVE	0.5	SERVING
MET RX PROTEIN PLUS	2	SCOOP
MET RX KETO PRO	2	SCOOP
NUTRI FORCE DRINK MIX, MRP	0.5	SERVING
EAS MYO. DEL. CH/PB BAR	0.5	BAR
EAS MYOPLEX + DELUXE	0.5	SERVING
EAS MYOPLEX LITE	0.75	SERVING
ADVANT EDGE QUICK STIR PROTEIN DRINK	0.75	SERVING
EAS NEUROGAIN	3.5	SCOOP
EAS PHOSPHAGEN HP	1	SCOOP
EAS PRECISION PROTEIN	1.5	SCOOP
EAS SIMPLY PROTEIN	2.75	SCOOP
EAS WHEY PROTEIN	1.5	SCOOP
EAS SUPPER SHAKE	0.33	SHAKE
VITAMIN WORLD DAILY RX, MRP	0.5	SHAKE
VITAMIN WORLD PROTOPLEX DELUXE, MRP	0.5	SHAKE
VITAMIN WORLD PRE. ENG. WHEY PROT.	1.75	SCOOP
PERFECT RX, MRP, CHOCOLATE	0.5	SHAKE
OPTI PRO	0.5	SHAKE
ARBY'S CHICK. SAND. R.DELX.LITE	0.5	BURGER
ARBY'S SIDE SALAD	1	SALAD
ARBY'S GARDEN SALAD	1	SALAD
ARBY'S RST. CHCK. SALAD	1	SALAD
ARBY'S RED. CAL. ITAL. DRESSING	1	PACKET
ARBY'S RED RANCH DRESSING	1	PACKET
MCD'S VINAG. LITE SALAD DR.	1	PACKET
MCD'S GARDEN SALAD	1	SALAD
MCD'S VINAG. LITE SALAD DR.	1	PACKET
P.HUT. HAND-TOSS CHEESE	0.5	SLICE
P.HUT. HAND-TOSS HAM	0.75	SLICE
P.HUT. HAND-TOSS VEG. LUV.	0.75	SLICE
P.HUT. HAND-TOSS PEPPERON	0.5	SLICE
P.HUT. THIN/CRISP CHEESE	0.75	SLICE
P.HUT. THIN/CRISP HAM	0.75	SLICE
P.HUT. THIN/CRISP VEG. LUV.	0.75	SLICE

P.HUT. THIN/CRISP PEPPERON	0.75	SLICE
SW 6" COLD SUB/VEGG. DELIT	1	SUB
SW 6" COLD SUB/TURK. BRST.	1	SUB
SW 6" COLD SUB/TURK.B/HAM	1	SUB
SW 6" COLD SUB/HAM	1	SUB
SW 6" COLD SUB/ROAST BEEF	1	SUB
SW 6" COLD SUB/SFOOD,CRAB	1	SUB
SW 6" COLD SUB/COLD CUT 3	1	SUB
SW 6" COLD SUB/TUNA	1	SUB
SW 6" HOT SUB/RST.CHICK.BR.	1	SUB
SW 6" HOT SUB/STAK/CHEESE	1	SUB
SW 6" HOT SUB/SUB MELT	1	SUB
SW VEGGIE DELITE SALAD	1	SALAD
SW TURKEY BREAST SALAD	1	SALAD
SW ROAST BEEF SALAD	1	SALAD
SW TURK. BRST/HAM SALAD	1	SALAD
SW RST. CHICK. BR. SALAD	0.75	SALAD
SW SEAFOOD/CRAB SALAD	0.75	SALAD
SW STEAK/CHEESE SALAD	0.75	SALAD
SW SUBWAY MELT SALAD	0.75	SALAD
SW COLD CUT 3 SALAD	0.75	SALAD
SW FAT FREE ITALIAN DRESS	1	OZ
SW FAT FREE FRENCH DRESS	1	OZ
SW FAT FREE RANCH DRESS	1	OZ
SW DELI STYLE TURKEY BR.	0.5	SNDWCH
SW DELI STYLE HAM	0.5	SNDWCH
SW DELI STYLE ROAST BEEF	0.5	SNDWCH
TB GRILLED STEAK SOFT TACO	0.55	TACO
WAHOO'S CHBROIL FISH TACO	0.75	TACO
WENDI'S SIDE SALAD	1	SALAD
WENDI'S FF FRENCH DRESSING	1	OZ
WENDI'S ITALIAN RED. F/C DRESS	1	OZ
WENDI'S SMALL CHILI	0.75	BOWL
WENDI'S GRILLED CHICK. FILLET	1	MEAT

1400 Calories/Day Eating Plan	
What Does Your Doctor Look Like Naked?	

Name: _____

Date: _____

Exercise: 30-40 min in a.m. before food		Write what you eat here:
Meal 1 Time: _____	1 Protein Source 2 Active Carbohydrates	
Meal 2 Time: _____	1 oz Raw Almonds	
Meal 3 Time: _____	1 Protein Source 1 Active Carbohydrates Free Carbohydrates (as much as you want)	
Meal 4 Time: _____	½ LOW CARB protein bar (OR) 1 scoop Whey Protein Powder in water	
Meal 5 Time:	1 Protein Source 0 Active Carbohydrates Free Carbohydrates (as much as you want)	
BedTime Meal (Optional)	Sugar Free Jell-O 1 cup	

Add fiber supplement in evening, such as Metamucil or other (sugar FREE).
Add spices, pepper, etc. as needed.
Try to eat every two to three hours.
Drink ¾ of a gallon of water EVERY DAY!
May have up to 2 diet pops (or) 2 cups a coffee a day.

Active Carbohydrates 1400 Calories

Fruit and Vegetables

APPLE	2.29	3 INCH
APPLESAUCE, MOTT'S	0.84	CUP
APRICOTS (CAN/DEL MONTE LITE)	1.54	CUP
APRICOTS (DRIED)	2.65	OZ
APRICOTS (FRESH 12/LB)	10.9	MEDIUM
ASPARAGUS	50	OZ
BANANA	1.76	MEDIUM
BLUEBERRIES (FRESH)	2.26	CUP
BRUSSELS SPROUTS, BOILED	3.09	CUP
CABBAGE, SHREDDED	10.3	CUP
CANTALOUPE	0.98	5 INCH
CARROT (FRESH)	16.7	OZ
CAULIFLOWER	7.13	CUP
CELERY	46.3	OZ
CHERRIES, FRESH, SWEET W/PIT	1.78	CUP
CHERRIES, DARK (CAN/DEL MONTE)	0.925	CUP
COLLARD GREENS (CAN)	3.09	CUP
COLLARD GREENS (FRESH)	15.4	CUP
CORN CAKE	5.3	CAKE
CORN (CAN/DEL MONTE NO SODIUM)	13.5	OZ
CUCUMBER, SLICED	13.2	CUP
EGGPLANT	8.4	CUP
FRUIT, MIXED FROZEN	2.06	CUP
GARLIC, 1 CLOVE	46	CLOVE
GARLIC, TRIMMED	4.4	OZ
GRAPES	1.63	CUP
GRAPE JUICE/VERYFINE	9.9	OZ
GRAPEFRUIT	2.01	4 INCH
GREEN BEANS (CAN/DEL MONTE NO SALT)	4.61	CUP
GREEN PEPPER	9.25	MEDIUM
KIWI	12.5	OZ
MUSHROOMS, FRESH	10.3	CUP
ONION, FRESH/CHOPPED	3.09	CUP
ORANGE, NAVAL	2.85	3 INCH

ORANGE, JUICE	13.5	OZ
PAPAYA	1.585	LB.
PAPAYA, PEELED/CUBED	3.44	CUP
PEACH, FRESH, SLICED	2.5	CUP
PEACH (CAN/DEL MONTE EXTRA LITE)	1.54	CUP
PEARS (CAN)	6.15	HALF
PEAS, BLACKEYED (CAN)	1.03	CUP
PEAS (CAN/DEL MONTE NO SODIUM)	13.5	OZ
PEAS, GREEN GIANT FROZEN, SWEET	1.77	CUP
PEAS, EDIBLE-PODDED	3.1	CUP
PINEAPPLE, FRESH/DICED	2.37	CUP
PINEAPPLE, DEL MONTE SNACK CAN (LITE)	2.65	3.5 OZ
PINEAPPLE (CAN/DOLE LITE SYRUP)	10.9	SLICE
PRUNES, DOLE, DRIED	2.65	OZ
PUMPKIN (CAN)	3.7	CUP
RAISENS	0.385	CUP
RED PEPPER	9.25	MEDIUM
STRAWBERRIES (FRESH)	1.9	PINT
STRAWBERRIES (FROZEN)	2.47	CUP
SQUASH, CAN, STOKLEY	1.85	CUP
SQUASH, FRESH BAKED	1.63	CUP
TANGERINE	5	2.5 INCH
TOMATO, CAN	17.2	OZ
TOMATO, FRESH	7.1	3 INCH
TOMATO, JUICE	29.5	OZ
VEGETABLES, MIXED (FROZEN)	2.5	CUP
WATERMELLON	1.22	1X10 INCH
ZUCCHINI, FRESH, SLICED	10.3	CUP

Yogurts and Desserts

DING DONG	1.16	DING
DREYERS FROZEN FAT FREE YOGURT	1.03	CUP
FRUIT ROLL-UP	2.65	ROLL-UP
POPCORN, WHITE	3.7	TBLSP
TCBY, SOFT SERVE/NONFAT/NO SUGAR	1.16	CUP
YOGURT, FAT FREE, MOUNTAIN HIGH	8	OZ
YOGURT, FAT FREE, DANNON	8	OZ
LUCERN, YOGURT, NONFAT, LITE	8	OZ

YOGURT, YOPLAIT, FAT FREE, LITE	6	OZ
YOGURT,YOPLAIT ORIGINAL/99% FAT FREE	6	OZ
YOGURT, HORIZON, FF / BLUEBERRY	6	OZ
PLANTER DRIED WALNUT PIECES	0.2	CUP
RAW ALMONDS, TOASTED	1	OZ
PECANS, DRIED	0.88	OZ
PEANUTS, DRY ROASTED	0.2	CUP
HOT CHOCOLATE	3	ENVEL.
ALMONDS, SHELLED	1	OZ

Cereals

CEREAL, CHEERIOS	1.69	CUP
CEREAL, COCOA KRISPIES	1.16	CUP
CEREAL, GRAPENUTS	0.462	CUP
CEREAL, HONEY NUT TOASTY O'S	1.68	CUP
CEREAL, WHEATIES	1.68	CUP
CEREAL, KELLOGG'S ALL BRAN	1.16	CUP
CEREAL, KELLOGG'S CORN FLAKES	1.68	CUP
CEREAL, KELLOGG'S RAISEN BRAN	1.09	CUP
CEREAL, KELLOGG'S CRACKLIN' OAT BRAN	0.7	CUP
CEREAL, NABISCO SHREDDED WHEAT	2.32	PIECE
CEREAL, NAB. SHREDDED WHEAT (SPOON)	1.09	CUP
CEREAL, RICE KRISPIES	2.1	CUP
CEREAL, BENEFIT NUTRITION, PROTEIN +	0.88	CUP
CREAM OF WHEAT	4.63	TBL/DRY
GRANOLA, CW POST HEARTY	0.44	CUP
GRANOLA, KELLOGG'S LOW FAT	3	CUP
OATMEAL (PRE-COOK MEASUREMENT)	0.66	CUP

Breads

BREAD, OROWHEAT LITE	4.63	SLICE
BREAD, SUSAN'S HOMEMADE/18 SLICES	2.05	SLICE
BREAD, SUSAN'S HOMEMADE	0.113	LOAF
BUN, WONDER REDUCED CALORIE LITE	2.31	BUN
CRACKER, ZESTA SALTINES	5.15	CRACKER
TORTILLA (CAROLYN)	1.09	TORT
TORTILLA, TORTILLA'S MEXICO, FLOUR	1.68	TORT

TORTILLA, TORTILLA'S MEXICO, CORN	2.06	TORT
TRISCUITS	1.32	OZ
WAFFLE, EGGO, HOMESTYLE	1.69	WAFFLE
WHOLE GRAIN/WHOLE WHEAT FLOUR	0.455	CUP

Rice/Potatoes/Beans

BLACK BEANS (BOILED)	0.82	CUP
BLACK BEANS (DRY)	0.66	CUP
CHICKPEAS/GARBANZO BEANS	0.22	CUP
KIDNEY BEANS (BOILED)	0.25	CUP
LIMA BEANS (BOILED)	0.89	CUP
NAVY BEANS (BOILED)	0.72	CUP
NAVY BEANS (CAN)	0.77	CUP
PINTO BEANS (BOILED)	0.79	CUP
PINTO BEANS (CAN)	0.975	CUP
PINTO BEANS (DRY)	0.309	CUP
PORK & BEANS/VAN CAMPS	0.84	CUP
POTATO, SWEET	1.57	5"X2"
POTATO	11	OZ
RICE CAKE	3.7	CAKE
RICE, WHITE, BASMATI	0.772	CUP (C)
RICE, BROWN LONG GRAIN	0.925	CUP (C)
RICE, INSTANT, MINUTE BRAND	0.58	CUP(UC)
RICE, WHITE, LONG GRAIN	0.29	CUP(UC)
SOYBEANS (BOILED)	0.75	CUP
YAM, BOILED OR BAKED	1.17	CUP

Pasta

MACARONI, DAVINI TWIST	0.7	CUP/DRY
MACARONI, HOSPITALITY ELBOW	0.385	CUP/DRY
MACARONI, AM. BEAUTY ELBOW	0.44	CUP/DRY
PASTA, CREAMETTE PLAIN	1.77	OZ
SPAGHETTI, EDEN WHOLE WHEAT	1.76	OZ/UC

Protein Sources 1400 Calories

White Meat

CHICKEN BREAST (HORMEL/CAN)	1.23	CAN
CHICKEN BREAST (SKINLESS)	6.18	OZ
CHICKEN (LEG W/SKIN & BONE)	0.7	
CHICKEN (THIGH W/SKIN & BONE)	1.21	
CHICKEN (LEG & THIGH W/SKIN & BONE)	0.443	
HAM, BAR S, XTRA LEAN, 96% FAT FREE	5.3	OZ
HAM, DAK CAN	6.15	OZ
PORK, SIRLOIN, LEAN W/ FAT	1.85	OZ
TURKEY BREAST (SKINLESS)	3.47	OZ
TURKEY BREAST (HORMEL/CAN)	1.06	CAN
TURKEY BRST/OVEN ROAST/SFWY/89% FF	7.4	OZ
VENISON/ANTELOPE	4.15	OZ

Red Meat

HAMBURGER (10% FAT)	3.3	OZ
HAMBURGER (15% FAT)	2.73	OZ
HAMBURGER (20% FAT)	2.65	OZ
HAMBURGER (27% FAT)	2.24	OZ
LAMB, SHOULDER	2.1	OZ
STEAK, BOTTOM ROUND	3.13	OZ
STEAK, BRISKET (FLAT HALF)	2.95	OZ
STEAK, CHUCK, ARM	3.04	OZ
STEAK, CHUCK, BLADE	2.6	OZ
STEAK, EYE ROUND	3.9	OZ
STEAK, FLANK	3.16	OZ
STEAK, NEW YORK STRIP	3.7	OZ
STEAK, PORTERHOUSE	3	OZ
STEAK, RIBEYE	2.91	OZ
STEAK, ROUND TIP	3.55	OZ
STEAK, SHANK (CROSSCUTS)	3.25	OZ
STEAK, T-BONE	3.05	OZ
STEAK, TENDERLOIN	3.1	OZ
STEAK, TOP LOIN	3.15	OZ
STEAK, TOP ROUND	3.64	OZ

STEAK, TOP SIRLOIN	3.38	OZ
STEAK, TYSON SEASONED BEEF STRIPS	3.95	OZ
TACO/BURRITO MEAT/SMART GROUND	0.96	CUP
OSCAR MAYER BACON	6.15	SLICE
LITTLE SIZZLER BROWN/SERVE SAUSAGE	2.4	LINK

Sea Food

BASS, FRESHWATER, DRY HEAT	4.5	OZ
BASS, STRIPED, DRY HEAT	5.3	OZ
COD, ATLANTIC, DRY HEAT	6.25	OZ
CRAB, ALASKA KING, MOIST HEAT	6.8	OZ
CRAB, BLUE, MOIST HEAT	6.4	OZ
FLOUNDER, DRY HEAT	5.6	OZ
HADDOCK, DRY HEAT	5.85	OZ
HALIBUT, DRY HEAT	4.67	OZ
LOBSTER, NORTHERN, MOIST HEAT	6.7	OZ
MAHI MAHI	7.6	OZ
ORANGE ROUGHY, DRY HEAT	7.33	OZ
PERCH, DRY HEAT	5.6	OZ
PERCH, OCEAN/ATLANTIC, DRY HEAT	5.4	OZ
SALMON, ATLANTIC, DRY HEAT	3.57	OZ
SHRIMP, MOIST HEAT	6.6	OZ
TROUT, DRY HEAT	3.45	OZ
TUNA BURGER, AHI/OMEGA FOODS	6.6	OZ
TUNA, LOW SODIUM, CAN	1.06	CAN
TUNA, WATER, CAN	1.23	CAN
TUNA, WHITE/LOW SALT, CAN (5 OZ)	1.06	CAN
TUNA, WHITE, CAN (5 OZ)	1.06	CAN
TUNA, FILLET/STEAK	4.2	OZ
WALLEYE, BAKED/BROILED/MICRO	5.5	OZ

Vegetarian

IVES VEG. COUSINE VEGGY DOG	3.08	DOG
SOY MILK (TRIS)	2	CUP
SOY MILK (SYLVIA)	1.75	CUP

Eggs/Dairy

1% COTTAGE CHEESE, NORDICA	1.16	CUP
2% COTTAGE CHEESE (LOW FAT)	0.925	CUP
COTTAGE CHEESE (LUCERNE FAT FREE)	1.16	CUP
COTT CHEESE MARIGOLD/DRY CURD	1.77	CUP
COTT CHEESE MARIGOLD/DRY CURD	28.3	TBLSP
COTT CHEESE BREAKSTONES FAT FREE	1.16	CUP
CHEDDER, SHREDDED, FAT FREE, KHF	1.03	CUP
CHEDDER, SHREDDED, 94% FAT FREE, HC	0.925	CUP
CHEESE, COLBY/MOZZARELLA	1.69	OZ
EGG WHITE	10.9	
EGG, WHOLE	2.46	
EGG BEATERS	1.54	CUP
MOZZARELLA SHREDDED, FAT FREE, KHF	0.92	CUP
SKIM MOZZARELLA STRING CHEESE	2.32	OZ

Free Carbs, Supplements, Fast Foods
1400 calories

Free Carbs

ASPARAGUS
BROCCOLI
CABBAGE
CAULIFLOWER
CELERY
CUCUMBER
GREEN BEANS
GREEN PEPPERS
GREEN SQUASH
LETTUCE, ICEBERG
LETTUCE, LEAF/SHREDDED
MUSHROOMS
ONION
PICKLES (DILL)
RADISH
RED PEPPERS

SPINACH (CAN/NO SALT)
SPINACH (FRESH)
TOMATO (EXCLUDING JUICE)
ZUCCHINI

Supplements/Fast Foods

ATKINS BAR	0.75	BAR
EAS ADVANTEDGE, C&C/LEM/BLUE	0.75	BAR
BAR, ZONE	0.75	BAR
BAR, PURE PROTEIN, 50 G.	1	BAR
BAR, W.W. PURE PROTEIN, 78 G.	0.5	BAR
BAR, PROTEIN REVOLUTION, PBJ	0.75	BAR
BAR, FIBAR, PEANUT BUTTER, 1.2 OZ	1.25	BAR
BAR, PREMIER 1, PROTEIN 8, CHOC/COCO	0.5	BAR
BAR, PREFERRED BAR, CHOC./FUDG/RAS	0.75	BAR
BAR, PREFERRED BAR, CHOC./FUDG/BROW	0.75	BAR
ALIVE, HI CARB POWDER	1	TBLSP
POWERADE	2	SERVING
PROTEIN,GNC P.P. EGG/WHEY	1.5	SERVING
PROTEIN. GNC P.PERF. WHEY	4	SCOOP
OPTIMUM NUTRITION WHEY	1.5	SCOOP
SYNTRAX WHEY PROTEIN	2	SCOOP
TRI PROTEIN PLUS POWDER	1.25	SERVING
HW STRAWBERRY PROT. POWD.	1.75	SCOOP
BIOCHEM WHEY PRO 290	2.25	SCOOP
HUMAN DEV. TECH. WHEY	1.25	SCOOP
NATURADE 100% SOY PROTEIN	0.5	CUP
SUPER GREEN PRO 96 - SOY	0.5	CUP
100% PURE WHEY, PROLAB	1.25	SCOOP
ECLIPSE BULK UP WHEY	1.75	SCOOP
VITAMIN WORLD WHEY 100%	1.5	SCOOP
ULT. NUT. PROSTAR WHEY	1.5	SCOOP
RED WINE	7	OZ
MET RX CH.RST.PNT.PRO + BAR	0.5	BAR
MET RX BAV. MINT. PRO + BAR	0.75	BAR
MET AFTER FX BAR	0.75	BAR
MET RX CH. CH. CHIP PRO + BAR	0.5	BAR
MET RX SOURCE ONE BAR	0.75	BAR

MET RX CHOC. GRAHCRK CHIP BAR	0.5	BAR
MET RX PEANUT BUTTER BAR	0.5	BAR
MET RX DRINK MIX, MRP	0.75	SERVING
MET RX PRO 50, ANABOLIC DRIVE	0.5	SERVING
MET RX PRO 60, ANABOLIC DRIVE	0.5	SERVING
MET RX PROTEIN PLUS	2.25	SCOOP
MET RX KETO PRO	2.25	SCOOP
NUTRI FORCE DRINK MIX, MRP	0.5	SERVING
EAS MYO. DEL. CH/PB BAR	0.5	BAR
EAS MYOPLEX + DELUXE	0.5	SERVING
EAS MYOPLEX LITE	0.75	SERVING
ADVANT EDGE QUICK STIR PROTEIN DRINK	0.75	SERVING
EAS NEUROGAIN	1	SCOOP
EAS PHOSPHAGEN HP	1.25	SCOOP
EAS PRECISION PROTEIN	1.75	SCOOP
EAS SIMPLY PROTEIN	3	SCOOP
EAS WHEY PROTEIN	1.5	SCOOP
EAS SUPPER SHAKE	0.33	SHAKE
VITAMIN WORLD DAILY RX, MRP	0.5	SHAKE
VITAMIN WORLD PROTOPLEX DELUXE, MRP	0.5	SHAKE
VITAMIN WORLD PRE. ENG. WHEY PROT.	1.75	SCOOP
PERFECT RX, MRP, CHOCOLATE	0.75	SHAKE
OPTI PRO	0.5	SHAKE
ARBY'S CHICK. SAND. R.DELX.LITE	0.5	BURGER
ARBY'S SIDE SALAD	1	SALAD
ARBY'S GARDEN SALAD	1	SALAD
ARBY'S RST. CHCK. SALAD	1	SALAD
ARBY'S RED. CAL. ITAL. DRESSING	1	PACKET
ARBY'S RED RANCH DRESSING	1	PACKET
MCD'S VINAG. LITE SALAD DR.	1	PACKET
MCD'S GARDEN SALAD	1	SALAD
MCD'S VINAG. LITE SALAD DR.	1	PACKET
P.HUT. HAND-TOSS CHEESE	0.5	SLICE
P.HUT. HAND-TOSS HAM	0.75	SLICE
P.HUT. HAND-TOSS VEG. LUV.	0.75	SLICE
P.HUT. HAND-TOSS PEPPERON	0.75	SLICE
P.HUT. THIN/CRISP CHEESE	0.75	SLICE
P.HUT. THIN/CRISP HAM	1	SLICE

P.HUT. THIN/CRISP VEG. LUV.	1	SLICE
P.HUT. THIN/CRISP PEPPERON	0.75	SLICE
SW 6" COLD SUB/VEGG. DELIT	1	SUB
SW 6" COLD SUB/TURK. BRST.	1	SUB
SW 6" COLD SUB/TURK.B/HAM	1	SUB
SW 6" COLD SUB/HAM	1	SUB
SW 6" COLD SUB/ROAST BEEF	1	SUB
SW 6" COLD SUB/SFOOD,CRAB	1	SUB
SW 6" COLD SUB/COLD CUT 3	1	SUB
SW 6" COLD SUB/TUNA	1	SUB
SW 6" HOT SUB/RST.CHICK.BR.	1	SUB
SW 6" HOT SUB/STAK/CHEESE	1	SUB
SW 6" HOT SUB/SUB MELT	1	SUB
SW VEGGIE DELITE SALAD	1	SALAD
SW TURKEY BREAST SALAD	1	SALAD
SW ROAST BEEF SALAD	1	SALAD
SW TURK. BRST/HAM SALAD	1	SALAD
SW RST. CHICK. BR. SALAD	0.75	SALAD
SW SEAFOOD/CRAB SALAD	0.75	SALAD
SW STEAK/CHEESE SALAD	0.75	SALAD
SW SUBWAY MELT SALAD	0.75	SALAD
SW COLD CUT 3 SALAD	0.75	SALAD
SW FAT FREE ITALIAN DRESS	1	OZ
SW FAT FREE FRENCH DRESS	1	OZ
SW FAT FREE RANCH DRESS	1	OZ
SW DELI STYLE TURKEY BR.	0.75	SNDWCH
SW DELI STYLE HAM	0.75	SNDWCH
SW DELI STYLE ROAST BEEF	0.75	SNDWCH
TB GRILLED STEAK SOFT TACO	0.75	TACO
WAHOO'S CHBROIL FISH TACO	0.5	TACO
WENDI'S SIDE SALAD	1	SALAD
WENDI'S FF FRENCH DRESSING	1	OZ
WENDI'S ITALIAN RED. F/C DRESS	1	OZ
WENDI'S SMALL CHILI	0.75	BOWL
WENDI'S GRILLED CHICK. FILLET	1	MEAT

1500 Calories/Day Eating Plan	
What Does Your Doctor Look Like Naked?	

Name: _____

Date: _____

Exercise: 30-40 min in a.m before food		
		Write what you eat here:
Meal 1 Time: _____	1 Protein Source 2 Active Carbohydrates	
Meal 2 Time: _____	1 oz Raw Almonds	
Meal 3 Time: _____	1 Protein Source 1 Active Carbohydrates Free Carbohydrates (as much as you want)	
Meal 4 Time: _____	½ LOW CARB protein bar (OR) 1 scoop Whey Protein Powder in water	
Meal 5 Time: _____	1 Protein Source 0 Active Carbohydrates Free Carbohydrates (as much as you want)	
Bedtime Meal (Optional)	Sugar Free Jell-O 1 cup	

Add fiber supplement in evening, such as Metamucil or other (sugar FREE).
Add spices, pepper, etc. as needed.
Try to eat every two to three hours.
Drink ¾ of a gallon of water EVERY DAY!
May have up to 2 diet pops (or) 2 cups a coffee a day.

Active Carbohydrates 1500 Calories

Fruit and Vegetables

APPLE	2.49	3 INCH
APPLESAUCE, MOTT'S	0.91	CUP
APRICOTS (CAN/DEL MONTE LITE)	1.68	CUP
APRICOTS (DRIED)	2.88	OZ
APRICOTS (FRESH 12/LB)	11.8	MEDIUM
ASPARAGUS	54.4	OZ
BANANA	1.92	MEDIUM
BLUEBERRIES (FRESH)	2.46	CUP
BRUSSELS SPROUTS, BOILED	3.35	CUP
CABBAGE, SHREDDED	11.2	CUP
CANTALOUPE	1.07	5 INCH
CARROT (FRESH)	18.1	OZ
CAULIFLOWER	7.75	CUP
CELERY	50	OZ
CHERRIES, FRESH, SWEET W/PIT	1.94	CUP
CHERRIES, DARK (CAN/DEL MONTE)	1	CUP
COLLARD GREENS (CAN)	3.36	CUP
COLLARD GREENS (FRESH)	16.8	CUP
CORN CAKE	5.75	CAKE
CORN (CAN/DEL MONTE NO SODIUM)	14.7	OZ
CUCUMBER, SLICED	14.4	CUP
EGGPLANT	9.1	CUP
FRUIT, MIXED FROZEN	2.24	CUP
GARLIC, 1 CLOVE	50	CLOVE
GARLIC, TRIMMED	4.8	OZ
GRAPES	1.77	CUP
GRAPE JUICE/VERYFINE	10.7	OZ
GRAPEFRUIT	2.19	4 INCH
GREEN BEANS (CAN/DEL MONTE NO SALT)	5	CUP
GREEN PEPPER	10	MEDIUM
KIWI	13.5	OZ
MUSHROOMS, FRESH	11.2	CUP
ONION, FRESH/CHOPPED	3.36	CUP
ORANGE, NAVAL	3.1	3 INCH

ORANGE, JUICE	14.6	OZ
PAPAYA	1.72	LB.
PAPAYA, PEELED/CUBED	3.74	CUP
PEACH, FRESH, SLICED	2.72	CUP
PEACH (CAN/DEL MONTE EXTRA LITE)	1.68	CUP
PEARS (CAN)	6.7	HALF
PEAS, BLACKEYED (CAN)	1.12	CUP
PEAS (CAN/DEL MONTE NO SODIUM)	14.7	OZ
PEAS, GREEN GIANT FROZEN, SWEET	1.92	CUP
PEAS, EDIBLE-PODDED	3.35	CUP
PINEAPPLE, FRESH/DICED	2.58	CUP
PINEAPPLE, DEL MONTE SNACK CAN (LITE)	2.88	3.5 OZ
PINEAPPLE (CAN/DOLE LITE SYRUP)	11.88	SLICE
PRUNES, DOLE, DRIED	2.88	OZ
PUMPKIN (CAN)	4	CUP
RAISINS	0.42	CUP
RED PEPPER	10	MEDIUM
STRAWBERRIES (FRESH)	2.08	PINT
STRAWBERRIES (FROZEN)	2.69	CUP
SQUASH, CAN, STOKLEY	2	CUP
SQUASH, FRESH BAKED	1.77	CUP
TANGERINE	5.45	2.5 INCH
TOMATO, CAN	18.8	OZ
TOMATO, FRESH	7.7	3 INCH
TOMATO, JUICE	32	OZ
VEGETABLES, MIXED (FROZEN)	2.24	CUP
WATERMELLON	1.32	1X10 INCH
ZUCCHINI, FRESH, SLICED	11.2	CUP

Yogurts and Desserts

DING DONG	1.26	DING
DREYERS FROZEN FAT FREE YOGURT	1.12	CUP
FRUIT ROLL-UP	2.88	ROLL-UP
POPCORN, WHITE	4	TBLSP
TCBY, SOFT SERVE/NONFAT/NO SUGAR	1.26	CUP
YOGURT, FAT FREE, MOUNTAIN HIGH	8	OZ
YOGURT, FAT FREE, DANNON	8	OZ
LUCERN, YOGURT, NONFAT, LITE	8	OZ

YOGURT, YOPLAIT, FAT FREE, LITE	6	OZ
YOGURT,YOPLAIT ORIGINAL/99% FAT FREE	6	OZ
YOGURT, HORIZON, FF / BLUEBERRY	6	OZ
PLANTER DRIED WALNUT PIECES	0.25	CUP
RAW ALMONDS, TOASTED	1.19	OZ
PECANS, DRIED	1	OZ
PEANUTS, DRY ROASTED	0.2	CUP
HOT CHOCOLATE	4	ENVEL.
ALMONDS, SHELLED	1	OZ

Cereals

CEREAL, CHEERIOS	1.83	CUP
CEREAL, COCOA KRISPIES	1.26	CUP
CEREAL, GRAPENUTS	0.5	CUP
CEREAL, HONEY NUT TOASTY O'S	1.83	CUP
CEREAL, WHEATIES	1.83	CUP
CEREAL, KELLOGG'S ALL BRAN	1.26	CUP
CEREAL, KELLOGG'S CORN FLAKES	1.83	CUP
CEREAL, KELLOGG'S RAISIN BRAN	1.18	CUP
CEREAL, KELLOGG'S CRACKLIN' OAT BRAN	0.76	CUP
CEREAL, NABISCO SHREDDED WHEAT	2.5	PIECE
CEREAL, NAB. SHREDDED WHEAT (SPOON)	1.18	CUP
CEREAL, RICE KRISPIES	2.29	CUP
CEREAL, BENEFIT NUTRITION, PROTEIN +	0.96	CUP
CREAM OF WHEAT	5	TBL/DRY
GRANOLA, CW POST HEARTY	0.48	CUP
GRANOLA, KELLOGG'S LOW FAT	4	CUP
OATMEAL (PRE-COOK MEASUREMENT)	0.72	CUP

Breads

BREAD, OROWHEAT LITE	5	SLICE
BREAD, SUSAN'S HOMEMADE/18 SLICES	2.22	SLICE
BREAD, SUSAN'S HOMEMADE	0.123	LOAF
BUN, WONDER REDUCED CALORIE LITE	2.5	BUN
CRACKER, ZESTA SALTINES	16.8	CRACKER
TORTILLA (CAROLYN)	1.18	TORT
TORTILLA, TORTILLA'S MEXICO, FLOUR	1.83	TORT

TORTILLA, TORTILLA'S MEXICO, CORN	2.24	TORT
TRISCUITS	1.44	OZ
WAFFLE, EGGO, HOMESTYLE	1.83	WAFFLE
WHOLE GRAIN/WHOLE WHEAT FLOUR	0.495	CUP

Rice/Potatoes/Beans

BLACK BEANS (BOILED)	0.89	CUP
BLACK BEANS (DRY)	0.72	CUP
CHICKPEAS/GARBANZO BEANS	0.25	CUP
KIDNEY BEANS (BOILED)	0.25	CUP
LIMA BEANS (BOILED)	0.568	CUP
NAVY BEANS (BOILED)	0.78	CUP
NAVY BEANS (CAN)	0.838	CUP
PINTO BEANS (BOILED)	0.86	CUP
PINTO BEANS (CAN)	1.06	CUP
PINTO BEANS (DRY)	0.335	CUP
PORK & BEANS/VAN CAMPS	0.91	CUP
POTATO, SWEET	1.71	5"X2"
POTATO	12	OZ
RICE CAKE	4	CAKE
RICE, WHITE, BASMATI	0.84	CUP (C)
RICE, BROWN LONG GRAIN	1	CUP (C)
RICE, INSTANT, MINUTE BRAND	0.63	CUP(UC)
RICE, WHITE, LONG GRAIN	0.315	CUP(UC)
SOYBEANS (BOILED)	0.75	CUP
YAM, BOILED OR BAKED	1.27	CUP

Pasta

MACARONI, DAVINI TWIST	0.765	CUP/DRY
MACARONI, HOSPITALITY ELBOW	0.42	CUP/DRY
MACARONI, AM. BEAUTY ELBOW	0.48	CUP/DRY
PASTA, CREAMETTE PLAIN	1.92	OZ
SPAGHETTI, EDEN WHOLE WHEAT	1.92	OZ/UC

Protein Sources 1500 Calories

White Meat

CHICKEN BREAST (HORMEL/CAN)	1.34	CAN
CHICKEN BREAST (SKINLESS)	6.7	OZ
CHICKEN (LEG W/ SKIN & BONE)	0.76	
CHICKEN (THIGH W/ SKIN & BONE)	1.32	
CHICKEN (LEG & THIGH W/ SKIN & BONE)	0.48	
HAM, BAR S, XTRA LEAN, 96% FAT FREE	5.75	OZ
HAM, DAK CAN	6.7	OZ
PORK, SIRLOIN, LEAN W/ FAT	2	OZ
TURKEY BREAST (SKINLESS)	3.76	OZ
TURKEY BREAST (HORMEL/CAN)	1.15	CAN
TURKEY BRST/OVEN ROAST/SFWY/89% FF	8	OZ
VENISON/ANTELOPE	4.5	OZ

Red Meat

HAMBURGER (10% FAT)	3.58	OZ
HAMBURGER (15% FAT)	2.96	OZ
HAMBURGER (20% FAT)	2.88	OZ
HAMBURGER (27% FAT)	2.44	OZ
LAMB, SHOULDER	2.29	OZ
STEAK, BOTTOM ROUND	3.4	OZ
STEAK, BRISKET (FLAT HALF)	3.2	OZ
STEAK, CHUCK, ARM	3.3	OZ
STEAK, CHUCK, BLADE	2.84	OZ
STEAK, EYE ROUND	4.22	OZ
STEAK, FLANK	3.44	OZ
STEAK, NEW YORK STRIP	4	OZ
STEAK, PORTERHOUSE	3.27	OZ
STEAK, RIBEYE	3.16	OZ
STEAK, ROUND TIP	3.85	OZ
STEAK, SHANK (CROSSCUTS)	3.53	OZ
STEAK, T-BONE	3.32	OZ
STEAK, TENDERLOIN	3.38	OZ
STEAK, TOP LOIN	3.44	OZ
STEAK, TOP ROUND	3.95	OZ

STEAK, TOP SIRLOIN	3.67	OZ
STEAK, TYSON SEASONED BEEF STRIPS	4.3	OZ
TACO/BURRITO MEAT/SMART GROUND	1.05	CUP
OSCAR MAYER BACON	6.7	SLICE
LITTLE SIZZLER BROWN/SERVE SAUSAGE	2.62	LINK

Sea Food

BASS, FRESHWATER, DRY HEAT	4.9	OZ
BASS, STRIPED, DRY HEAT	5.75	OZ
COD, ATLANTIC, DRY HEAT	6.8	OZ
CRAB, ALASKA KING, MOIST HEAT	7.38	OZ
CRAB, BLUE, MOIST HEAT	6.95	OZ
FLOUNDER, DRY HEAT	6.1	OZ
HADDOCK, DRY HEAT	6.35	OZ
HALIBUT, DRY HEAT	5.08	OZ
LOBSTER, NORTHERN, MOIST HEAT	7.3	OZ
MAHI MAHI	8.3	OZ
ORANGE ROUGHY, DRY HEAT	7.9	OZ
PERCH, DRY HEAT	6.1	OZ
PERCH, OCEAN/ATLANTIC, DRY HEAT	5.86	OZ
SALMON, ATLANTIC, DRY HEAT	3.87	OZ
SHRIMP, MOIST HEAT	7.2	OZ
TROUT, DRY HEAT	3.75	OZ
TUNA BURGER, AHI / OMEGA FOODS	7.2	OZ
TUNA, LOW SODIUM, CAN	1.15	CAN
TUNA, WATER, CAN	1.34	CAN
TUNA, WHITE / LOW SALT, CAN (5 OZ)	1.15	CAN
TUNA, WHITE, CAN (5 OZ)	1.15	CAN
TUNA, FILLET/STEAK	4.57	OZ
WALLEYE, BAKED/BROILED/MICRO	5.97	OZ

Vegetarian

IVES VEG. COUSINE VEGGY DOG	3.35	DOG
SOY MILK (TRIS)	2.25	CUP
SOY MILK (SYLVIA)	2	CUP

Eggs/Dairy

1% COTTAGE CHEESE, NORDICA	1.26	CUP
2% COTTAGE CHEESE (LOW FAT)	1	CUP
COTTAGE CHEESE (LUCERNE FAT FREE)	1.26	CUP
COTT CHEESE MARIGOLD/DRY CURD	1.92	CUP
COTT CHEESE MARIGOLD/DRY CURD	30.5	TBLSP
COTT CHEESE BREAKSTONES FAT FREE	1.26	CUP
CHEDDER, SHREDDED, FAT FREE, KHF	1.12	CUP
CHEDDER, SHREDDED, 94% FAT FREE, HC	1	CUP
CHEESE, COLBY/MOZZARELLA	1.83	OZ
EGG WHITE	11.8	
EGG, WHOLE	2.69	
EGG BEATERS	1.68	CUP
MOZZARELLA SHREDDED, FAT FREE, KHF	1	CUP
SKIM MOZZARELLA STRING CHEESE	2.5	OZ

Free Carbs, Supplements, Fast Foods
1500 calories

Free Carbs
ASPARAGUS
BROCCOLI
CABBAGE
CAULIFLOWER
CELERY
CUCUMBER
GREEN BEANS
GREEN PEPPERS
GREEN SQUASH
LETTUCE, ICEBERG
LETTUCE, LEAF/SHREDDED
MUSHROOMS
ONION
PICKLES (DILL)
RADISH

RED PEPPERS
SPINACH (CAN/NO SALT)
SPINACH (FRESH)
TOMATO (EXCLUDING JUICE)
ZUCCHINI

Supplements/Fast Foods

ATKINS BAR	0.75	BAR
EAS ADVANTEDGE, C&C/LEM/BLUE	0.75	BAR
BAR, ZONE	0.88	BAR
BAR, PURE PROTEIN, 50 G.	1	BAR
BAR, W.W. PURE PROTEIN, 78 G.	0.5	BAR
BAR, PROTEIN REVOLUTION, PBJ	0.88	BAR
BAR, FIBAR, PEANUT BUTTER, 1.2 OZ	1.33	BAR
BAR, PREMIER 1, PROTEIN 8, CHOC/COCO	0.75	BAR
BAR, PREFERRED BAR, CHOC./FUDG/RAS	0.88	BAR
BAR, PREFERRED BAR, CHOC./FUDG/BROW	0.88	BAR
ALIVE, HI CARB POWDER	5	TBLSP
POWERADE	2	SERVING
PROTEIN,GNC P.P. EGG/WHEY	1.5	SERVING
PROTEIN. GNC P.PERF. WHEY	4	SCOOP
OPTIMUM NUTRITION WHEY	1.75	SCOOP
SYNTRAX WHEY PROTEIN	2.25	SCOOP
TRI PROTEIN PLUS POWDER	1.5	SERVING
HW STRAWBERRY PROT. POWD.	2	SCOOP
BIOCHEM WHEY PRO 290	2.5	SCOOP
HUMAN DEV. TECH. WHEY	1.5	SCOOP
NATURADE 100% SOY PROTEIN	0.5	CUP
SUPER GREEN PRO 96 - SOY	0.5	CUP
100% PURE WHEY, PROLAB	0.75	SCOOP
ECLIPSE BULK UP WHEY	2	SCOOP
VITAMIN WORLD WHEY 100%	1.75	SCOOP
ULT. NUT. PROSTAR WHEY	1.75	SCOOP
RED WINE	8	OZ
MET RX CH.RST.PNT.PRO + BAR	0.5	BAR
MET RX BAV. MINT. PRO + BAR	0.75	BAR
MET AFTER FX BAR	0.75	BAR
MET RX CH. CH. CHIP PRO + BAR	0.75	BAR

MET RX SOURCE ONE BAR	0.75	BAR
MET RX CHOC. GRAHCRK CHIP BAR	0.5	BAR
MET RX PEANUT BUTTER BAR	0.5	BAR
MET RX DRINK MIX, MRP	0.75	SERVING
MET RX PRO 50, ANABOLIC DRIVE	0.75	SERVING
MET RX PRO 60, ANABOLIC DRIVE	0.5	SERVING
MET RX PROTEIN PLUS	2.5	SCOOP
MET RX KETO PRO	2.5	SCOOP
NUTRI FORCE DRINK MIX, MRP	0.75	SERVING
EAS MYO. DEL. CH/PB BAR	0.5	BAR
EAS MYOPLEX + DELUXE	0.5	SERVING
EAS MYOPLEX LITE	0.75	SERVING
ADVANT EDGE QUICK STIR PROTEIN DRINK	0.75	SERVING
EAS NEUROGAIN	4	SCOOP
EAS PHOSPHAGEN HP	1	SCOOP
EAS PRECISION PROTEIN	1.75	SCOOP
EAS SIMPLY PROTEIN	3	SCOOP
EAS WHEY PROTEIN	1.75	SCOOP
EAS SUPPER SHAKE	0.33	SHAKE
VITAMIN WORLD DAILY RX, MRP	0.75	SHAKE
VITAMIN WORLD PROTOPLEX DELUXE, MRP	0.5	SHAKE
VITAMIN WORLD PRE. ENG. WHEY PROT.	2	SCOOP
PERFECT RX, MRP, CHOCOLATE	0.75	SHAKE
OPTI PRO	0.75	SHAKE
ARBY'S CHICK. SAND. R.DELX.LITE	0.5	BURGER
ARBY'S SIDE SALAD	1	SALAD
ARBY'S GARDEN SALAD	1	SALAD
ARBY'S RST. CHCK. SALAD	1	SALAD
ARBY'S RED. CAL. ITAL. DRESSING	1	PACKET
ARBY'S RED RANCH DRESSING	1	PACKET
MCD'S VINAG. LITE SALAD DR.	1	PACKET
MCD'S GARDEN SALAD	1	SALAD
MCD'S VINAG. LITE SALAD DR.	1	PACKET
P.HUT. HAND-TOSS CHEESE	0.75	SLICE
P.HUT. HAND-TOSS HAM	0.75	SLICE
P.HUT. HAND-TOSS VEG. LUV.	0.75	SLICE
P.HUT. HAND-TOSS PEPPERON	0.75	SLICE
P.HUT. THIN/CRISP CHEESE	1	SLICE

P.HUT. THIN/CRISP HAM	1	SLICE
P.HUT. THIN/CRISP VEG. LUV.	1	SLICE
P.HUT. THIN/CRISP PEPPERON	0.75	SLICE
SW 6" COLD SUB/VEGG. DELIT	1	SUB
SW 6" COLD SUB/TURK. BRST.	1	SUB
SW 6" COLD SUB/TURK.B/HAM	1	SUB
SW 6" COLD SUB/HAM	1	SUB
SW 6" COLD SUB/ROAST BEEF	1	SUB
SW 6" COLD SUB/SFOOD,CRAB	1	SUB
SW 6" COLD SUB/COLD CUT 3	1	SUB
SW 6" COLD SUB/TUNA	1	SUB
SW 6" HOT SUB/RST.CHICK.BR.	1	SUB
SW 6" HOT SUB/STAK/CHEESE	1	SUB
SW 6" HOT SUB/SUB MELT	1	SUB
SW VEGGIE DELITE SALAD	1	SALAD
SW TURKEY BREAST SALAD	1	SALAD
SW ROAST BEEF SALAD	1	SALAD
SW TURK. BRST/HAM SALAD	1	SALAD
SW RST. CHICK. BR. SALAD	1	SALAD
SW SEAFOOD/CRAB SALAD	1	SALAD
SW STEAK/CHEESE SALAD	0.75	SALAD
SW SUBWAY MELT SALAD	1	SALAD
SW COLD CUT 3 SALAD	1	SALAD
SW FAT FREE ITALIAN DRESS	1	OZ
SW FAT FREE FRENCH DRESS	1	OZ
SW FAT FREE RANCH DRESS	1	OZ
SW DELI STYLE TURKEY BR.	0.75	SNDWCH
SW DELI STYLE HAM	0.75	SNDWCH
SW DELI STYLE ROAST BEEF	0.75	SNDWCH
TB GRILLED STEAK SOFT TACO	0.75	TACO
WAHOO'S CHBROIL FISH TACO	1	TACO
WENDI'S SIDE SALAD	1	SALAD
WENDI'S FF FRENCH DRESSING	1	OZ
WENDI'S ITALIAN RED. F/C DRESS	1	OZ
WENDI'S SMALL CHILI	1	BOWL
WENDI'S GRILLED CHICK. FILLET	1.5	MEAT

1600 Calories/Day Eating Plan		
What Does Your Doctor Look Like Naked?		
Name: _____ Date: _____		
Exercise: 30-40 min in a.m. before food		Write what you eat here:
Meal 1 Time: _____	1 Protein Source 2 Active Carbohydrates	
Meal 2 Time:	1.5 oz Raw Almonds	
Meal 3 Time: _____	1 Protein Source 1 Active Carbohydrates Free Carbohydrates (as much as you want)	
Meal 4 Time: _____	½ LOW CARB protein bar (OR) 1.5 scoops Whey Protein Powder in water	
Meal 5 Time: _____	1 Protein Source 0 Active Carbohydrates Free Carbohydrates (as much as you want)	
BEDTIME Meal (Optional)	Sugar Free Jell-O 1 cup	
Add fiber supplement in evening, such as Metamucil or other (sugar FREE). Add spices, pepper, etc. as needed. Try to eat every two to three hours. Drink 1 gallon of water EVERY DAY! May have up to 2 diet pops (or) 2 cups a coffee a day.		

Active Carbohydrates 1600 Calories

Fruit and Vegetables

APPLE	2.494	3 INCH
APPLESAUCE, MOTT'S	0.91	CUP
APRICOTS (CAN/DEL MONTE LITE)	1.68	CUP
APRICOTS (DRIED)	2.88	OZ
APRICOTS (FRESH 12/LB)	11.8	MEDIUM
ASPARAGUS	54.4	OZ
BANANA	1.92	MEDIUM
BLUEBERRIES (FRESH)	2.46	CUP
BRUSSELS SPROUTS, BOILED	3.35	CUP
CABBAGE, SHREDDED	11.2	CUP
CANTALOUPE	1.07	5 INCH
CARROT (FRESH)	18.1	OZ
CAULIFLOWER	7.75	CUP
CELERY	50	OZ
CHERRIES, FRESH, SWEET W/PIT	1.94	CUP
CHERRIES, DARK (CAN/DEL MONTE)	1	CUP
COLLARD GREENS (CAN)	3.36	CUP
COLLARD GREENS (FRESH)	16.8	CUP
CORN CAKE	5.75	CAKE
CORN (CAN/DEL MONTE NO SODIUM)	14.7	OZ
CUCUMBER, SLICED	14.4	CUP
EGGPLANT	9.1	CUP
FRUIT, MIXED FROZEN	2.24	CUP
GARLIC, 1 CLOVE	50	CLOVE
GARLIC, TRIMMED	4.8	OZ
GRAPES	1.77	CUP
GRAPE JUICE/VERYFINE	10.7	OZ
GRAPEFRUIT	2.19	4 INCH
GREEN BEANS (CAN/DEL MONTE NO SALT)	5	CUP
GREEN PEPPER	10	MEDIUM
KIWI	13.5	OZ
MUSHROOMS, FRESH	11.2	CUP
ONION, FRESH/CHOPPED	3.36	CUP
ORANGE, NAVAL	3.1	3 INCH

ORANGE, JUICE	14.6	OZ
PAPAYA	1.72	LB.
PAPAYA, PEELED/CUBED	3.74	CUP
PEACH, FRESH, SLICED	2.72	CUP
PEACH (CAN/DEL MONTE EXTRA LITE)	1.68	CUP
PEARS (CAN)	6.7	HALF
PEAS, BLACKEYED (CAN)	1.12	CUP
PEAS (CAN/DEL MONTE NO SODIUM)	14.7	OZ
PEAS, GREEN GIANT FROZEN, SWEET	1.92	CUP
PEAS, EDIBLE-PODDED	3.35	CUP
PINEAPPLE, FRESH/DICED	2.58	CUP
PINEAPPLE, DEL MONTE SNACK CAN (LITE)	2.88	3.5 OZ
PINEAPPLE (CAN/DOLE LITE SYRUP)	11.88	SLICE
PRUNES, DOLE, DRIED	2.88	OZ
PUMPKIN (CAN)	4	CUP
RAISINS	0.42	CUP
RED PEPPER	10	MEDIUM
STRAWBERRIES (FRESH)	2.08	PINT
STRAWBERRIES (FROZEN)	2.69	CUP
SQUASH, CAN, STOKLEY	2	CUP
SQUASH, FRESH BAKED	1.77	CUP
TANGERINE	5.45	2.5 INCH
TOMATO, CAN	18.8	OZ
TOMATO, FRESH	7.7	3 INCH
TOMATO, JUICE	32	OZ
VEGETABLES, MIXED (FROZEN)	2.24	CUP
WATERMELLON	1.32	1X10 INCH
ZUCCHINI, FRESH, SLICED	11.2	CUP

Yogurts and Desserts

DING DONG	1.26	DING
DREYERS FROZEN FAT FREE YOGURT	1.12	CUP
FRUIT ROLL-UP	2.88	ROLL-UP
POPCORN, WHITE	4	TBLSP
TCBY, SOFT SERVE/NONFAT/NO SUGAR	1.26	CUP
YOGURT, FAT FREE, MOUNTAIN HIGH	8	OZ
YOGURT, FAT FREE, DANNON	8	OZ
LUCERN, YOGURT, NONFAT, LITE	8	OZ

YOGURT, YOPLAIT, FAT FREE, LITE	8	OZ
YOGURT,YOPLAIT ORIGINAL/99% FAT FREE	6	OZ
YOGURT, HORIZON, FF / BLUEBERRY	6	OZ
PLANTER DRIED WALNUT PIECES	0.25	CUP
RAW ALMONDS, TOASTED	1.19	OZ
PECANS, DRIED	1	OZ
PEANUTS, DRY ROASTED	0.2	CUP
HOT CHOCOLATE	4	ENVEL.
ALMONDS, SHELLED	1	OZ

Cereals

CEREAL, CHEERIOS	1.83	CUP
CEREAL, COCOA KRISPIES	1.26	CUP
CEREAL, GRAPENUTS	0.5	CUP
CEREAL, HONEY NUT TOASTY O'S	1.83	CUP
CEREAL, WHEATIES	1.83	CUP
CEREAL, KELLOGG'S ALL BRAN	1.26	CUP
CEREAL, KELLOGG'S CORN FLAKES	1.83	CUP
CEREAL, KELLOGG'S RAISIN BRAN	1.18	CUP
CEREAL, KELLOGG'S CRACKLIN' OAT BRAN	0.76	CUP
CEREAL, NABISCO SHREDDED WHEAT	2.5	PIECE
CEREAL, NAB. SHREDDED WHEAT (SPOON)	1.18	CUP
CEREAL, RICE KRISPIES	2.29	CUP
CEREAL, BENEFIT NUTRITION, PROTEIN +	0.96	CUP
CREAM OF WHEAT	5	TBL/DRY
GRANOLA, CW POST HEARTY	0.48	CUP
GRANOLA, KELLOGG'S LOW FAT	4	CUP
OATMEAL (PRE-COOK MEASUREMENT)	0.72	CUP

Breads

BREAD, OROWHEAT LITE	5	SLICE
BREAD, SUSAN'S HOMEMADE/18 SLICES	2.22	SLICE
BREAD, SUSAN'S HOMEMADE	0.123	LOAF
BUN, WONDER REDUCED CALORIE LITE	2.5	BUN
CRACKER, ZESTA SALTINES	16.8	CRACKER
TORTILLA (CAROLYN)	1.18	TORT
TORTILLA, TORTILLA'S MEXICO, FLOUR	1.83	TORT

TORTILLA, TORTILLA'S MEXICO, CORN	2.24	TORT
TRISCUITS	1.44	OZ
WAFFLE, EGGO, HOMESTYLE	1.83	WAFFLE
WHOLE GRAIN/WHOLE WHEAT FLOUR	0.495	CUP

Rice/Potatoes/Beans

BLACK BEANS (BOILED)	0.89	CUP
BLACK BEANS (DRY)	0.72	CUP
CHICKPEAS/GARBANZO BEANS	0.25	CUP
KIDNEY BEANS (BOILED)	0.25	CUP
LIMA BEANS (BOILED)	0.97	CUP
NAVY BEANS (BOILED)	0.78	CUP
NAVY BEANS (CAN)	0.838	CUP
PINTO BEANS (BOILED)	0.86	CUP
PINTO BEANS (CAN)	1.06	CUP
PINTO BEANS (DRY)	0.335	CUP
PORK & BEANS/VAN CAMPS	0.91	CUP
POTATO, SWEET	1.71	5"X2"
POTATO	12	OZ
RICE CAKE	4	CAKE
RICE, WHITE, BASMATI	0.84	CUP (C)
RICE, BROWN LONG GRAIN	1	CUP (C)
RICE, INSTANT, MINUTE BRAND	0.63	CUP(UC)
RICE, WHITE, LONG GRAIN	0.315	CUP(UC)
SOYBEANS (BOILED)	0.75	CUP
YAM, BOILED OR BAKED	1.27	CUP

Pasta

MACARONI, DAVINI TWIST	0.765	CUP/DRY
MACARONI, HOSPITALITY ELBOW	0.42	CUP/DRY
MACARONI, AM. BEAUTY ELBOW	0.48	CUP/DRY
PASTA, CREAMETTE PLAIN	1.92	OZ
SPAGHETTI, EDEN WHOLE WHEAT	1.92	OZ/UC

Protein Sources 1600 Calories

White Meat

CHICKEN BREAST (HORMEL/CAN)	1.34	CAN
CHICKEN BREAST (SKINLESS)	6.7	OZ
CHICKEN (LEG W/ SKIN & BONE)	0.76	
CHICKEN (THIGH W/ SKIN & BONE)	1.32	
CHICKEN (LEG & THIGH W/ SKIN & BONE)	0.48	
HAM, BAR S, XTRA LEAN, 96% FAT FREE	5.75	OZ
HAM, DAK CAN	6.7	OZ
PORK, SIRLOIN, LEAN W/ FAT	2	OZ
TURKEY BREAST (SKINLESS)	3.76	OZ
TURKEY BREAST (HORMEL/CAN)	1.15	CAN
TURKEY BRST/OVEN ROAST/SFWY/89% FF	8	OZ
VENISON / ANTELOPE	4.5	OZ

Red Meat

HAMBURGER (10% FAT)	3.58	OZ
HAMBURGER (15% FAT)	2.96	OZ
HAMBURGER (20% FAT)	2.88	OZ
HAMBURGER (27% FAT)	2.44	OZ
LAMB, SHOULDER	2.29	OZ
STEAK, BOTTOM ROUND	3.4	OZ
STEAK, BRISKET (FLAT HALF)	3.2	OZ
STEAK, CHUCK, ARM	3.3	OZ
STEAK, CHUCK, BLADE	2.84	OZ
STEAK, EYE ROUND	4.22	OZ
STEAK, FLANK	3.44	OZ
STEAK, NEW YORK STRIP	4	OZ
STEAK, PORTERHOUSE	3.27	OZ
STEAK, RIBEYE	3.16	OZ
STEAK, ROUND TIP	3.85	OZ
STEAK, SHANK (CROSSCUTS)	3.53	OZ
STEAK, T-BONE	3.32	OZ
STEAK, TENDERLOIN	3.38	OZ
STEAK, TOP LOIN	3.44	OZ
STEAK, TOP ROUND	3.95	OZ

STEAK, TOP SIRLOIN	3.67	OZ
STEAK, TYSON SEASONED BEEF STRIPS	4.3	OZ
TACO/BURRITO MEAT/SMART GROUND	1.05	CUP
OSCAR MAYER BACON	6.7	SLICE
LITTLE SIZZLER BROWN/SERVE SAUSAGE	2.62	LINK

Sea Food

BASS, FRESHWATER, DRY HEAT	4.9	OZ
BASS, STRIPED, DRY HEAT	5.75	OZ
COD, ATLANTIC, DRY HEAT	6.8	OZ
CRAB, ALASKA KING, MOIST HEAT	7.38	OZ
CRAB, BLUE, MOIST HEAT	6.95	OZ
FLOUNDER, DRY HEAT	6.1	OZ
HADDOCK, DRY HEAT	6.35	OZ
HALIBUT, DRY HEAT	5.08	OZ
LOBSTER, NORTHERN, MOIST HEAT	7.3	OZ
MAHI MAHI	8.3	OZ
ORANGE ROUGHY, DRY HEAT	7.9	OZ
PERCH, DRY HEAT	6.1	OZ
PERCH, OCEAN/ATLANTIC, DRY HEAT	5.86	OZ
SALMON, ATLANTIC, DRY HEAT	3.87	OZ
SHRIMP, MOIST HEAT	7.2	OZ
TROUT, DRY HEAT	3.75	OZ
TUNA BURGER, AHI / OMEGA FOODS	7.2	OZ
TUNA, LOW SODIUM, CAN	1.15	CAN
TUNA, WATER, CAN	1.34	CAN
TUNA, WHITE / LOW SALT, CAN (5 OZ)	1.15	CAN
TUNA, WHITE, CAN (5 OZ)	1.15	CAN
TUNA, FILLET/STEAK	4.57	OZ
WALLEYE, BAKED/BROILED/MICRO	5.97	OZ

Vegetarian

IVES VEG. COUSINE VEGGY DOG	3.35	DOG
SOY MILK (TRIS)	2.25	CUP
SOY MILK (SYLVIA)	2	CUP

Eggs/Dairy

1% COTTAGE CHEESE, NORDICA	1.26	CUP
2% COTTAGE CHEESE (LOW FAT)	1	CUP
COTTAGE CHEESE (LUCERNE FAT FREE)	1.26	CUP
COTT CHEESE MARIGOLD/DRY CURD	1.92	CUP
COTT CHEESE MARIGOLD/DRY CURD	30.5	TBLSP
COTT CHEESE BREAKSTONES FAT FREE	1.26	CUP
CHEDDER, SHREDDED, FAT FREE, KHF	1.12	CUP
CHEDDER, SHREDDED, 94% FAT FREE, HC	1	CUP
CHEESE, COLBY/MOZZARELLA	1.83	OZ
EGG WHITE	11.8	
EGG, WHOLE	2.69	
EGG BEATERS	1.68	CUP
MOZZARELLA SHREDDED, FAT FREE, KHF	1	CUP
SKIM MOZZARELLA STRING CHEESE	2.5	OZ

Free Carbs, Supplements, Fast Foods
1600 calories

Free Carbs

ASPARAGUS
BROCCOLI
CABBAGE
CAULIFLOWER
CELERY
CUCUMBER
GREEN BEANS
GREEN PEPPERS
GREEN SQUASH
LETTUCE, ICEBERG
LETTUCE, LEAF/SHREDDED
MUSHROOMS
ONION
PICKLES (DILL)
RADISH

RED PEPPERS
SPINACH (CAN/NO SALT)
SPINACH (FRESH)
TOMATO (EXCLUDING JUICE)
ZUCCHINI

Supplements/Fast Foods

ATKINS BAR	0.75	BAR
EAS ADVANTEDGE, C&C/LEM/BLUE	0.75	BAR
BAR, ZONE	0.88	BAR
BAR, PURE PROTEIN, 50 G.	1	BAR
BAR, W.W. PURE PROTEIN, 78 G.	0.5	BAR
BAR, PROTEIN REVOLUTION, PBJ	0.88	BAR
BAR, FIBAR, PEANUT BUTTER, 1.2 OZ	1.33	BAR
BAR, PREMIER 1, PROTEIN 8, CHOC/COCO	0.75	BAR
BAR, PREFERRED BAR, CHOC./FUDG/RAS	0.88	BAR
BAR, PREFERRED BAR, CHOC./FUDG/BROW	0.88	BAR
ALIVE, HI CARB POWDER	5	TBLSP
POWERADE	2	SERVING
PROTEIN,GNC P.P. EGG/WHEY	1.5	SERVING
PROTEIN. GNC P.PERF. WHEY	1.5	SCOOP
OPTIMUM NUTRITION WHEY	1.75	SCOOP
SYNTRAX WHEY PROTEIN	2.25	SCOOP
TRI PROTEIN PLUS POWDER	1.5	SERVING
HW STRAWBERRY PROT. POWD.	2	SCOOP
BIOCHEM WHEY PRO 290	2.5	SCOOP
HUMAN DEV. TECH. WHEY	1.5	SCOOP
NATURADE 100% SOY PROTEIN	0.5	CUP
SUPER GREEN PRO 96 - SOY	0.5	CUP
100% PURE WHEY, PROLAB	1.5	SCOOP
ECLIPSE BULK UP WHEY	2	SCOOP
VITAMIN WORLD WHEY 100%	1.75	SCOOP
ULT. NUT. PROSTAR WHEY	1.75	SCOOP
RED WINE	8	OZ
MET RX CH.RST.PNT.PRO + BAR	0.5	BAR
MET RX BAV. MINT. PRO + BAR	0.75	BAR
MET AFTER FX BAR	0.75	BAR
MET RX CH. CH. CHIP PRO + BAR	0.75	BAR

MET RX SOURCE ONE BAR	0.75	BAR
MET RX CHOC. GRAHCRK CHIP BAR	0.5	BAR
MET RX PEANUT BUTTER BAR	0.5	BAR
MET RX DRINK MIX, MRP	0.75	SERVING
MET RX PRO 50, ANABOLIC DRIVE	0.75	SERVING
MET RX PRO 60, ANABOLIC DRIVE	0.5	SERVING
MET RX PROTEIN PLUS	2.5	SCOOP
MET RX KETO PRO	2.5	SCOOP
NUTRI FORCE DRINK MIX, MRP	0.75	SERVING
EAS MYO. DEL. CH/PB BAR	3	BAR
EAS MYOPLEX + DELUXE	0.5	SERVING
EAS MYOPLEX LITE	0.75	SERVING
ADVANT EDGE QUICK STIR PROTEIN DRINK	0.75	SERVING
EAS NEUROGAIN	4	SCOOP
EAS PHOSPHAGEN HP	1	SCOOP
EAS PRECISION PROTEIN	1.75	SCOOP
EAS SIMPLY PROTEIN	3	SCOOP
EAS WHEY PROTEIN	1.75	SCOOP
EAS SUPPER SHAKE	0.33	SHAKE
VITAMIN WORLD DAILY RX, MRP	0.75	SHAKE
VITAMIN WORLD PROTOPLEX DELUXE, MRP	0.5	SHAKE
VITAMIN WORLD PRE. ENG. WHEY PROT.	2	SCOOP
PERFECT RX, MRP, CHOCOLATE	0.75	SHAKE
OPTI PRO	0.75	SHAKE
ARBY'S CHICK. SAND. R.DELX.LITE	0.5	BURGER
ARBY'S SIDE SALAD	1	SALAD
ARBY'S GARDEN SALAD	1	SALAD
ARBY'S RST. CHCK. SALAD	1	SALAD
ARBY'S RED. CAL. ITAL. DRESSING	1	PACKET
ARBY'S RED RANCH DRESSING	1	PACKET
MCD'S VINAG. LITE SALAD DR.	1	PACKET
MCD'S GARDEN SALAD	1	SALAD
MCD'S VINAG. LITE SALAD DR.	1	PACKET
P.HUT. HAND-TOSS CHEESE	0.75	SLICE
P.HUT. HAND-TOSS HAM	0.75	SLICE
P.HUT. HAND-TOSS VEG. LUV.	0.75	SLICE
P.HUT. HAND-TOSS PEPPERON	0.75	SLICE
P.HUT. THIN/CRISP CHEESE	1	SLICE

P.HUT. THIN/CRISP HAM	1	SLICE
P.HUT. THIN/CRISP VEG. LUV.	1	SLICE
P.HUT. THIN/CRISP PEPPERON	0.75	SLICE
SW 6" COLD SUB/VEGG. DELIT	1	SUB
SW 6" COLD SUB/TURK. BRST.	1	SUB
SW 6" COLD SUB/TURK.B/HAM	1	SUB
SW 6" COLD SUB/HAM	1	SUB
SW 6" COLD SUB/ROAST BEEF	1	SUB
SW 6" COLD SUB/SFOOD,CRAB	1	SUB
SW 6" COLD SUB/COLD CUT 3	1	SUB
SW 6" COLD SUB/TUNA	1	SUB
SW 6" HOT SUB/RST.CHICK.BR.	1	SUB
SW 6" HOT SUB/STAK/CHEESE	1	SUB
SW 6" HOT SUB/SUB MELT	1	SUB
SW VEGGIE DELITE SALAD	1	SALAD
SW TURKEY BREAST SALAD	1	SALAD
SW ROAST BEEF SALAD	1	SALAD
SW TURK. BRST/HAM SALAD	1	SALAD
SW RST. CHICK. BR. SALAD	1	SALAD
SW SEAFOOD/CRAB SALAD	1	SALAD
SW STEAK/CHEESE SALAD	0.75	SALAD
SW SUBWAY MELT SALAD	1	SALAD
SW COLD CUT 3 SALAD	1	SALAD
SW FAT FREE ITALIAN DRESS	1	OZ
SW FAT FREE FRENCH DRESS	1	OZ
SW FAT FREE RANCH DRESS	1	OZ
SW DELI STYLE TURKEY BR.	0.75	SNDWCH
SW DELI STYLE HAM	0.75	SNDWCH
SW DELI STYLE ROAST BEEF	0.75	SNDWCH
TB GRILLED STEAK SOFT TACO	0.75	TACO
WAHOO'S CHBROIL FISH TACO	1	TACO
WENDI'S SIDE SALAD	1	SALAD
WENDI'S FF FRENCH DRESSING	1	OZ
WENDI'S ITALIAN RED. F/C DRESS	1	OZ
WENDI'S SMALL CHILI	1	BOWL
WENDI'S GRILLED CHICK. FILLET	1	MEAT

1700 Calories/Day Eating Plan		
What Does Your Doctor Look Like Naked?		
Name: _____ Date: _____		
Exercise: 30-40 min in a.m. before food		Write what you eat here:
Meal 1 Time: _____	2 Protein Source 2 Active Carbohydrates	
Meal 2 Time: _____	1.5 oz Raw Almonds	
Meal 3 Time: _____	1 Protein Source 2 Active Carbohydrates Free Carbohydrates (as much as you want)	
Meal 4 Time: _____	1/2 LOW CARB protein bar (OR) 1.5 scoops Whey Protein Powder in water	
Meal 5 Time: _____	1 Protein Source 0 Active Carbohydrates Free Carbohydrates (as much as you want)	
BEDTIME Meal (Optional)	Sugar Free Jell-O 1 cup	
Add fiber supplement in evening , SUCH AS Metamucil or other (sugar FREE). Add spices, pepper, etc. as needed. Try to eat every two to three hours. Drink 1 gallon of water EVERY DAY! May have up to 2 diet pops (or) 2 cups a coffee a day.		

Active Carbohydrates 1700 Calories

Fruit and Vegetables

APPLE	6.7	3 INCH
APPLESAUCE, MOTT'S	0.76	CUP
APRICOTS (CAN/DEL MONTE LITE)	1.4	CUP
APRICOTS (DRIED)	2.4	OZ
APRICOTS (FRESH 12/LB)	9.9	MEDIUM
ASPARAGUS	45.5	OZ
BANANA	1.6	MEDIUM
BLUEBERRIES (FRESH)	2.05	CUP
BRUSSELS SPROUTS, BOILED	2.8	CUP
CABBAGE, SHREDDED	9.3	CUP
CANTALOUPE	0.9	5 INCH
CARROT (FRESH)	15.2	OZ
CAULIFLOWER	42	CUP
CELERY	29.5	OZ
CHERRIES, FRESH, SWEET W/PIT	1.62	CUP
CHERRIES, DARK (CAN/DEL MONTE)	0.84	CUP
COLLARD GREENS (CAN)	2.8	CUP
COLLARD GREENS (FRESH)	14	CUP
CORN CAKE	4.8	CAKE
CORN (CAN/DEL MONTE NO SODIUM)	12.3	OZ
CUCUMBER, SLICED	12	CUP
EGGPLANT	7.6	CUP
FRUIT, MIXED FROZEN	1.86	CUP
GARLIC, 1 CLOVE	42	CLOVE
GARLIC, TRIMMED	4	OZ
GRAPES	1.48	CUP
GRAPE JUICE/VERYFINE	1.48	OZ
GRAPEFRUIT	1.83	4 INCH
GREEN BEANS (CAN/DEL MONTE NO SALT)	4.2	CUP
GREEN PEPPER	8.4	MEDIUM
KIWI	11.4	OZ
MUSHROOMS, FRESH	9.4	CUP
ONION, FRESH/CHOPPED	2.81	CUP
ORANGE, NAVAL	2.6	3 INCH
ORANGE, JUICE	12.2	OZ

PAPAYA	1.44	LB.
PAPAYA, PEELED/CUBED	3.1	CUP
PEACH, FRESH, SLICED	2.28	CUP
PEACH (CAN/DEL MONTE EXTRA LITE)	1.4	CUP
PEARS (CAN)	5.6	HALF
PEAS, BLACKEYED (CAN)	0.93	CUP
PEAS (CAN/DEL MONTE NO SODIUM)	12.3	OZ
PEAS, GREEN GIANT FROZEN, SWEET	1.6	CUP
PEAS, EDIBLE-PODDED	2.8	CUP
PINEAPPLE, FRESH/DICED	2.15	CUP
PINEAPPLE, DEL MONTE SNACK CAN (LITE)	2.4	3.5 OZ
PINEAPPLE (CAN/DOLE LITE SYRUP)	9.9	SLICE
PRUNES, DOLE, DRIED	2.4	OZ
PUMPKIN (CAN)	3.35	CUP
RAISINS	0.35	CUP
RED PEPPER	8.4	MEDIUM
STRAWBERRIES (FRESH)	1.75	PINT
STRAWBERRIES (FROZEN)	2.25	CUP
SQUASH, CAN, STOKLEY	1.68	CUP
SQUASH, FRESH BAKED	1.48	CUP
TANGERINE	4.55	2.5 INCH
TOMATO, CAN	15.7	OZ
TOMATO, FRESH	6.45	3 INCH
TOMATO, JUICE	27	OZ
VEGETABLES, MIXED (FROZEN)	1.87	CUP
WATERMELLON	1.1	1X10 INCH
ZUCCHINI, FRESH, SLICED	9.3	CUP

Yogurts and Desserts

DING DONG	1.05	DING
DREYERS FROZEN FAT FREE YOGURT	0.9	CUP
FRUIT ROLL-UP	2.4	ROLL-UP
POPCORN, WHITE	3.35	TBLSP
TCBY, SOFT SERVE/NONFAT/NO SUGAR	1.05	CUP
YOGURT, FAT FREE, MOUNTAIN HIGH	8	OZ
YOGURT, FAT FREE, DANNON	8	OZ
LUCERN, YOGURT, NONFAT, LITE	8	OZ
YOGURT, YOPLAIT, FAT FREE, LITE	6	OZ

YOGURT,YOPLAIT ORIGINAL/99% FAT FREE	6	OZ
YOGURT, HORIZON, FF / BLUEBERRY	6	OZ
PLANTER DRIED WALNUT PIECES	0.2	CUP
RAW ALMONDS, TOASTED	1	OZ
PECANS, DRIED	0.88	OZ
PEANUTS, DRY ROASTED	0.2	CUP
HOT CHOCOLATE	3	ENVEL.
ALMONDS, SHELLED	1	OZ

Cereals

CEREAL, CHEERIOS	1.53	CUP
CEREAL, COCOA KRISPIES	1.05	CUP
CEREAL, GRAPENUTS	0.42	CUP
CEREAL, HONEY NUT TOASTY O'S	1.53	CUP
CEREAL, WHEATIES	1.53	CUP
CEREAL, KELLOGG'S ALL BRAN	1.05	CUP
CEREAL, KELLOGG'S CORN FLAKES	1.53	CUP
CEREAL, KELLOGG'S RAISIN BRAN	1	CUP
CEREAL, KELLOGG'S CRACKLIN' OAT BRAN	0.64	CUP
CEREAL, NABISCO SHREDDED WHEAT	2.1	PIECE
CEREAL, NAB. SHREDDED WHEAT (SPOON)	0.99	CUP
CEREAL, RICE KRISPIES	1.9	CUP
CEREAL, BENEFIT NUTRITION, PROTEIN +	0.8	CUP
CREAM OF WHEAT	4.2	TBL/DRY
GRANOLA, CW POST HEARTY	0.4	CUP
GRANOLA, KELLOGG'S LOW FAT	2	CUP
OATMEAL (PRE-COOK MEASUREMENT)	0.6	CUP

Breads

BREAD, OROWHEAT LITE	4.2	SLICE
BREAD, SUSAN'S HOMEMADE/18 SLICES	1.86	SLICE
BREAD, SUSAN'S HOMEMADE	0.103	LOAF
BUN, WONDER REDUCED CALORIE LITE	2.1	BUN
CRACKER, ZESTA SALTINES	14	CRACKER
TORTILLA (CAROLYN)	0.99	TORT
TORTILLA, TORTILLA'S MEXICO, FLOUR	1.53	TORT
TORTILLA, TORTILLA'S MEXICO, CORN	1.87	TORT

TRISCUITS	1.2	OZ
WAFFLE, EGGO, HOMESTYLE	1.53	WAFFLE
WHOLE GRAIN/WHOLE WHEAT FLOUR	0.412	CUP

Rice/Potatoes/Beans

BLACK BEANS (BOILED)	0.74	CUP
BLACK BEANS (DRY)	0.6	CUP
CHICKPEAS / GARBANZO BEANS	0.22	CUP
KIDNEY BEANS (BOILED)	0.25	CUP
LIMA BEANS (BOILED)	0.81	CUP
NAVY BEANS (BOILED)	0.65	CUP
NAVY BEANS (CAN)	0.7	CUP
PINTO BEANS (BOILED)	0.72	CUP
PINTO BEANS (CAN)	0.88	CUP
PINTO BEANS (DRY)	0.28	CUP
PORK & BEANS / VAN CAMPS	0.76	CUP
POTATO, SWEET	1.43	5"X2"
POTATO	10	OZ
RICE CAKE	3.35	CAKE
RICE, WHITE, BASMATI	0.7	CUP (C)
RICE, BROWN LONG GRAIN	0.84	CUP (C)
RICE, INSTANT, MINUTE BRAND	0.525	CUP(UC)
RICE, WHITE, LONG GRAIN	0.263	CUP(UC)
SOYBEANS (BOILED)	0.66	CUP
YAM, BOILED OR BAKED	1.06	CUP

Pasta

MACARONI, DAVINI TWIST	0.64	CUP/DRY
MACARONI, HOSPITALITY ELBOW	0.35	CUP/DRY
MACARONI, AM. BEAUTY ELBOW	0.4	CUP/DRY
PASTA, CREAMETTE PLAIN	1.6	OZ
SPAGHETTI, EDEN WHOLE WHEAT	1.6	OZ/UC

Protein Sources 1700 Calories

White Meat

CHICKEN BREAST (HORMEL/CAN)	1.12	CAN
CHICKEN BREAST (SKINLESS)	5.6	OZ
CHICKEN (LEG W/ SKIN & BONE)	0.64	
CHICKEN (THIGH W/ SKIN & BONE)	1.1	
CHICKEN (LEG & THIGH W/ SKIN & BONE)	0.4	
HAM, BAR S, XTRA LEAN, 96% FAT FREE	4.25	OZ
HAM, DAK CAN	5.6	OZ
PORK, SIRLOIN, LEAN W/ FAT	1.68	OZ
TURKEY BREAST (SKINLESS)	3.14	OZ
TURKEY BREAST (HORMEL/CAN)	0.96	CAN
TURKEY BRST/OVEN ROAST/SFWY/89% FF	6.7	OZ
VENISON / ANTELOPE	3.75	OZ

Red Meat

HAMBURGER (10 % FAT)	3	OZ
HAMBURGER (15 % FAT)	2.48	OZ
HAMBURGER (20 % FAT)	2.4	OZ
HAMBURGER (27 % FAT)	2.04	OZ
LAMB, SHOULDER	1.92	OZ
STEAK, BOTTOM ROUND	2.84	OZ
STEAK, BRISKET (FLAT HALF)	2.68	OZ
STEAK, CHUCK, ARM	2.77	OZ
STEAK, CHUCK, BLADE	2.38	OZ
STEAK, EYE ROUND	3.53	OZ
STEAK, FLANK	2.87	OZ
STEAK, NEW YORK STRIP	3.35	OZ
STEAK, PORTERHOUSE	2.74	OZ
STEAK, RIBEYE	2.65	OZ
STEAK, ROUND TIP	3.22	OZ
STEAK, SHANK (CROSSCUTS)	2.95	OZ
STEAK, T-BONE	2.8	OZ
STEAK, TENDERLOIN	2.83	OZ
STEAK, TOP LOIN	2.88	OZ
STEAK, TOP ROUND	3.3	OZ

STEAK, TOP SIRLOIN	3.06	OZ
STEAK, TYSON SEASONED BEEF STRIPS	3.6	OZ
TACO/BURRITO MEAT/SMART GROUND	0.88	CUP
OSCAR MAYER BACON	5.6	SLICE
LITTLE SIZZLER BROWN/SERVE SAUSAGE	2.2	LINK

Sea Food

BASS, FRESHWATER, DRY HEAT	4.08	OZ
BASS, STRIPED, DRY HEAT	4.8	OZ
COD, ATLANTIC, DRY HEAT	5.65	OZ
CRAB, ALASKA KING, MOIST HEAT	6.15	OZ
CRAB, BLUE, MOIST HEAT	5.8	OZ
FLOUNDER, DRY HEAT	5.1	OZ
HADDOCK, DRY HEAT	5.3	OZ
HALIBUT, DRY HEAT	4.25	OZ
LOBSTER, NORTHERN, MOIST HEAT	6.1	OZ
MAHI MAHI	6.9	OZ
ORANGE ROUGHY, DRY HEAT	6.6	OZ
PERCH, DRY HEAT	5.1	OZ
PERCH, OCEAN/ATLANTIC, DRY HEAT	5.1	OZ
SALMON, ATLANTIC, DRY HEAT	3.25	OZ
SHRIMP, MOIST HEAT	6	OZ
TROUT, DRY HEAT	3.1	OZ
TUNA BURGER, AHI / OMEGA FOODS	6	OZ
TUNA, LOW SODIUM, CAN	0.96	CAN
TUNA, WATER, CAN	1.12	CAN
TUNA, WHITE / LOW SALT, CAN (5 OZ)	0.96	CAN
TUNA, WHITE, CAN (5 OZ)	0.96	CAN
TUNA, FILLET/STEAK	3.8	OZ
WALLEYE, BAKED/BROILED/MICRO	5	OZ

Vegetarian

IVES VEG. COUSINE VEGGY DOG	2.8	DOG
SOY MILK (TRIS)	1.8	CUP
SOY MILK (SYLVIA)	1.5	CUP

Eggs/Dairy

1 % COTTAGE CHEESE, NORDICA	1.05	CUP
2 % COTTAGE CHEESE (LOW FAT)	0.84	CUP
COTTAGE CHEESE (LUCERNE FAT FREE)	1.05	CUP
COTT CHEESE MARIGOLD/DRY CURD	1.6	CUP
COTT CHEESE MARIGOLD/DRY CURD	25.7	TBLSP
COTT CHEESE BREAKSTONES FAT FREE	1.05	CUP
CHEDDER, SHREDDED, FAT FREE, KHF	0.93	CUP
CHEDDER, SHREDDED, 94% FAT FREE, HC	0.84	CUP
CHEESE, COLBY/MOZZARELLA	1.53	OZ
EGG WHITE	9.9	
EGG, WHOLE	2.25	
EGG BEATERS	1.4	CUP
MOZZARELLA SHREDDED, FAT FREE, KHF	0.84	CUP
SKIM MOZZARELLA STRING CHEESE	2.1	OZ

Free Carbs, Supplements, Fast Foods
1700 calories

Free Carbs

ASPARAGUS
BROCCOLI
CABBAGE
CAULIFLOWER
CELERY
CUCUMBER
GREEN BEANS
GREEN PEPPERS
GREEN SQUASH
LETTUCE, ICEBERG
LETTUCE, LEAF/SHREDDED
MUSHROOMS
ONION
PICKLES (DILL)
RADISH
RED PEPPERS

SPINACH (CAN/NO SALT)
SPINACH (FRESH)
TOMATO (EXCLUDING JUICE)
ZUCCHINI

Supplements/Fast Foods

ATKINS BAR	0.75	BAR
EAS ADVANTEDGE, C&C/LEM/BLUE	0.75	BAR
BAR, ZONE	0.75	BAR
BAR, PURE PROTEIN, 50 G.	0.75	BAR
BAR, W.W. PURE PROTEIN, 78 G.	0.5	BAR
BAR, PROTEIN REVOLUTION, PBJ	0.5	BAR
BAR, FIBAR, PEANUT BUTTER, 1.2 OZ	1	BAR
BAR, PREMIER 1, PROTEIN 8, CHOC/COCO	0.5	BAR
BAR, PREFERRED BAR, CHOC./FUDG/RAS	0.5	BAR
BAR, PREFERRED BAR, CHOC./FUDG/BROW	0.5	BAR
ALIVE, HI CARB POWDER	3	TBLSP
POWERADE	2	SERVING
PROTEIN,GNC P.P. EGG/WHEY	1.25	SERVING
PROTEIN. GNC P.PERF. WHEY	4	SCOOP
OPTIMUM NUTRITION WHEY	1.5	SCOOP
SYNTRAX WHEY PROTEIN	1.75	SCOOP
TRI PROTEIN PLUS POWDER	1	SERVING
HW STRAWBERRY PROT. POWD.	1.5	SCOOP
BIOCHEM WHEY PRO 290	2	SCOOP
HUMAN DEV. TECH. WHEY	1.25	SCOOP
NATURADE 100% SOY PROTEIN	0.5	CUP
SUPER GREEN PRO 96 - SOY	0.5	CUP
100% PURE WHEY, PROLAB	1.25	SCOOP
ECLIPSE BULK UP WHEY	1.75	SCOOP
VITAMIN WORLD WHEY 100%	1.25	SCOOP
ULT. NUT. PROSTAR WHEY	1.25	SCOOP
RED WINE	6.5	OZ
MET RX CH.RST.PNT.PRO + BAR	0.5	BAR
MET RX BAV. MINT. PRO + BAR	0.5	BAR
MET AFTER FX BAR	0.5	BAR
MET RX CH. CH. CHIP PRO + BAR	0.5	BAR
MET RX SOURCE ONE BAR	0.55	BAR

MET RX CHOC. GRAHCRK CHIP BAR	0.5	BAR
MET RX PEANUT BUTTER BAR	0.5	BAR
MET RX DRINK MIX, MRP	0.5	SERVING
MET RX PRO 50, ANABOLIC DRIVE	0.5	SERVING
MET RX PRO 60, ANABOLIC DRIVE	0.5	SERVING
MET RX PROTEIN PLUS	2	SCOOP
MET RX KETO PRO	2	SCOOP
NUTRI FORCE DRINK MIX, MRP	0.5	SERVING
EAS MYO. DEL. CH/PB BAR	2	BAR
EAS MYOPLEX + DELUXE	14	SERVING
EAS MYOPLEX LITE	0.5	SERVING
ADVANT EDGE QUICK STIR PROTEIN DRINK	0.75	SERVING
EAS NEUROGAIN	3.5	SCOOP
EAS PHOSPHAGEN HP	1	SCOOP
EAS PRECISION PROTEIN	1.5	SCOOP
EAS SIMPLY PROTEIN	2.75	SCOOP
EAS WHEY PROTEIN	1.5	SCOOP
EAS SUPPER SHAKE	0.33	SHAKE
VITAMIN WORLD DAILY RX, MRP	0.5	SHAKE
VITAMIN WORLD PROTOPLEX DELUXE, MRP	0.5	SHAKE
VITAMIN WORLD PRE. ENG. WHEY PROT.	1.75	SCOOP
PERFECT RX, MRP, CHOCOLATE	0.5	SHAKE
OPTI PRO	0.5	SHAKE
ARBY'S CHICK. SAND. R.DELX.LITE	0.5	BURGER
ARBY'S SIDE SALAD	1	SALAD
ARBY'S GARDEN SALAD	1	SALAD
ARBY'S RST. CHCK. SALAD	1	SALAD
ARBY'S RED. CAL. ITAL. DRESSING	1	PACKET
ARBY'S RED RANCH DRESSING	1	PACKET
MCD'S VINAG. LITE SALAD DR.	1	PACKET
MCD'S GARDEN SALAD	1	SALAD
MCD'S VINAG. LITE SALAD DR.	1	PACKET
P.HUT. HAND-TOSS CHEESE	0.5	SLICE
P.HUT. HAND-TOSS HAM	0.75	SLICE
P.HUT. HAND-TOSS VEG. LUV.	0.75	SLICE
P.HUT. HAND-TOSS PEPPERON	0.5	SLICE
P.HUT. THIN/CRISP CHEESE	0.75	SLICE
P.HUT. THIN/CRISP HAM	0.75	SLICE

P.HUT. THIN/CRISP VEG. LUV.	0.75	SLICE
P.HUT. THIN/CRISP PEPPERON	0.75	SLICE
SW 6" COLD SUB/VEGG. DELIT	1	SUB
SW 6" COLD SUB/TURK. BRST.	1	SUB
SW 6" COLD SUB/TURK.B/HAM	1	SUB
SW 6" COLD SUB/HAM	1	SUB
SW 6" COLD SUB/ROAST BEEF	1	SUB
SW 6" COLD SUB/SFOOD,CRAB	1	SUB
SW 6" COLD SUB/COLD CUT 3	1	SUB
SW 6" COLD SUB/TUNA	1	SUB
SW 6" HOT SUB/RST.CHICK.BR.	1	SUB
SW 6" HOT SUB/STAK/CHEESE	1	SUB
SW 6" HOT SUB/SUB MELT	1	SUB
SW VEGGIE DELITE SALAD	1	SALAD
SW TURKEY BREAST SALAD	1	SALAD
SW ROAST BEEF SALAD	1	SALAD
SW TURK. BRST/HAM SALAD	1	SALAD
SW RST. CHICK. BR. SALAD	1	SALAD
SW SEAFOOD/CRAB SALAD	1	SALAD
SW STEAK/CHEESE SALAD	0.75	SALAD
SW SUBWAY MELT SALAD	0.75	SALAD
SW COLD CUT 3 SALAD	0.75	SALAD
SW FAT FREE ITALIAN DRESS	1	OZ
SW FAT FREE FRENCH DRESS	1	OZ
SW FAT FREE RANCH DRESS	1	OZ
SW DELI STYLE TURKEY BR.	0.5	SNDWCH
SW DELI STYLE HAM	0.5	SNDWCH
SW DELI STYLE ROAST BEEF	0.5	SNDWCH
TB GRILLED STEAK SOFT TACO	0.55	TACO
WAHOO'S CHBROIL FISH TACO	0.75	TACO
WENDI'S SIDE SALAD	1	SALAD
WENDI'S FF FRENCH DRESSING	1	OZ
WENDI'S ITALIAN RED. F/C DRESS	1	OZ
WENDI'S SMALL CHILI	0.75	BOWL
WENDI'S GRILLED CHICK. FILLET	1	MEAT

1800 Calories/Day Eating Plan		
What Does Your Doctor Look Like Naked?		
Name: _____ Date: _____		
Exercise: 30-40 min in a.m. before food		Write what you eat here:
Meal 1 Time: _____	2 Protein Source 2 Active Carbohydrates	
Meal 2 Time: _____	1.5 oz Raw Almonds	
Meal 3 Time: _____	1 Protein Source 2 Active Carbohydrates Free Carbohydrates (as much as you want)	
Meal 4 Time: _____	½ LOW CARB protein bar (OR) 1.5 scoops Whey Protein Powder in water	
Meal 5 Time: _____	1 Protein Source 0 Active Carbohydrates Free Carbohydrates (as much as you want)	
BEDTIME Meal (Optional)	Sugar Free Jell-O 1 cup	
Add fiber supplement in evening, such as Metamucil or other (sugar FREE). Add spices, pepper, etc. as needed. Try to eat every two to three hours. Drink 1 gallon of water EVERY DAY! May have up to 2 diet pops (or) 2 cups a coffee a day.		

Active Carbohydrates 1800 Calories

Fruit and Vegetables

APPLE	7.15	3 INCH
APPLESAUCE, MOTT'S	0.81	CUP
APRICOTS (CAN/DEL MONTE LITE)	1.49	CUP
APRICOTS (DRIED)	2.55	OZ
APRICOTS (FRESH 12/LB)	10.5	MEDIUM
ASPARAGUS	48	OZ
BANANA	1.7	MEDIUM
BLUEBERRIES (FRESH)	2.18	CUP
BRUSSELS SPROUTS, BOILED	2.97	CUP
CABBAGE, SHREDDED	9.9	CUP
CANTALOUPE	0.95	5 INCH
CARROT (FRESH)	16.1	OZ
CAULIFLOWER	6.85	CUP
CELERY	44.5	OZ
CHERRIES, FRESH, SWEET W/PIT	1.72	CUP
CHERRIES, DARK (CAN/DEL MONTE)	0.89	CUP
COLLARD GREENS (CAN)	2.97	CUP
COLLARD GREENS (FRESH)	14.9	CUP
CORN CAKE	5.1	CAKE
CORN (CAN/DEL MONTE NO SODIUM)	13	OZ
CUCUMBER, SLICED	12.7	CUP
EGGPLANT	8.1	CUP
FRUIT, MIXED FROZEN	1.98	CUP
GARLIC, 1 CLOVE	44.5	CLOVE
GARLIC, TRIMMED	4.25	OZ
GRAPES	1.57	CUP
GRAPE JUICE/VERYFINE	9.5	OZ
GRAPEFRUIT	1.94	4 INCH
GREEN BEANS (CAN/DEL MONTE NO SALT)	4.45	CUP
GREEN PEPPER	8.9	MEDIUM
KIWI	12	OZ
MUSHROOMS, FRESH	9.9	CUP
ONION, FRESH/CHOPPED	2.97	CUP
ORANGE, NAVAL	2.75	3 INCH

ORANGE, JUICE	13	OZ
PAPAYA	1.525	LB.
PAPAYA, PEELED/CUBED	3.3	CUP
PEACH, FRESH, SLICED	2.41	CUP
PEACH (CAN/DEL MONTE EXTRA LITE)	1.49	CUP
PEARS (CAN)	5.9	HALF
PEAS, BLACKEYED (CAN)	0.99	CUP
PEAS (CAN/DEL MONTE NO SODIUM)	13	OZ
PEAS, GREEN GIANT FROZEN, SWEET	1.7	CUP
PEAS, EDIBLE-PODDED	2.97	CUP
PINEAPPLE, FRESH/DICED	2.29	CUP
PINEAPPLE, DEL MONTE SNACK CAN (LITE)	2.53	3.5 OZ
PINEAPPLE (CAN/DOLE LITE SYRUP)	10.5	SLICE
PRUNES, DOLE, DRIED	2.55	OZ
PUMPKIN (CAN)	3.57	CUP
RAISINS	0.37	CUP
RED PEPPER	8.9	MEDIUM
STRAWBERRIES (FRESH)	1.84	PINT
STRAWBERRIES (FROZEN)	2.38	CUP
SQUASH, CAN, STOKLEY	1.78	CUP
SQUASH, FRESH BAKED	1.57	CUP
TANGERINE	4.83	2.5 INCH
TOMATO, CAN	16.7	OZ
TOMATO, FRESH	6.85	3 INCH
TOMATO, JUICE	28.5	OZ
VEGETABLES, MIXED (FROZEN)	1.98	CUP
WATERMELLON	1.17	1X10 INCH
ZUCCHINI, FRESH, SLICED	9.9	CUP

Yogurts and Desserts

DING DONG	1.11	DING
DREYERS FROZEN FAT FREE YOGURT	0.99	CUP
FRUIT ROLL-UP	2.55	ROLL-UP
POPCORN, WHITE	3.57	TBLSP
TCBY, SOFT SERVE/NONFAT/NO SUGAR	1.11	CUP
YOGURT, FAT FREE, MOUNTAIN HIGH	8	OZ
YOGURT, FAT FREE, DANNON	8	OZ
LUCERN, YOGURT, NONFAT, LITE	8	OZ

YOGURT, YOPLAIT, FAT FREE, LITE	6	OZ
YOGURT,YOPLAIT ORIGINAL/99% FAT FREE	6	OZ
YOGURT, HORIZON, FF / BLUEBERRY	6	OZ
PLANTER DRIED WALNUT PIECES	0.2	CUP
RAW ALMONDS, TOASTED	1	OZ
PECANS, DRIED	0.75	OZ
PEANUTS, DRY ROASTED	0.2	CUP
HOT CHOCOLATE	3.5	ENVEL.
ALMONDS, SHELLED	1	OZ

Cereals

CEREAL, CHEERIOS	1.62	CUP
CEREAL, COCOA KRISPIES	1.11	CUP
CEREAL, GRAPENUTS	0.445	CUP
CEREAL, HONEY NUT TOASTY O'S	1.62	CUP
CEREAL, WHEATIES	1.62	CUP
CEREAL, KELLOGG'S ALL BRAN	1.11	CUP
CEREAL, KELLOGG'S CORN FLAKES	1.62	CUP
CEREAL, KELLOGG'S RAISIN BRAN	1.05	CUP
CEREAL, KELLOGG'S CRACKLIN' OAT BRAN	0.7	CUP
CEREAL, NABISCO SHREDDED WHEAT	2.23	PIECE
CEREAL, NAB. SHREDDED WHEAT (SPOON)	1.05	CUP
CEREAL, RICE KRISPIES	2.03	CUP
CEREAL, BENEFIT NUTRITION, PROTEIN +	0.85	CUP
CREAM OF WHEAT	4.45	TBL/DRY
GRANOLA, CW POST HEARTY	0.425	CUP
GRANOLA, KELLOGG'S LOW FAT	2	CUP
OATMEAL (PRE-COOK MEASUREMENT)	0.636	CUP

Breads

BREAD, OROWHEAT LITE	4.47	SLICE
BREAD, SUSAN'S HOMEMADE/18 SLICES	1.97	SLICE
BREAD, SUSAN'S HOMEMADE	0.11	LOAF
BUN, WONDER REDUCED CALORIE LITE	2.23	BUN
CRACKER, ZESTA SALTINES	14.9	CRACKER
TORTILLA (CAROLYN)	1.05	TORT
TORTILLA, TORTILLA'S MEXICO, FLOUR	1.62	TORT

TORTILLA, TORTILLA'S MEXICO, CORN	1.98	TORT
TRISCUITS	1.27	OZ
WAFFLE, EGGO, HOMESTYLE	1.17	WAFFLE
WHOLE GRAIN/WHOLE WHEAT FLOUR	0.438	CUP

Rice/Potatoes/Beans

BLACK BEANS (BOILED)	0.79	CUP
BLACK BEANS (DRY)	0.636	CUP
CHICKPEAS / GARBANZO BEANS	0.25	CUP
KIDNEY BEANS (BOILED)	0.25	CUP
LIMA BEANS (BOILED)	0.86	CUP
NAVY BEANS (BOILED)	0.69	CUP
NAVY BEANS (CAN)	0.745	CUP
PINTO BEANS (BOILED)	0.76	CUP
PINTO BEANS (CAN)	0.94	CUP
PINTO BEANS (DRY)	0.297	CUP
PORK & BEANS / VAN CAMPS	0.81	CUP
POTATO, SWEET	1.51	5"X2"
POTATO	10.6	OZ
RICE CAKE	3.56	CAKE
RICE, WHITE, BASMATI	0.745	CUP (C)
RICE, BROWN LONG GRAIN	0.89	CUP (C)
RICE, INSTANT, MINUTE BRAND	0.558	CUP(UC)
RICE, WHITE, LONG GRAIN	0.279	CUP(UC)
SOYBEANS (BOILED)	0.5	CUP
YAM, BOILED OR BAKED	1.13	CUP

Pasta

MACARONI, DAVINI TWIST	0.68	CUP/DRY
MACARONI, HOSPITALITY ELBOW	0.37	CUP/DRY
MACARONI, AM. BEAUTY ELBOW	0.425	CUP/DRY
PASTA, CREAMETTE PLAIN	1.7	OZ
SPAGHETTI, EDEN WHOLE WHEAT	1.7	OZ/UC

Protein Sources 1800 Calories

White Meat

CHICKEN BREAST (HORMEL/CAN)	1.19	CAN
CHICKEN BREAST (SKINLESS)	5.95	OZ
CHICKEN (LEG W/ SKIN & BONE)	0.675	
CHICKEN (THIGH W/ SKIN & BONE)	1.165	
CHICKEN (LEG & THIGH W/ SKIN & BONE)	0.428	
HAM, BAR S, XTRA LEAN, 96% FAT FREE	5.1	OZ
HAM, DAK CAN	5.95	OZ
PORK, SIRLOIN, LEAN W/ FAT	1.78	OZ
TURKEY BREAST (SKINLESS)	3.33	OZ
TURKEY BREAST (HORMEL/CAN)	1.02	CAN
TURKEY BRST/OVEN ROAST/SFWY/89% FF	7.1	OZ
VENISON / ANTELOPE	3.98	OZ

Red Meat

HAMBURGER (10% FAT)	3.16	OZ
HAMBURGER (15% FAT)	2.62	OZ
HAMBURGER (20% FAT)	2.55	OZ
HAMBURGER (27% FAT)	2.16	OZ
LAMB, SHOULDER	2.03	OZ
STEAK, BOTTOM ROUND	3.01	OZ
STEAK, BRISKET (FLAT HALF)	2.84	OZ
STEAK, CHUCK, ARM	2.92	OZ
STEAK, CHUCK, BLADE	2.52	OZ
STEAK, EYE ROUND	3.74	OZ
STEAK, FLANK	3.04	OZ
STEAK, NEW YORK STRIP	3.57	OZ
STEAK, PORTERHOUSE	2.9	OZ
STEAK, RIBEYE	2.8	OZ
STEAK, ROUND TIP	3.42	OZ
STEAK, SHANK (CROSSCUTS)	3.14	OZ
STEAK, T-BONE	2.94	OZ
STEAK, TENDERLOIN	2.99	OZ
STEAK, TOP LOIN	3.05	OZ
STEAK, TOP ROUND	3.5	OZ

STEAK, TOP SIRLOIN	3.24	OZ
STEAK, TYSON SEASONED BEEF STRIPS	3.83	OZ
TACO/BURRITO MEAT/SMART GROUND	0.93	CUP
OSCAR MAYER BACON	5.95	SLICE
LITTLE SIZZLER BROWN/SERVE SAUSAGE	2.32	LINK

Sea Food

BASS, FRESHWATER, DRY HEAT	4.33	OZ
BASS, STRIPED, DRY HEAT	5.1	OZ
COD, ATLANTIC, DRY HEAT	6	OZ
CRAB, ALASKA KING, MOIST HEAT	6.53	OZ
CRAB, BLUE, MOIST HEAT	6.15	OZ
FLOUNDER, DRY HEAT	5.4	OZ
HADDOCK, DRY HEAT	5.65	OZ
HALIBUT, DRY HEAT	4.5	OZ
LOBSTER, NORTHERN, MOIST HEAT	6.45	OZ
MAHI MAHI	7.35	OZ
ORANGE ROUGHY, DRY HEAT	7.05	OZ
PERCH, DRY HEAT	5.4	OZ
PERCH, OCEAN/ATLANTIC, DRY HEAT	5.2	OZ
SALMON, ATLANTIC, DRY HEAT	3.44	OZ
SHRIMP, MOIST HEAT	6.36	OZ
TROUT, DRY HEAT	3.33	OZ
TUNA BURGER, AHI / OMEGA FOODS	6.38	OZ
TUNA, LOW SODIUM, CAN	1.02	CAN
TUNA, WATER, CAN	1.19	CAN
TUNA, WHITE / LOW SALT, CAN (5 OZ)	1.02	CAN
TUNA, WHITE, CAN (5 OZ)	1.02	CAN
TUNA, FILLET/STEAK	4.05	OZ
WALLEYE, BAKED/BROILED/MICRO	5.3	OZ

Vegetarian

IVES VEG. COUSINE VEGGY DOG	2.98	DOG
SOY MILK (TRIS)	2	CUP
SOY MILK (SYLVIA)	1.75	CUP

Eggs/Dairy

1% COTTAGE CHEESE, NORDICA	1.12	CUP
2% COTTAGE CHEESE (LOW FAT)	0.89	CUP
COTTAGE CHEESE (LUCERNE FAT FREE)	1.11	CUP
COTT CHEESE MARIGOLD/DRY CURD	1.7	CUP
COTT CHEESE MARIGOLD/DRY CURD	27.2	TBLSP
COTT CHEESE BREAKSTONES FAT FREE	1.11	CUP
CHEDDER, SHREDDED, FAT FREE, KHF	0.99	CUP
CHEDDER, SHREDDED, 94% FAT FREE, HC	0.89	CUP
CHEESE, COLBY/MOZZARELLA	1.62	OZ
EGG WHITE	10.5	
EGG, WHOLE	2.38	
EGG BEATERS	1.49	CUP
MOZZARELLA SHREDDED, FAT FREE, KHF	0.89	CUP
SKIM MOZZARELLA STRING CHEESE	2.23	OZ

Free Carbs, Supplements, Fast Foods
1800 calories

Free Carbs

ASPARAGUS
BROCCOLI
CABBAGE
CAULIFLOWER
CELERY
CUCUMBER
GREEN BEANS
GREEN PEPPERS
GREEN SQUASH
LETTUCE, ICEBERG
LETTUCE, LEAF/SHREDDED
MUSHROOMS
ONION
PICKLES (DILL)
RADISH
RED PEPPERS

SPINACH (CAN/NO SALT)
SPINACH (FRESH)
TOMATO (EXCLUDING JUICE)
ZUCCHINI

Supplements/Fast Foods

ATKINS BAR	0.75	BAR
EAS ADVANTEDGE, C&C/LEM/BLUE	0.75	BAR
BAR, ZONE	0.75	BAR
BAR, PURE PROTEIN, 50 G.	0.75	BAR
BAR, W.W. PURE PROTEIN, 78 G.	0.5	BAR
BAR, PROTEIN REVOLUTION, PBJ	0.75	BAR
BAR, FIBAR, PEANUT BUTTER, 1.2 OZ	1.25	BAR
BAR, PREMIER 1, PROTEIN 8, CHOC/COCO	0.5	BAR
BAR, PREFERRED BAR, CHOC./FUDG/RAS	0.75	BAR
BAR, PREFERRED BAR, CHOC./FUDG/BROW	0.75	BAR
ALIVE, HI CARB POWDER	4	TBLSP
POWERADE	2	SERVING
PROTEIN,GNC P.P. EGG/WHEY	1.25	SERVING
PROTEIN. GNC P.PERF. WHEY	4	SCOOP
OPTIMUM NUTRITION WHEY	1.5	SCOOP
SYNTRAX WHEY PROTEIN	1.75	SCOOP
TRI PROTEIN PLUS POWDER	1.25	SERVING
HW STRAWBERRY PROT. POWD.	1.75	SCOOP
BIOCHEM WHEY PRO 290	2	SCOOP
HUMAN DEV. TECH. WHEY	1.25	SCOOP
NATURADE 100% SOY PROTEIN	0.5	CUP
SUPER GREEN PRO 96 - SOY	0.5	CUP
100% PURE WHEY, PROLAB	1.25	SCOOP
ECLIPSE BULK UP WHEY	1.75	SCOOP
VITAMIN WORLD WHEY 100%	1.5	SCOOP
ULT. NUT. PROSTAR WHEY	1.5	SCOOP
RED WINE	7	OZ
MET RX CH.RST.PNT.PRO + BAR	0.5	BAR
MET RX BAV. MINT. PRO + BAR	0.5	BAR
MET AFTER FX BAR	0.5	BAR
MET RX CH. CH. CHIP PRO + BAR	0.5	BAR
MET RX SOURCE ONE BAR	0.75	BAR

MET RX CHOC. GRAHCRK CHIP BAR	0.5	BAR
MET RX PEANUT BUTTER BAR	0.5	BAR
MET RX DRINK MIX, MRP	0.5	SERVING
MET RX PRO 50, ANABOLIC DRIVE	0.5	SERVING
MET RX PRO 60, ANABOLIC DRIVE	0.5	SERVING
MET RX PROTEIN PLUS	2.5	SCOOP
MET RX KETO PRO	2.25	SCOOP
NUTRI FORCE DRINK MIX, MRP	0.5	SERVING
EAS MYO. DEL. CH/PB BAR	0.5	BAR
EAS MYOPLEX + DELUXE	0.5	SERVING
EAS MYOPLEX LITE	0.75	SERVING
ADVANT EDGE QUICK STIR PROTEIN DRINK	0.75	SERVING
EAS NEUROGAIN	3.5	SCOOP
EAS PHOSPHAGEN HP	1	SCOOP
EAS PRECISION PROTEIN	1.75	SCOOP
EAS SIMPLY PROTEIN	3	SCOOP
EAS WHEY PROTEIN	1.5	SCOOP
EAS SUPPER SHAKE	0.33	SHAKE
VITAMIN WORLD DAILY RX, MRP	0.5	SHAKE
VITAMIN WORLD PROTOPLEX DELUXE, MRP	0.5	SHAKE
VITAMIN WORLD PRE. ENG. WHEY PROT.	2	SCOOP
PERFECT RX, MRP, CHOCOLATE	0.5	SHAKE
OPTI PRO	0.5	SHAKE
ARBY'S CHICK. SAND. R.DELX.LITE	0.5	BURGER
ARBY'S SIDE SALAD	1	SALAD
ARBY'S GARDEN SALAD	1	SALAD
ARBY'S RST. CHCK. SALAD	1	SALAD
ARBY'S RED. CAL. ITAL. DRESSING	1	PACKET
ARBY'S RED RANCH DRESSING	1	PACKET
MCD'S VINAG. LITE SALAD DR.	1	PACKET
MCD'S GARDEN SALAD	1	SALAD
MCD'S VINAG. LITE SALAD DR.	1	PACKET
P.HUT. HAND-TOSS CHEESE	0.75	SLICE
P.HUT. HAND-TOSS HAM	0.75	SLICE
P.HUT. HAND-TOSS VEG. LUV.	0.75	SLICE
P.HUT. HAND-TOSS PEPPERON	0.75	SLICE
P.HUT. THIN/CRISP CHEES	0.75	SLICE
P.HUT. THIN/CRISP HAM	0.75	SLICE

P.HUT. THIN/CRISP VEG. LUV.	0.75	SLICE
P.HUT. THIN/CRISP PEPPERON	0.75	SLICE
SW 6" COLD SUB/VEGG. DELIT	1	SUB
SW 6" COLD SUB/TURK. BRST.	1	SUB
SW 6" COLD SUB/TURK.B/HAM	1	SUB
SW 6" COLD SUB/HAM	1	SUB
SW 6" COLD SUB/ROAST BEEF	1	SUB
SW 6" COLD SUB/SFOOD,CRAB	1	SUB
SW 6" COLD SUB/COLD CUT 3	1	SUB
SW 6" COLD SUB/TUNA	1	SUB
SW 6" HOT SUB/RST.CHICK.BR.	1	SUB
SW 6" HOT SUB/STAK/CHEESE	1	SUB
SW 6" HOT SUB/SUB MELT	1	SUB
SW VEGGIE DELITE SALAD	1	SALAD
SW TURKEY BREAST SALAD	1	SALAD
SW ROAST BEEF SALAD	1	SALAD
SW TURK. BRST/HAM SALAD	1	SALAD
SW RST. CHICK. BR. SALAD	0.75	SALAD
SW SEAFOOD/CRAB SALAD	0.75	SALAD
SW STEAK/CHEESE SALAD	0.5	SALAD
SW SUBWAY MELT SALAD	0.5	SALAD
SW COLD CUT 3 SALAD	0.5	SALAD
SW FAT FREE ITALIAN DRESS	1	OZ
SW FAT FREE FRENCH DRESS	1	OZ
SW FAT FREE RANCH DRESS	1	OZ
SW DELI STYLE TURKEY BR.	0.5	SNDWCH
SW DELI STYLE HAM	0.5	SNDWCH
SW DELI STYLE ROAST BEEF	0.5	SNDWCH
TB GRILLED STEAK SOFT TACO	0.5	TACO
WAHOO'S CHBROIL FISH TACO	0.5	TACO
WENDI'S SIDE SALAD	1	SALAD
WENDI'S FF FRENCH DRESSING	1	OZ
WENDI'S ITALIAN RED. F/C DRESS	1	OZ
WENDI'S SMALL CHILI	0.75	BOWL
WENDI'S GRILLED CHICK. FILLET	1.5	MEAT

1900 Calories/Day Eating Plan		
What Does Your Doctor Look Like Naked?		

Name: _____

Date: _____

Exercise: 30-40 min in a.m. before food		Write what you eat here:
Meal 1 Time: _____	2 Protein Source 2 Active Carbohydrates	
Meal 2 Time: _____	1.5 oz Raw Almonds	
Meal 3 Time: _____	1 Protein Source 2 Active Carbohydrates Free Carbohydrates (as much as you want)	
Meal 4 Time: _____	½ LOW CARB protein bar (OR) 1.5 scoops Whey Protein Powder in water	
Meal 5 Time: _____	1 Protein Source 0 Active Carbohydrates Free Carbohydrates (as much as you want)	
Bedtime Meal (Optional)	Sugar Free Jell-O 1 cup	

Add fiber supplement in evening, such as Metamucil or other (sugar FREE).
Add spices, pepper, etc. as needed.
Try to eat every two to three hours.
Drink 1 gallon of water EVERY DAY!
May have up to 2 diet pops (or) 2 cups a coffee a day.

Active Carbohydrates 1900 Calories

Fruit and Vegetables

APPLE	2.35	3 INCH
APPLESAUCE, MOTT'S	0.865	CUP
APRICOTS (CAN/DEL MONTE LITE)	1.59	CUP
APRICOTS (DRIED)	2.72	OZ
APRICOTS (FRESH 12/LB)	11.2	MEDIUM
ASPARAGUS	51.5	OZ
BANANA	1.81	MEDIUM
BLUEBERRIES (FRESH)	2.32	CUP
BRUSSELS SPROUTS, BOILED	3.18	CUP
CABBAGE, SHREDDED	10.6	CUP
CANTALOUPE	1.01	5 INCH
CARROT (FRESH)	17.2	OZ
CAULIFLOWER	7.34	CUP
CELERY	47.5	OZ
CHERRIES, FRESH, SWEET W/PIT	1.83	CUP
CHERRIES, DARK (CAN/DEL MONTE)	0.95	CUP
COLLARD GREENS (CAN)	3.18	CUP
COLLARD GREENS (FRESH)	15.9	CUP
CORN CAKE	5.45	CAKE
CORN (CAN/DEL MONTE NO SODIUM)	13.9	OZ
CUCUMBER, SLICED	13.6	CUP
EGGPLANT	8.65	CUP
FRUIT, MIXED FROZEN	2.12	CUP
GARLIC, 1 CLOVE	47.5	CLOVE
GARLIC, TRIMMED	4.53	OZ
GRAPES	1.67	CUP
GRAPE JUICE/VERYFINE	10.18	OZ
GRAPEFRUIT	2.07	4 INCH
GREEN BEANS (CAN/DEL MONTE NO SALT)	4.75	CUP
GREEN PEPPER	9.5	MEDIUM
KIWI	12.8	OZ
MUSHROOMS, FRESH	10.6	CUP
ONION, FRESH/CHOPPED	3.17	CUP
ORANGE, NAVAL	2.93	3 INCH

ORANGE, JUICE	13.85	OZ
PAPAYA	1.63	LB.
PAPAYA, PEELED/CUBED	3.52	CUP
PEACH, FRESH, SLICED	2.58	CUP
PEACH (CAN/DEL MONTE EXTRA LITE)	1.59	CUP
PEARS (CAN)	6.35	HALF
PEAS, BLACKEYED (CAN)	1.06	CUP
PEAS (CAN/DEL MONTE NO SODIUM)	13.9	OZ
PEAS, GREEN GIANT FROZEN, SWEET	1.84	CUP
PEAS, EDIBLE-PODDED	3.18	CUP
PINEAPPLE, FRESH/DICED	2.44	CUP
PINEAPPLE, DEL MONTE SNACK CAN (LITE)	2.72	3.5 OZ
PINEAPPLE (CAN/DOLE LITE SYRUP)	11.2	SLICE
PRUNES, DOLE, DRIED	2.72	OZ
PUMPKIN (CAN)	3.8	CUP
RAISINS	0.397	CUP
RED PEPPER	9.5	MEDIUM
STRAWBERRIES (FRESH)	1.96	PINT
STRAWBERRIES (FROZEN)	2.54	CUP
SQUASH, CAN, STOKLEY	1.9	CUP
SQUASH, FRESH BAKED	1.67	CUP
TANGERINE	5.15	2.5 INCH
TOMATO, CAN	17.8	OZ
TOMATO, FRESH	7.33	3 INCH
TOMATO, JUICE	30.4	OZ
VEGETABLES, MIXED (FROZEN)	2.12	CUP
WATERMELLON	1.25	1X10 INCH
ZUCCHINI, FRESH, SLICED	10.6	CUP

Yogurts and Desserts

DING DONG	1.19	DING
DREYERS FROZEN FAT FREE YOGURT	1.06	CUP
FRUIT ROLL-UP	2.72	ROLL-UP
POPCORN, WHITE	3.8	TBLSP
TCBY, SOFT SERVE/NONFAT/NO SUGAR	1.19	CUP
YOGURT, FAT FREE, MOUNTAIN HIGH	8	OZ
YOGURT, FAT FREE, DANNON	8	OZ
LUCERN, YOGURT, NONFAT, LITE	8	OZ

YOGURT, YOPLAIT, FAT FREE, LITE	6	OZ
YOGURT, YOPLAIT ORIGINAL/99% FAT FREE	6	OZ
YOGURT, HORIZON, FF / BLUEBERRY	6	OZ
PLANTER DRIED WALNUT PIECES	0.2	CUP
RAW ALMONDS, TOASTED	1	OZ
PECANS, DRIED	0.88	OZ
PEANUTS, DRY ROASTED	0.2	CUP
HOT CHOCOLATE	3	ENVEL.
ALMONDS, SHELLED	1	OZ

Cereals

CEREAL, CHEERIOS	1.73	CUP
CEREAL, COCOA KRISPIES	1.19	CUP
CEREAL, GRAPENUTS	0.475	CUP
CEREAL, HONEY NUT TOASTY O'S	1.73	CUP
CEREAL, WHEATIES	1.73	CUP
CEREAL, KELLOGG'S ALL BRAN	1.19	CUP
CEREAL, KELLOGG'S CORN FLAKES	1.73	CUP
CEREAL, KELLOGG'S RAISIN BRAN	1.12	CUP
CEREAL, KELLOGG'S CRACKLIN' OAT BRAN	0.72	CUP
CEREAL, NABISCO SHREDDED WHEAT	2.38	PIECE
CEREAL, NAB. SHREDDED WHEAT (SPOON)	1.12	CUP
CEREAL, RICE KRISPIES	2.17	CUP
CEREAL, BENEFIT NUTRITION, PROTEIN +	0.91	CUP
CREAM OF WHEAT	4.75	TBL/DRY
GRANOLA, CW POST HEARTY	0.453	CUP
GRANOLA, KELLOGG'S LOW FAT	4	CUP
OATMEAL (PRE-COOK MEASUREMENT)	0.68	CUP

Breads

BREAD, OROWHEAT LITE	4.75	SLICE
BREAD, SUSAN'S HOMEMADE/18 SLICES	2.1	SLICE
BREAD, SUSAN'S HOMEMADE	0.117	LOAF
BUN, WONDER REDUCED CALORIE LITE	2.38	BUN
CRACKER, ZESTA SALTINES	15.9	CRACKER
TORTILLA, (CAROLYN)	1.12	TORT
TORTILLA, TORTILLA'S MEXICO, FLOUR	1.73	TORT

TORTILLA, TORTILLA'S MEXICO, CORN	2.12	TORT
TRISCUITS	1.36	OZ
WAFFLE, EGGO, HOMESTYLE	1.73	WAFFLE
WHOLE GRAIN/WHOLE WHEAT FLOUR	0.467	CUP

Rice/Potatoes/Beans

BLACK BEANS (BOILED)	0.845	CUP
BLACK BEANS (DRY)	0.68	CUP
CHICKPEAS/GARBANZO BEANS	0.22	CUP
KIDNEY BEANS (BOILED)	0.25	CUP
LIMA BEANS (BOILED)	0.915	CUP
NAVY BEANS (BOILED)	0.74	CUP
NAVY BEANS (CAN)	0.795	CUP
PINTO BEANS (BOILED)	0.815	CUP
PINTO BEANS (CAN)	1	CUP
PINTO BEANS (DRY)	0.318	CUP
PORK & BEANS/VAN CAMPS	0.865	CUP
POTATO, SWEET	1.615	5"X2"
POTATO	11.3	OZ
RICE CAKE	3.8	CAKE
RICE, WHITE, BASMATI	0.795	CUP (C)
RICE, BROWN LONG GRAIN	0.95	CUP (C)
RICE, INSTANT, MINUTE BRAND	0.595	CUP(UC)
RICE, WHITE, LONG GRAIN	0.297	CUP(UC)
SOYBEANS (BOILED)	0.75	CUP
YAM, BOILED OR BAKED	1.2	CUP

Pasta

MACARONI, DAVINI TWIST	0.725	CUP/DRY
MACARONI, HOSPITALITY ELBOW	0.396	CUP/DRY
MACARONI, AM. BEAUTY ELBOW	0.454	CUP/DRY
PASTA, CREAMETTE PLAIN	1.81	OZ
SPAGHETTI, EDEN WHOLE WHEAT	1.81	OZ/UC

Protein Sources 1900 Calories

White Meat

CHICKEN BREAST (HORMEL/CAN)	1.27	CAN
CHICKEN BREAST (SKINLESS)	6.35	OZ
CHICKEN (LEG W/ SKIN & BONE)	0.72	
CHICKEN (THIGH W/ SKIN & BONE)	1.245	
CHICKEN (LEG & THIGH W/ SKIN & BONE)	0.455	
HAM, BAR S, XTRA LEAN, 96% FAT FREE	5.45	OZ
HAM, DAK CAN	6.34	OZ
PORK, SIRLOIN, LEAN W/ FAT	1.9	OZ
TURKEY BREAST (SKINLESS)	3.56	OZ
TURKEY BREAST (HORMEL/CAN)	1.09	CAN
TURKEY BRST/OVEN ROAST/SFWY/89% FF	7.6	OZ
VENISON / ANTELOPE	4.25	OZ

Red Meat

HAMBURGER (10% FAT)	3.39	OZ
HAMBURGER (15% FAT)	2.8	OZ
HAMBURGER (20% FAT)	2.72	OZ
HAMBURGER (27% FAT)	2.3	OZ
LAMB, SHOULDER	2.17	OZ
STEAK, BOTTOM ROUND	3.21	OZ
STEAK, BRISKET (FLAT HALF)	3.02	OZ
STEAK, CHUCK, ARM	3.12	OZ
STEAK, CHUCK, BLADE	2.69	OZ
STEAK, EYE ROUND	4	OZ
STEAK, FLANK	3.25	OZ
STEAK, NEW YORK STRIP	3.8	OZ
STEAK, PORTERHOUSE	3.09	OZ
STEAK, RIBEYE	2.99	OZ
STEAK, ROUND TIP	3.64	OZ
STEAK, SHANK (CROSSCUTS)	3.35	OZ
STEAK, T-BONE	3.14	OZ
STEAK, TENDERLOIN	3.2	OZ
STEAK, TOP LOIN	3.25	OZ
STEAK, TOP ROUND	3.74	OZ

STEAK, TOP SIRLOIN	3.47	OZ
STEAK, TYSON SEASONED BEEF STRIPS	4.08	OZ
TACO/BURRITO MEAT/SMART GROUND	0.99	CUP
OSCAR MAYER BACON	6.34	SLICE
LITTLE SIZZLER BROWN/SERVE SAUSAGE	2.47	LINK

Sea Food

BASS, FRESHWATER, DRY HEAT	4.6	OZ
BASS, STRIPED, DRY HEAT	5.45	OZ
COD, ATLANTIC, DRY HEAT	6.43	OZ
CRAB, ALASKA KING, MOIST HEAT	7	OZ
CRAB, BLUE, MOIST HEAT	6.58	OZ
FLOUNDER, DRY HEAT	5.78	OZ
HADDOCK, DRY HEAT	6	OZ
HALIBUT, DRY HEAT	4.8	OZ
LOBSTER, NORTHERN, MOIST HEAT	6.9	OZ
MAHI MAHI	7.84	OZ
ORANGE ROUGHY, DRY HEAT	7.52	OZ
PERCH, DRY HEAT	5.78	OZ
PERCH, OCEAN/ATLANTIC, DRY HEAT	5.55	OZ
SALMON, ATLANTIC, DRY HEAT	3.66	OZ
SHRIMP, MOIST HEAT	6.8	OZ
TROUT, DRY HEAT	3.55	OZ
TUNA BURGER, AHI/OMEGA FOODS	6.8	OZ
TUNA, LOW SODIUM, CAN	1.09	CAN
TUNA, WATER, CAN	1.27	CAN
TUNA, WHITE / LOW SALT, CAN (5 OZ)	1.09	CAN
TUNA, WHITE, CAN (5 OZ)	1.09	CAN
TUNA, FILLET/STEAK	4.32	OZ
WALLEYE, BAKED/BROILED/MICRO	5.63	OZ

Vegetarian

IVES VEG. COUSINE VEGGY DOG	3.17	DOG
SOY MILK (TRIS)	2	CUP
SOY MILK (SYLVIA)	1.75	CUP

Eggs/Dairy

1% COTTAGE CHEESE, NORDICA	1.19	CUP
2% COTTAGE CHEESE (LOW FAT)	0.95	CUP
COTTAGE CHEESE (LUCERNE FAT FREE)	1.19	CUP
COTT CHEESE MARIGOLD/DRY CURD	1.81	CUP
COTT CHEESE MARIGOLD/DRY CURD	29	TBLSP
COTT CHEESE BREAKSTONES FAT FREE	1.19	CUP
CHEDDER, SHREDDED, FAT FREE, KHF	1.06	CUP
CHEDDER, SHREDDED, 94% FAT FREE, HC	0.95	CUP
CHEESE, COLBY/MOZZARELLA	1.73	OZ
EGG WHITE	11.2	
EGG, WHOLE	2.54	
EGG BEATERS	1.59	CUP
MOZZARELLA SHREDDED, FAT FREE, KHF	0.95	CUP
SKIM MOZZARELLA STRING CHEESE	2.38	OZ

Free Carbs, Supplements, Fast Foods
1900 calories

Free Carbs

ASPARAGUS
BROCCOLI
CABBAGE
CAULIFLOWER
CELERY
CUCUMBER
GREEN BEANS
GREEN PEPPERS
GREEN SQUASH
LETTUCE, ICEBERG
LETTUCE, LEAF/SHREDDED
MUSHROOMS
ONION
PICKLES (DILL)
RADISH

RED PEPPERS
SPINACH (CAN/NO SALT)
SPINACH (FRESH)
TOMATO (EXCLUDING JUICE)
ZUCCHINI

Supplements/Fast Foods

ATKINS BAR	0.75	BAR
EAS ADVANTEDGE, C&C/LEM/BLUE	0.75	BAR
BAR, ZONE	0.75	BAR
BAR, PURE PROTEIN, 50 G.	1	BAR
BAR, W.W. PURE PROTEIN, 78 G.	0.5	BAR
BAR, PROTEIN REVOLUTION, PBJ	0.75	BAR
BAR, FIBAR, PEANUT BUTTER, 1.2 OZ	1.25	BAR
BAR, PREMIER 1, PROTEIN 8, CHOC/COCO	0.5	BAR
BAR, PREFERRED BAR, CHOC./FUDG/RAS	0.75	BAR
BAR, PREFERRED BAR, CHOC./FUDG/BROW	0.75	BAR
ALIVE, HI CARB POWDER	3	TBLSP
POWERADE	2	SERVING
PROTEIN,GNC P.P. EGG/WHEY	1.5	SERVING
PROTEIN. GNC P.PERF. WHEY	4	SCOOP
OPTIMUM NUTRITION WHEY	1.5	SCOOP
SYNTRAX WHEY PROTEIN	2	SCOOP
TRI PROTEIN PLUS POWDER	1.25	SERVING
HW STRAWBERRY PROT. POWD.	1.75	SCOOP
BIOCHEM WHEY PRO 290	2.25	SCOOP
HUMAN DEV. TECH. WHEY	1.25	SCOOP
NATURADE 100% SOY PROTEIN	0.5	CUP
SUPER GREEN PRO 96 - SOY	0.5	CUP
100% PURE WHEY, PROLAB	1.25	SCOOP
ECLIPSE BULK UP WHEY	1.75	SCOOP
VITAMIN WORLD WHEY 100%	1.5	SCOOP
ULT. NUT. PROSTAR WHEY	1.5	SCOOP
RED WINE	7	OZ
MET RX CH.RST.PNT.PRO + BAR	0.5	BAR
MET RX BAV. MINT. PRO + BAR	0.75	BAR
MET AFTER FX BAR	0.75	BAR
MET RX CH. CH. CHIP PRO + BAR	0.5	BAR

MET RX SOURCE ONE BAR	0.75	BAR
MET RX CHOC. GRAHCRK CHIP BAR	0.5	BAR
MET RX PEANUT BUTTER BAR	0.5	BAR
MET RX DRINK MIX, MRP	0.75	SERVING
MET RX PRO 50, ANABOLIC DRIVE	0.5	SERVING
MET RX PRO 60, ANABOLIC DRIVE	0.5	SERVING
MET RX PROTEIN PLUS	2.25	SCOOP
MET RX KETO PRO	2.25	SCOOP
NUTRI FORCE DRINK MIX, MRP	0.5	SERVING
EAS MYO. DEL. CH/PB BAR	0.5	BAR
EAS MYOPLEX + DELUXE	0.5	SERVING
EAS MYOPLEX LITE	0.75	SERVING
ADVANT EDGE QUICK STIR PROTEIN DRINK	0.75	SERVING
EAS NEUROGAIN	3.5	SCOOP
EAS PHOSPHAGEN HP	1	SCOOP
EAS PRECISION PROTEIN	1.75	SCOOP
EAS SIMPLY PROTEIN	3	SCOOP
EAS WHEY PROTEIN	1.5	SCOOP
EAS SUPPER SHAKE	0.33	SHAKE
VITAMIN WORLD DAILY RX, MRP	0.5	SHAKE
VITAMIN WORLD PROTOPLEX DELUXE, MRP	0.5	SHAKE
VITAMIN WORLD PRE. ENG. WHEY PROT.	1.75	SCOOP
PERFECT RX, MRP, CHOCOLATE	0.75	SHAKE
OPTI PRO	0.5	SHAKE
ARBY'S CHICK. SAND. R.DELX.LITE	0.5	BURGER
ARBY'S SIDE SALAD	1	SALAD
ARBY'S GARDEN SALAD	1	SALAD
ARBY'S RST. CHCK. SALAD	1	SALAD
ARBY'S RED. CAL. ITAL. DRESSING	1	PACKET
ARBY'S RED RANCH DRESSING	1	PACKET
MCD'S VINAG. LITE SALAD DR.	1	PACKET
MCD'S GARDEN SALAD	1	SALAD
MCD'S VINAG. LITE SALAD DR.	1	PACKET
P.HUT. HAND-TOSS CHEESE	0.75	SLICE
P.HUT. HAND-TOSS HAM	0.75	SLICE
P.HUT. HAND-TOSS VEG. LUV.	0.75	SLICE
P.HUT. HAND-TOSS PEPPERON	0.75	SLICE
P.HUT. THIN/CRISP CHEESE	0.75	SLICE

P.HUT. THIN/CRISP HAM	1	SLICE
P.HUT. THIN/CRISP VEG. LUV.	1	SLICE
P.HUT. THIN/CRISP PEPPERON	0.75	SLICE
SW 6" COLD SUB/VEGG. DELIT	1	SUB
SW 6" COLD SUB/TURK. BRST.	1	SUB
SW 6" COLD SUB/TURK.B/HAM	1	SUB
SW 6" COLD SUB/HAM	1	SUB
SW 6" COLD SUB/ROAST BEEF	1	SUB
SW 6" COLD SUB/SFOOD,CRAB	1	SUB
SW 6" COLD SUB/COLD CUT 3	1	SUB
SW 6" COLD SUB/TUNA	1	SUB
SW 6" HOT SUB/RST.CHICK.BR.	1	SUB
SW 6" HOT SUB/STAK/CHEESE	1	SUB
SW 6" HOT SUB/SUB MELT	1	SUB
SW VEGGIE DELITE SALAD	1	SALAD
SW TURKEY BREAST SALAD	1	SALAD
SW ROAST BEEF SALAD	1	SALAD
SW TURK. BRST/HAM SALAD	1	SALAD
SW RST. CHICK. BR. SALAD	1	SALAD
SW SEAFOOD/CRAB SALAD	1	SALAD
SW STEAK/CHEESE SALAD	0.75	SALAD
SW SUBWAY MELT SALAD	1	SALAD
SW COLD CUT 3 SALAD	1	SALAD
SW FAT FREE ITALIAN DRESS	1	OZ
SW FAT FREE FRENCH DRESS	1	OZ
SW FAT FREE RANCH DRESS	1	OZ
SW DELI STYLE TURKEY BR.	0.75	SNDWCH
SW DELI STYLE HAM	0.75	SNDWCH
SW DELI STYLE ROAST BEEF	0.75	SNDWCH
TB GRILLED STEAK SOFT TACO	0.75	TACO
WAHOO'S CHBROIL FISH TACO	0.5	TACO
WENDI'S SIDE SALAD	1	SALAD
WENDI'S FF FRENCH DRESSING	1	OZ
WENDI'S ITALIAN RED. F/C DRESS	1	OZ
WENDI'S SMALL CHILI	0.75	BOWL
WENDI'S GRILLED CHICK. FILLET	1	MEAT

2000 Calories/Day Eating Plan		
What Does Your Doctor Look Like Naked?		
Name: _____		
Date: _____		
Exercise: 30-40 min in a.m. before food		
		Write what you eat here:
Meal 1 Time: _____	2 Protein Source 2 Active Carbohydrates	
Meal 2 Time: _____	1.5 oz Raw Almonds	
Meal 3 Time: _____	1 Protein Source 2 Active Carbohydrates Free Carbohydrates (as much as you want)	
Meal 4 Time: _____	1 LOW CARB protein bar (OR) 1.5 scoops Whey Protein Powder in water	
Meal 5 Time: _____	1 Protein Source 0 Active Carbohydrates Free Carbohydrates (as much as you want)	
Bedtime Meal (Optional)	Sugar Free Jell-O 1 cup	

Add fiber supplement in evening, such as Metamucil or other (sugar FREE).
Add spices, pepper, etc. as needed.
Try to eat every two to three hours.
Drink 1 ¼ gallons of water EVERY DAY!
May have up to 2 diet pops (or) 2 cups a coffee a day.

Active Carbohydrates 2000 Calories

Fruit and Vegetables

APPLE	2.29	3 INCH
APPLESAUCE, MOTT'S	0.84	CUP
APRICOTS (CAN/DEL MONTE LITE)	1.54	CUP
APRICOTS (DRIED)	2.65	OZ
APRICOTS (FRESH 12/LB)	10.9	MEDIUM
ASPARAGUS	50	OZ
BANANA	1.76	MEDIUM
BLUEBERRIES (FRESH)	2.26	CUP
BRUSSELS SPROUTS, BOILED	3.09	CUP
CABBAGE, SHREDDED	10.3	CUP
CANTALOUPE	0.98	5 INCH
CARROT (FRESH)	16.7	OZ
CAULIFLOWER	7.13	CUP
CELERY	46.3	OZ
CHERRIES, FRESH, SWEET W/PIT	1.78	CUP
CHERRIES, DARK (CAN/DEL MONTE)	0.925	CUP
COLLARD GREENS (CAN)	3.09	CUP
COLLARD GREENS (FRESH)	15.4	CUP
CORN CAKE	5.3	CAKE
CORN (CAN/DEL MONTE NO SODIUM)	13.5	OZ
CUCUMBER, SLICED	13.2	CUP
EGGPLANT	8.4	CUP
FRUIT, MIXED FROZEN	2.06	CUP
GARLIC, 1 CLOVE	46	CLOVE
GARLIC, TRIMMED	4.4	OZ
GRAPES	1.63	CUP
GRAPE JUICE/VERYFINE	9.9	OZ
GRAPEFRUIT	2.01	4 INCH
GREEN BEANS (CAN/DEL MONTE NO SALT)	4.61	CUP
GREEN PEPPER	9.25	MEDIUM
KIWI	12.5	OZ
MUSHROOMS, FRESH	10.3	CUP
ONION, FRESH/CHOPPED	3.09	CUP
ORANGE, NAVAL	2.85	3 INCH

ORANGE, JUICE	13.5	OZ
PAPAYA	1.585	LB.
PAPAYA, PEELED/CUBED	3.44	CUP
PEACH, FRESH, SLICED	2.5	CUP
PEACH (CAN/DEL MONTE EXTRA LITE)	1.54	CUP
PEARS (CAN)	6.15	HALF
PEAS, BLACKEYED (CAN)	1.03	CUP
PEAS (CAN/DEL MONTE NO SODIUM)	13.5	OZ
PEAS, GREEN GIANT FROZEN, SWEET	1.77	CUP
PEAS, EDIBLE-PODDED	3.1	CUP
PINEAPPLE, FRESH/DICED	2.37	CUP
PINEAPPLE, DEL MONTE SNACK CAN (LITE)	2.65	3.5 OZ
PINEAPPLE (CAN/DOLE LITE SYRUP)	10.9	SLICE
PRUNES, DOLE, DRIED	2.65	OZ
PUMPKIN (CAN)	3.7	CUP
RAISENS	0.385	CUP
RED PEPPER	9.25	MEDIUM
STRAWBERRIES (FRESH)	1.9	PINT
STRAWBERRIES (FROZEN)	2.47	CUP
SQUASH, CAN, STOKLEY	1.85	CUP
SQUASH, FRESH BAKED	1.63	CUP
TANGERINE	5	2.5 INCH
TOMATO, CAN	17.2	OZ
TOMATO, FRESH	7.1	3 INCH
TOMATO, JUICE	29.5	OZ
VEGETABLES, MIXED (FROZEN)	2.5	CUP
WATERMELLON	1.22	1X10 INCH
ZUCCHINI, FRESH, SLICED	10.3	CUP

Yogurts and Desserts

DING DONG	1.16	DING
DREYERS FROZEN FAT FREE YOGURT	1.03	CUP
FRUIT ROLL-UP	2.65	ROLL-UP
POPCORN, WHITE	3.7	TBLSP
TCBY, SOFT SERVE/NONFAT/NO SUGAR	1.16	CUP
YOGURT, FAT FREE, MOUNTAIN HIGH	8	OZ
YOGURT, FAT FREE, DANNON	8	OZ
LUCERN, YOGURT, NONFAT, LITE	8	OZ

YOGURT, YOPLAIT, FAT FREE, LITE	6	OZ
YOGURT,YOPLAIT ORIGINAL/99% FAT FREE	6	OZ
YOGURT, HORIZON, FF / BLUEBERRY	6	OZ
PLANTER DRIED WALNUT PIECES	0.2	CUP
RAW ALMONDS, TOASTED	1	OZ
PECANS, DRIED	0.88	OZ
PEANUTS, DRY ROASTED	0.2	CUP
HOT CHOCOLATE	3	ENVEL.
ALMONDS, SHELLED	1	OZ

Cereals

CEREAL, CHEERIOS	1.69	CUP
CEREAL, COCOA KRISPIES	1.16	CUP
CEREAL, GRAPENUTS	0.462	CUP
CEREAL, HONEY NUT TOASTY O'S	1.68	CUP
CEREAL, WHEATIES	1.68	CUP
CEREAL, KELLOGG'S ALL BRAN	1.16	CUP
CEREAL, KELLOGG'S CORN FLAKES	1.68	CUP
CEREAL, KELLOGG'S RAISEN BRAN	1.09	CUP
CEREAL, KELLOGG'S CRACKLIN' OAT BRAN	0.7	CUP
CEREAL, NABISCO SHREDDED WHEAT	2.32	PIECE
CEREAL, NAB. SHREDDED WHEAT (SPOON)	1.09	CUP
CEREAL, RICE KRISPIES	2.1	CUP
CEREAL, BENEFIT NUTRITION, PROTEIN +	0.88	CUP
CREAM OF WHEAT	4.63	TBL/DRY
GRANOLA, CW POST HEARTY	0.44	CUP
GRANOLA, KELLOGG'S LOW FAT	3	CUP
OATMEAL (PRE-COOK MEASUREMENT)	0.66	CUP

Breads

BREAD, OROWHEAT LITE	4.63	SLICE
BREAD, SUSAN'S HOMEMADE/18 SLICES	2.05	SLICE
BREAD, SUSAN'S HOMEMADE	0.113	LOAF
BUN, WONDER REDUCED CALORIE LITE	2.31	BUN
CRACKER, ZESTA SALTINES	5.15	CRACKER
TORTILLA (CAROLYN)	1.09	TORT
TORTILLA, TORTILLA'S MEXICO, FLOUR	1.68	TORT

TORTILLA, TORTILLA'S MEXICO, CORN	2.06	TORT
TRISCUITS	1.32	OZ
WAFFLE, EGGO, HOMESTYLE	1.69	WAFFLE
WHOLE GRAIN/WHOLE WHEAT FLOUR	0.455	CUP

Rice/Potatoes/Beans

BLACK BEANS (BOILED)	0.82	CUP
BLACK BEANS (DRY)	0.66	CUP
CHICKPEAS / GARBANZO BEANS	0.22	CUP
KIDNEY BEANS (BOILED)	0.25	CUP
LIMA BEANS (BOILED)	0.89	CUP
NAVY BEANS (BOILED)	0.72	CUP
NAVY BEANS (CAN)	0.77	CUP
PINTO BEANS (BOILED)	0.79	CUP
PINTO BEANS (CAN)	0.975	CUP
PINTO BEANS (DRY)	0.309	CUP
PORK & BEANS / VAN CAMPS	0.84	CUP
POTATO, SWEET	1.57	5"X2"
POTATO	11	OZ
RICE CAKE	3.7	CAKE
RICE, WHITE, BASMATI	0.772	CUP (C)
RICE, BROWN LONG GRAIN	0.925	CUP (C)
RICE, INSTANT, MINUTE BRAND	0.58	CUP(UC)
RICE, WHITE, LONG GRAIN	0.29	CUP(UC)
SOYBEANS (BOILED)	0.75	CUP
YAM, BOILED OR BAKED	1.17	CUP

Pasta

MACARONI, DAVINI TWIST	0.7	CUP/DRY
MACARONI, HOSPITALITY ELBOW	0.385	CUP/DRY
MACARONI, AM. BEAUTY ELBOW	0.44	CUP/DRY
PASTA, CREAMETTE PLAIN	1.77	OZ
SPAGHETTI, EDEN WHOLE WHEAT	1.76	OZ/UC

Protein Sources 2000 Calories

White Meat

CHICKEN BREAST (HORMEL/CAN)	1.23	CAN
CHICKEN BREAST (SKINLESS)	6.18	OZ
CHICKEN (LEG W/ SKIN & BONE)	0.7	
CHICKEN (THIGH W/ SKIN & BONE)	1.21	
CHICKEN (LEG & THIGH W/ SKIN & BONE)	0.443	
HAM, BAR S, XTRA LEAN, 96% FAT FREE	5.3	OZ
HAM, DAK CAN	6.15	OZ
PORK, SIRLOIN, LEAN W/ FAT	1.85	OZ
TURKEY BREAST (SKINLESS)	3.47	OZ
TURKEY BREAST (HORMEL/CAN)	1.06	CAN
TURKEY BRST/OVEN ROAST/SFWY/89% FF	7.4	OZ
VENISON / ANTELOPE	4.15	OZ

Red Meat

HAMBURGER(10% FAT)	3.3	OZ
HAMBURGER(15% FAT)	2.73	OZ
HAMBURGER(20% FAT)	2.65	OZ
HAMBURGER(27% FAT)	2.24	OZ
LAMB, SHOULDER	2.1	OZ
STEAK, BOTTOM ROUND	3.13	OZ
STEAK, BRISKET (FLAT HALF)	2.95	OZ
STEAK, CHUCK, ARM	3.04	OZ
STEAK, CHUCK, BLADE	2.6	OZ
STEAK, EYE ROUND	3.9	OZ
STEAK, FLANK	3.16	OZ
STEAK, NEW YORK STRIP	3.7	OZ
STEAK, PORTERHOUSE	3	OZ
STEAK, RIBEYE	2.91	OZ
STEAK, ROUND TIP	3.55	OZ
STEAK, SHANK (CROSSCUTS)	3.25	OZ
STEAK, T-BONE	3.05	OZ
STEAK, TENDERLOIN	3.1	OZ
STEAK, TOP LOIN	3.15	OZ
STEAK, TOP ROUND	3.64	OZ

STEAK, TOP SIRLOIN	3.38	OZ
STEAK, TYSON SEASONED BEEF STRIPS	3.95	OZ
TACO/BURRITO MEAT/SMART GROUND	0.96	CUP
OSCAR MAYER BACON	6.15	SLICE
LITTLE SIZZLER BROWN/SERVE SAUSAGE	2.4	LINK

Sea Food

BASS, FRESHWATER, DRY HEAT	4.5	OZ
BASS, STRIPED, DRY HEAT	5.3	OZ
COD, ATLANTIC, DRY HEAT	6.25	OZ
CRAB, ALASKA KING, MOIST HEAT	6.8	OZ
CRAB, BLUE, MOIST HEAT	6.4	OZ
FLOUNDER, DRY HEAT	5.6	OZ
HADDOCK, DRY HEAT	5.85	OZ
HALIBUT, DRY HEAT	4.67	OZ
LOBSTER, NORTHERN, MOIST HEAT	6.7	OZ
MAHI MAHI	7.6	OZ
ORANGE ROUGHY, DRY HEAT	7.33	OZ
PERCH, DRY HEAT	5.6	OZ
PERCH, OCEAN/ATLANTIC, DRY HEAT	5.4	OZ
SALMON, ATLANTIC, DRY HEAT	3.57	OZ
SHRIMP, MOIST HEAT	6.6	OZ
TROUT, DRY HEAT	3.45	OZ
TUNA BURGER, AHI / OMEGA FOODS	6.6	OZ
TUNA, LOW SODIUM, CAN	1.06	CAN
TUNA, WATER, CAN	1.23	CAN
TUNA, WHITE / LOW SALT, CAN (5 OZ)	1.06	CAN
TUNA, WHITE, CAN (5 OZ)	1.06	CAN
TUNA, FILLET/STEAK	4.2	OZ
WALLEYE, BAKED/BROILED/MICRO	5.5	OZ

Vegetarian

IVES VEG. COUSINE VEGGY DOG	3.08	DOG
SOY MILK (TRIS)	2	CUP
SOY MILK (SYLVIA)	1.75	CUP

Eggs/Dairy

1% COTTAGE CHEESE, NORDICA	1.16	CUP
2% COTTAGE CHEESE (LOW FAT)	0.925	CUP
COTTAGE CHEESE (LUCERNE FAT FREE)	1.16	CUP
COTT CHEESE MARIGOLD/DRY CURD	1.77	CUP
COTT CHEESE MARIGOLD/DRY CURD	28.3	TBLSP
COTT CHEESE BREAKSTONES FAT FREE	1.16	CUP
CHEDDER, SHREDDED, FAT FREE, KHF	1.03	CUP
CHEDDER, SHREDDED, 94% FAT FREE, HC	0.925	CUP
CHEESE, COLBY/MOZZARELLA	1.69	OZ
EGG WHITE	10.9	
EGG, WHOLE	2.46	
EGG BEATERS	1.54	CUP
MOZZARELLA SHREDDED, FAT FREE, KHF	0.92	CUP
SKIM MOZZARELLA STRING CHEESE	2.32	OZ

Free Carbs, Supplements, Fast Foods
2000 calories

Free Carbs

ASPARAGUS
BROCCOLI
CABBAGE
CAULIFLOWER
CELERY
CUCUMBER
GREEN BEANS
GREEN PEPPERS
GREEN SQUASH
LETTUCE, ICEBERG
LETTUCE, LEAF/SHREDDED
MUSHROOMS
ONION
PICKLES (DILL)
RADISH

RED PEPPERS
SPINACH (CAN/NO SALT)
SPINACH (FRESH)
TOMATO (EXCLUDING JUICE)
ZUCCHINI

Supplements/Fast Foods

ATKINS BAR	0.75	BAR
EAS ADVANTEDGE, C&C/LEM/BLUE	0.75	BAR
BAR, ZONE	0.75	BAR
BAR, PURE PROTEIN, 50 G.	1	BAR
BAR, W.W. PURE PROTEIN, 78 G.	0.5	BAR
BAR, PROTEIN REVOLUTION, PBJ	0.75	BAR
BAR, FIBAR, PEANUT BUTTER, 1.2 OZ	1.25	BAR
BAR, PREMIER 1, PROTEIN 8, CHOC/COCO	0.5	BAR
BAR, PREFERRED BAR, CHOC./FUDG/RAS	0.75	BAR
BAR, PREFERRED BAR, CHOC./FUDG/BROW	0.75	BAR
ALIVE, HI CARB POWDER	1	TBLSP
POWERADE	2	SERVING
PROTEIN,GNC P.P. EGG/WHEY	1.5	SERVING
PROTEIN. GNC P.PERF. WHEY	4	SCOOP
OPTIMUM NUTRITION WHEY	1.5	SCOOP
SYNTRAX WHEY PROTEIN	2	SCOOP
TRI PROTEIN PLUS POWDER	1.25	SERVING
HW STRAWBERRY PROT. POWD.	1.75	SCOOP
BIOCHEM WHEY PRO 290	2.25	SCOOP
HUMAN DEV. TECH. WHEY	1.25	SCOOP
NATURADE 100% SOY PROTEIN	0.5	CUP
SUPER GREEN PRO 96 - SOY	0.5	CUP
100% PURE WHEY, PROLAB	1.25	SCOOP
ECLIPSE BULK UP WHEY	1.75	SCOOP
VITAMIN WORLD WHEY 100%	1.5	SCOOP
ULT. NUT. PROSTAR WHEY	1.5	SCOOP
RED WINE	7	OZ
MET RX CH.RST.PNT.PRO + BAR	0.5	BAR
MET RX BAV. MINT. PRO + BAR	0.75	BAR
MET AFTER FX BAR	0.75	BAR
MET RX CH. CH. CHIP PRO + BAR	0.5	BAR

MET RX SOURCE ONE BAR	0.75	BAR
MET RX CHOC. GRAHCRK CHIP BAR	0.5	BAR
MET RX PEANUT BUTTER BAR	0.5	BAR
MET RX DRINK MIX, MRP	0.75	SERVING
MET RX PRO 50, ANABOLIC DRIVE	0.5	SERVING
MET RX PRO 60, ANABOLIC DRIVE	0.5	SERVING
MET RX PROTEIN PLUS	2.25	SCOOP
MET RX KETO PRO	2.25	SCOOP
NUTRI FORCE DRINK MIX, MRP	0.5	SERVING
EAS MYO. DEL. CH/PB BAR	0.5	BAR
EAS MYOPLEX + DELUXE	0.5	SERVING
EAS MYOPLEX LITE	0.75	SERVING
ADVANT EDGE QUICK STIR PROTEIN DRINK	0.75	SERVING
EAS NEUROGAIN	1	SCOOP
EAS PHOSPHAGEN HP	1.25	SCOOP
EAS PRECISION PROTEIN	1.75	SCOOP
EAS SIMPLY PROTEIN	3	SCOOP
EAS WHEY PROTEIN	1.5	SCOOP
EAS SUPPER SHAKE	0.33	SHAKE
VITAMIN WORLD DAILY RX, MRP	0.5	SHAKE
VITAMIN WORLD PROTOPLEX DELUXE, MRP	0.5	SHAKE
VITAMIN WORLD PRE. ENG. WHEY PROT.	1.75	SCOOP
PERFECT RX, MRP, CHOCOLATE	0.75	SHAKE
OPTI PRO	0.5	SHAKE
ARBY'S CHICK. SAND. R.DELX.LITE	0.5	BURGER
ARBY'S SIDE SALAD	1	SALAD
ARBY'S GARDEN SALAD	1	SALAD
ARBY'S RST. CHCK. SALAD	1	SALAD
ARBY'S RED. CAL. ITAL. DRESSING	1	PACKET
ARBY'S RED RANCH DRESSING	1	PACKET
MCD'S VINEG. LITE SALAD DR.	1	PACKET
MCD'S GARDEN SALAD	1	SALAD
MCD'S VINEG. LITE SALAD DR.	1	PACKET
P.HUT. HAND-TOSS CHEESE	0.5	SLICE
P.HUT. HAND-TOSS HAM	0.75	SLICE
P.HUT. HAND-TOSS VEG. LUV.	0.75	SLICE
P.HUT. HAND-TOSS PEPPERON	0.75	SLICE
P.HUT. THIN/CRISP CHEESE	0.75	SLICE

P.HUT. THIN/CRISP HAM	1	SLICE
P.HUT. THIN/CRISP VEG. LUV.	1	SLICE
P.HUT. THIN/CRISP PEPPERON	0.75	SLICE
SW 6" COLD SUB/VEGG. DELIT	1	SUB
SW 6" COLD SUB/TURK. BRST.	1	SUB
SW 6" COLD SUB/TURK.B/HAM	1	SUB
SW 6" COLD SUB/HAM	1	SUB
SW 6" COLD SUB/ROAST BEEF	1	SUB
SW 6" COLD SUB/SFOOD,CRAB	1	SUB
SW 6" COLD SUB/COLD CUT 3	1	SUB
SW 6" COLD SUB/TUNA	1	SUB
SW 6" HOT SUB/RST.CHICK.BR.	1	SUB
SW 6" HOT SUB/STAK/CHEESE	1	SUB
SW 6" HOT SUB/SUB MELT	1	SUB
SW VEGGIE DELITE SALAD	1	SALAD
SW TURKEY BREAST SALAD	1	SALAD
SW ROAST BEEF SALAD	1	SALAD
SW TURK. BRST/HAM SALAD	1	SALAD
SW RST. CHICK. BR. SALAD	0.75	SALAD
SW SEAFOOD/CRAB SALAD	0.75	SALAD
SW STEAK/CHEESE SALAD	0.75	SALAD
SW SUBWAY MELT SALAD	0.75	SALAD
SW COLD CUT 3 SALAD	0.75	SALAD
SW FAT FREE ITALIAN DRESS	1	OZ
SW FAT FREE FRENCH DRESS	1	OZ
SW FAT FREE RANCH DRESS	1	OZ
SW DELI STYLE TURKEY BR.	0.75	SNDWCH
SW DELI STYLE HAM	0.75	SNDWCH
SW DELI STYLE ROAST BEEF	0.75	SNDWCH
TB GRILLED STEAK SOFT TACO	0.75	TACO
WAHOO'S CHBROIL FISH TACO	0.5	TACO
WENDI'S SIDE SALAD	1	SALAD
WENDI'S FF FRENCH DRESSING	1	OZ
WENDI'S ITALIAN RED. F/C DRESS	1	OZ
WENDI'S SMALL CHILI	0.75	BOWL
WENDI'S GRILLED CHICK. FILLET	1	MEAT

2100 Calories/Day Eating Plan	
What Does Your Doctor Look Like Naked?	
Name: _____	
Date: _____	

Exercise: 30-40 min in a.m. before food		Write what you eat here:
Meal 1 Time: _____	2 Protein Source 2 Active Carbohydrates	
Meal 2 Time: _____	1.5 oz Raw Almonds	
Meal 3 Time: _____	1 Protein Source 2 Active Carbohydrates Free Carbohydrates (as much as you want)	
Meal 4 Time: _____	1 LOW CARB protein bar (OR) 2 scoops Whey Protein Powder in water	
Meal 5 Time: _____	1 Protein Source 0 Active Carbohydrates Free Carbohydrates (as much as you want)	
BEDTIME Meal (Optional)	Sugar Free Jell-O 1 cup	

Add fiber supplement in evening, such as Metamucil or other (sugar FREE).
Add spices, pepper, etc. as needed.
Try to eat every two to three hours.
Drink 1¼ gallons of water EVERY DAY!
May have up to 2 diet pops (or) 2 cups a coffee a day.

Active Carbohydrates 2100 Calories

Fruit and Vegetables

APPLE	2.49	3 INCH
APPLESAUCE, MOTT'S	0.91	CUP
APRICOTS (CAN/DEL MONTE LITE)	1.68	CUP
APRICOTS (DRIED)	2.88	OZ
APRICOTS (FRESH 12/LB)	11.8	MEDIUM
ASPARAGUS	54.4	OZ
BANANA	1.92	MEDIUM
BLUEBERRIES (FRESH)	2.46	CUP
BRUSSELS SPROUTS, BOILED	3.35	CUP
CABBAGE, SHREDDED	11.2	CUP
CANTALOUPE	1.07	5 INCH
CARROT (FRESH)	18.1	OZ
CAULIFLOWER	7.75	CUP
CELERY	50	OZ
CHERRIES, FRESH, SWEET W/PIT	1.94	CUP
CHERRIES, DARK (CAN/DEL MONTE)	1	CUP
COLLARD GREENS (CAN)	3.36	CUP
COLLARD GREENS (FRESH)	16.8	CUP
CORN CAKE	5.75	CAKE
CORN (CAN/DEL MONTE NO SODIUM)	14.7	OZ
CUCUMBER, SLICED	14.4	CUP
EGGPLANT	9.1	CUP
FRUIT, MIXED FROZEN	2.24	CUP
GARLIC, 1 CLOVE	50	CLOVE
GARLIC, TRIMMED	4.8	OZ
GRAPES	1.77	CUP
GRAPE JUICE/VERYFINE	10.7	OZ
GRAPEFRUIT	2.19	4 INCH
GREEN BEANS (CAN/DEL MONTE NO SALT)	5	CUP
GREEN PEPPER	10	MEDIUM
KIWI	13.5	OZ
MUSHROOMS, FRESH	11.2	CUP
ONION, FRESH/CHOPPED	3.36	CUP
ORANGE, NAVAL	3.1	3 INCH

ORANGE, JUICE	14.6	OZ
PAPAYA	1.72	LB.
PAPAYA, PEELED/CUBED	3.74	CUP
PEACH, FRESH, SLICED	2.72	CUP
PEACH (CAN/DEL MONTE EXTRA LITE)	1.68	CUP
PEARS (CAN)	6.7	HALF
PEAS, BLACKEYED (CAN)	1.12	CUP
PEAS (CAN/DEL MONTE NO SODIUM)	14.7	OZ
PEAS, GREEN GIANT FROZEN, SWEET	1.92	CUP
PEAS, EDIBLE-PODDED	3.35	CUP
PINEAPPLE, FRESH/DICED	2.58	CUP
PINEAPPLE, DEL MONTE SNACK CAN (LITE)	2.88	3.5 OZ
PINEAPPLE (CAN/DOLE LITE SYRUP)	11.88	SLICE
PRUNES, DOLE, DRIED	2.88	OZ
PUMPKIN (CAN)	4	CUP
RAISINS	0.42	CUP
RED PEPPER	10	MEDIUM
STRAWBERRIES (FRESH)	2.08	PINT
STRAWBERRIES (FROZEN)	2.69	CUP
SQUASH, CAN, STOKLEY	2	CUP
SQUASH, FRESH BAKED	1.77	CUP
TANGERINE	5.45	2.5 INCH
TOMATO, CAN	18.8	OZ
TOMATO, FRESH	7.7	3 INCH
TOMATO, JUICE	32	OZ
VEGETABLES, MIXED (FROZEN)	2.24	CUP
WATERMELLON	1.32	1X10 INCH
ZUCCHINI, FRESH, SLICED	11.2	CUP

Yogurts and Desserts

DING DONG	1.26	DING
DREYERS FROZEN FAT FREE YOGURT	1.12	CUP
FRUIT ROLL-UP	2.88	ROLL-UP
POPCORN, WHITE	4	TBLSP
TCBY, SOFT SERVE/NONFAT/NO SUGAR	1.26	CUP
YOGURT, FAT FREE, MOUNTAIN HIGH	8	OZ
YOGURT, FAT FREE, DANNON	8	OZ
LUCERN, YOGURT, NONFAT, LITE	8	OZ

YOGURT, YOPLAIT, FAT FREE, LITE	6	OZ
YOGURT, YOPLAIT ORIGINAL/99% FAT FREE	6	OZ
YOGURT, HORIZON, FF / BLUEBERRY	6	OZ
PLANTER DRIED WALNUT PIECES	0.25	CUP
RAW ALMONDS, TOASTED	1.19	OZ
PECANS, DRIED	1	OZ
PEANUTS, DRY ROASTED	0.2	CUP
HOT CHOCOLATE	4	ENVEL.
ALMONDS, SHELLED	1	OZ

Cereals

CEREAL, CHEERIOS	1.83	CUP
CEREAL, COCOA KRISPIES	1.26	CUP
CEREAL, GRAPENUTS	0.5	CUP
CEREAL, HONEY NUT TOASTY O'S	1.83	CUP
CEREAL, WHEATIES	1.83	CUP
CEREAL, KELLOGG'S ALL BRAN	1.26	CUP
CEREAL, KELLOGG'S CORN FLAKES	1.83	CUP
CEREAL, KELLOGG'S RAISIN BRAN	1.18	CUP
CEREAL, KELLOGG'S CRACKLIN' OAT BRAN	0.76	CUP
CEREAL, NABISCO SHREDDED WHEAT	2.5	PIECE
CEREAL, NAB. SHREDDED WHEAT (SPOON)	1.18	CUP
CEREAL, RICE KRISPIES	2.29	CUP
CEREAL, BENEFIT NUTRITION, PROTEIN +	0.96	CUP
CREAM OF WHEAT	5	TBL/DRY
GRANOLA, CW POST HEARTY	0.48	CUP
GRANOLA, KELLOGG'S LOW FAT	4	CUP
OATMEAL (PRE-COOK MEASUREMENT)	0.72	CUP

Breads

BREAD, OROWHEAT LITE	5	SLICE
BREAD, SUSAN'S HOMEMADE/18 SLICES	2.22	SLICE
BREAD, SUSAN'S HOMEMADE	0.123	LOAF
BUN, WONDER REDUCED CALORIE LITE	2.5	BUN
CRACKER, ZESTA SALTINES	16.8	CRACKER
TORTILLA (CAROLYN)	1.18	TORT
TORTILLA, TORTILLA'S MEXICO, FLOUR	1.83	TORT

TORTILLA, TORTILLA'S MEXICO, CORN	2.24	TORT
TRISCUITS	1.44	OZ
WAFFLE, EGGO, HOMESTYLE	1.83	WAFFLE
WHOLE GRAIN/WHOLE WHEAT FLOUR	0.495	CUP

Rice/Potatoes/Beans

BLACK BEANS (BOILED)	0.89	CUP
BLACK BEANS (DRY)	0.72	CUP
CHICKPEAS/GARBANZO BEANS	0.25	CUP
KIDNEY BEANS (BOILED)	0.25	CUP
LIMA BEANS (BOILED)	0.568	CUP
NAVY BEANS (BOILED)	0.78	CUP
NAVY BEANS (CAN)	0.838	CUP
PINTO BEANS (BOILED)	0.86	CUP
PINTO BEANS (CAN)	1.06	CUP
PINTO BEANS (DRY)	0.335	CUP
PORK & BEANS/VAN CAMPS	0.91	CUP
POTATO, SWEET	1.71	5"X2"
POTATO	12	OZ
RICE CAKE	4	CAKE
RICE, WHITE, BASMATI	0.84	CUP (C)
RICE, BROWN LONG GRAIN	1	CUP (C)
RICE, INSTANT, MINUTE BRAND	0.63	CUP(UC)
RICE, WHITE, LONG GRAIN	0.315	CUP(UC)
SOYBEANS (BOILED)	0.75	CUP
YAM, BOILED OR BAKED	1.27	CUP

Pasta

MACARONI, DAVINI TWIST	0.765	CUP/DRY
MACARONI, HOSPITALITY ELBOW	0.42	CUP/DRY
MACARONI, AM. BEAUTY ELBOW	0.48	CUP/DRY
PASTA, CREAMETTE PLAIN	1.92	OZ
SPAGHETTI, EDEN WHOLE WHEAT	1.92	OZ/UC

Protein Sources 2100 Calories

White Meat

CHICKEN BREAST (HORMEL/CAN)	1.34	CAN
CHICKEN BREAST (SKINLESS)	6.7	OZ
CHICKEN (LEG W/SKIN & BONE)	0.76	
CHICKEN (THIGH W/SKIN & BONE)	1.32	
CHICKEN (LEG & THIGH W/SKIN & BONE)	0.48	
HAM, BAR S, XTRA LEAN, 96% FAT FREE	5.75	OZ
HAM, DAK CAN	6.7	OZ
PORK, SIRLOIN, LEAN W/FAT	2	OZ
TURKEY BREAST (SKINLESS)	3.76	OZ
TURKEY BREAST (HORMEL/CAN)	1.15	CAN
TURKEY BRST/OVEN ROAST/SFWY/89% FF	8	OZ
VENISON/ANTELOPE	4.5	OZ

Red Meat

HAMBURGER (10% FAT)	3.58	OZ
HAMBURGER (15% FAT)	2.96	OZ
HAMBURGER (20% FAT)	2.88	OZ
HAMBURGER (27% FAT)	2.44	OZ
LAMB, SHOULDER	2.29	OZ
STEAK, BOTTOM ROUND	3.4	OZ
STEAK, BRISKET (FLAT HALF)	3.2	OZ
STEAK, CHUCK, ARM	3.3	OZ
STEAK, CHUCK, BLADE	2.84	OZ
STEAK, EYE ROUND	4.22	OZ
STEAK, FLANK	3.44	OZ
STEAK, NEW YORK STRIP	4	OZ
STEAK, PORTERHOUSE	3.27	OZ
STEAK, RIBEYE	3.16	OZ
STEAK, ROUND TIP	3.85	OZ
STEAK, SHANK (CROSSCUTS)	3.53	OZ
STEAK, T-BONE	3.32	OZ
STEAK, TENDERLOIN	3.38	OZ
STEAK, TOP LOIN	3.44	OZ
STEAK, TOP ROUND	3.95	OZ

STEAK, TOP SIRLOIN	3.67	OZ
STEAK, TYSON SEASONED BEEF STRIPS	4.3	OZ
TACO/BURRITO MEAT/SMART GROUND	1.05	CUP
OSCAR MAYER BACON	6.7	SLICE
LITTLE SIZZLER BROWN/SERVE SAUSAGE	2.62	LINK

Sea Food

BASS, FRESHWATER, DRY HEAT	4.9	OZ
BASS, STRIPED, DRY HEAT	5.75	OZ
COD, ATLANTIC, DRY HEAT	6.8	OZ
CRAB, ALASKA KING, MOIST HEAT	7.38	OZ
CRAB, BLUE, MOIST HEAT	6.95	OZ
FLOUNDER, DRY HEAT	6.1	OZ
HADDOCK, DRY HEAT	6.35	OZ
HALIBUT, DRY HEAT	5.08	OZ
LOBSTER, NORTHERN, MOIST HEAT	7.3	OZ
MAHI MAHI	8.3	OZ
ORANGE ROUGHY, DRY HEAT	7.9	OZ
PERCH, DRY HEAT	6.1	OZ
PERCH, OCEAN/ATLANTIC, DRY HEAT	5.86	OZ
SALMON, ATLANTIC, DRY HEAT	3.87	OZ
SHRIMP, MOIST HEAT	7.2	OZ
TROUT, DRY HEAT	3.75	OZ
TUNA BURGER, AHI / OMEGA FOODS	7.2	OZ
TUNA, LOW SODIUM, CAN	1.15	CAN
TUNA, WATER, CAN	1.34	CAN
TUNA, WHITE/NONFAT, CAN (5 OZ)	1.15	CAN
TUNA, WHITE, CAN (5 OZ)	1.15	CAN
TUNA, FILLET/STEAK	4.57	OZ
WALLEYE, BAKED/BROILED/MICRO	5.97	OZ

Vegetarian

IVES VEG. COUSINE VEGGY DOG	3.35	DOG
SOY MILK (TRIS)	2.25	CUP
SOY MILK (SYLVIA)	2	CUP

Eggs/Dairy

1% COTTAGE CHEESE, NORDICA	1.26	CUP
2% COTTAGE CHEESE (LOW FAT)	1	CUP
COTTAGE CHEESE (LUCERNE FAT FREE)	1.26	CUP
COTT CHEESE MARIGOLD/DRY CURD	1.92	CUP
COTT CHEESE MARIGOLD/DRY CURD	30.5	TBLSP
COTT CHEESE BREAKSTONES FAT FREE	1.26	CUP
CHEDDER, SHREDDED, FAT FREE, KHF	1.12	CUP
CHEDDER, SHREDDED, 94% FAT FREE, HC	1	CUP
CHEESE, COLBY/MOZZARELLA	1.83	OZ
EGG WHITE	11.8	
EGG, WHOLE	2.69	
EGG BEATERS	1.68	CUP
MOZZARELLA SHREDDED, FAT FREE, KHF	1	CUP
SKIM MOZZARELLA STRING CHEESE	2.5	OZ

Free Carbs, Supplements, Fast Foods
2100 calories

Free Carbs
ASPARAGUS
BROCCOLI
CABBAGE
CAULIFLOWER
CELERY
CUCUMBER
GREEN BEANS
GREEN PEPPERS
GREEN SQUASH
LETTUCE, ICEBERG
LETTUCE, LEAF/SHREDDED
MUSHROOMS
ONION
PICKLES (DILL)
RADISH

RED PEPPERS
SPINACH (CAN/NO SALT)
SPINACH (FRESH)
TOMATO (EXCLUDING JUICE)
ZUCCHINI

Supplements/Fast Foods

ATKINS BAR	0.75	BAR
EAS ADVANTEDGE, C&C/LEM/BLUE	0.75	BAR
BAR, ZONE	0.88	BAR
BAR, PURE PROTEIN, 50 G.	1	BAR
BAR, W.W. PURE PROTEIN, 78 G.	0.5	BAR
BAR, PROTEIN REVOLUTION, PBJ	0.88	BAR
BAR, FIBAR, PEANUT BUTTER, 1.2 OZ	1.33	BAR
BAR, PREMIER 1, PROTEIN 8, CHOC/COCO	0.75	BAR
BAR, PREFERRED BAR, CHOC./FUDG/RAS	0.88	BAR
BAR, PREFERRED BAR, CHOC./FUDG/BROW	0.88	BAR
ALIVE, HI CARB POWDER	5	TBLSP
POWERADE	2	SERVING
PROTEIN,GNC P.P. EGG/WHEY	1.5	SERVING
PROTEIN. GNC P.PERF. WHEY	4	SCOOP
OPTIMUM NUTRITION WHEY	1.75	SCOOP
SYNTRAX WHEY PROTEIN	2.25	SCOOP
TRI PROTEIN PLUS POWDER	1.5	SERVING
HW STRAWBERRY PROT. POWD.	2	SCOOP
BIOCHEM WHEY PRO 290	2.5	SCOOP
HUMAN DEV. TECH. WHEY	1.5	SCOOP
NATURADE 100% SOY PROTEIN	0.5	CUP
SUPER GREEN PRO 96 - SOY	0.5	CUP
100% PURE WHEY, PROLAB	0.75	SCOOP
ECLIPSE BULK UP WHEY	2	SCOOP
VITAMIN WORLD WHEY 100%	1.75	SCOOP
ULT. NUT. PROSTAR WHEY	1.75	SCOOP
RED WINE	8	OZ
MET RX CH.RST.PNT.PRO + BAR	0.5	BAR
MET RX BAV. MINT. PRO + BAR	0.75	BAR
MET AFTER FX BAR	0.75	BAR
MET RX CH. CH. CHIP PRO + BAR	0.75	BAR

MET RX SOURCE ONE BAR	0.75	BAR
MET RX CHOC. GRAHCRK CHIP BAR	0.5	BAR
MET RX PEANUT BUTTER BAR	0.5	BAR
MET RX DRINK MIX, MRP	0.75	SERVING
MET RX PRO 50, ANABOLIC DRIVE	0.75	SERVING
MET RX PRO 60, ANABOLIC DRIVE	0.5	SERVING
MET RX PROTEIN PLUS	2.5	SCOOP
MET RX KETO PRO	2.5	SCOOP
NUTRI FORCE DRINK MIX, MRP	0.75	SERVING
EAS MYO. DEL. CH/PB BAR	0.5	BAR
EAS MYOPLEX + DELUXE	0.5	SERVING
EAS MYOPLEX LITE	0.75	SERVING
ADVANT EDGE QUICK STIR PROTEIN DRINK	0.75	SERVING
EAS NEUROGAIN	4	SCOOP
EAS PHOSPHAGEN HP	1	SCOOP
EAS PRECISION PROTEIN	1.75	SCOOP
EAS SIMPLY PROTEIN	3	SCOOP
EAS WHEY PROTEIN	1.75	SCOOP
EAS SUPPER SHAKE	0.33	SHAKE
VITAMIN WORLD DAILY RX, MRP	0.75	SHAKE
VITAMIN WORLD PROTOPLEX DELUXE, MRP	0.5	SHAKE
VITAMIN WORLD PRE. ENG. WHEY PROT.	2	SCOOP
PERFECT RX, MRP, CHOCOLATE	0.75	SHAKE
OPTI PRO	0.75	SHAKE
ARBY'S CHICK. SAND. R.DELX.LITE	0.5	BURGER
ARBY'S SIDE SALAD	1	SALAD
ARBY'S GARDEN SALAD	1	SALAD
ARBY'S RST. CHCK. SALAD	1	SALAD
ARBY'S RED. CAL. ITAL. DRESSING	1	PACKET
ARBY'S RED RANCH DRESSING	1	PACKET
MCD'S VINEG. LITE SALAD DR.	1	PACKET
MCD'S GARDEN SALAD	1	SALAD
MCD'S VINEG. LITE SALAD DR.	1	PACKET
P.HUT. HAND-TOSS CHEESE	0.75	SLICE
P.HUT. HAND-TOSS HAM	0.75	SLICE
P.HUT. HAND-TOSS VEG. LUV.	0.75	SLICE
P.HUT. HAND-TOSS PEPPERON	0.75	SLICE
P.HUT. THIN/CRISP CHEESE	1	SLICE

P.HUT. THIN/CRISP HAM	1	SLICE
P.HUT. THIN/CRISP VEG. LUV.	1	SLICE
P.HUT. THIN/CRISP PEPPERON	0.75	SLICE
SW 6" COLD SUB/VEGG. DELIT	1	SUB
SW 6" COLD SUB/TURK. BRST.	1	SUB
SW 6" COLD SUB/TURK.B/HAM	1	SUB
SW 6" COLD SUB/HAM	1	SUB
SW 6" COLD SUB/ROAST BEEF	1	SUB
SW 6" COLD SUB/SFOOD,CRAB	1	SUB
SW 6" COLD SUB/COLD CUT 3	1	SUB
SW 6" COLD SUB/TUNA	1	SUB
SW 6" HOT SUB/RST.CHICK.BR.	1	SUB
SW 6" HOT SUB/STAK/CHEESE	1	SUB
SW 6" HOT SUB/SUB MELT	1	SUB
SW VEGGIE DELITE SALAD	1	SALAD
SW TURKEY BREAST SALAD	1	SALAD
SW ROAST BEEF SALAD	1	SALAD
SW TURK. BRST/HAM SALAD	1	SALAD
SW RST. CHICK. BR. SALAD	1	SALAD
SW SEAFOOD/CRAB SALAD	1	SALAD
SW STEAK/CHEESE SALAD	0.75	SALAD
SW SUBWAY MELT SALAD	1	SALAD
SW COLD CUT 3 SALAD	1	SALAD
SW FAT FREE ITALIAN DRESS	1	OZ
SW FAT FREE FRENCH DRESS	1	OZ
SW FAT FREE RANCH DRESS	1	OZ
SW DELI STYLE TURKEY BR.	0.75	SNDWCH
SW DELI STYLE HAM	0.75	SNDWCH
SW DELI STYLE ROAST BEEF	0.75	SNDWCH
TB GRILLED STEAK SOFT TACO	0.75	TACO
WAHOO'S CHBROIL FISH TACO	1	TACO
WENDI'S SIDE SALAD	1	SALAD
WENDI'S FF FRENCH DRESSING	1	OZ
WENDI'S ITALIAN RED. F/C DRESS	1	OZ
WENDI'S SMALL CHILI	1	BOWL
WENDI'S GRILLED CHICK. FILLET	1.5	MEAT

	2200 Calories/Day Eating Plan	
	What Does Your Doctor Look Like Naked?	

Name: _____

Date: _____

Exercise: 30-40 min in a.m. before food		
		Write what you eat here:
Meal 1 Time: _____	2 Protein Source 3 Active Carbohydrates	
Meal 2 Time: _____	1.5 oz Raw Almonds	
Meal 3 Time: _____	1 Protein Source 2 Active Carbohydrates Free Carbohydrates (as much as you want)	
Meal 4 Time: _____	1 LOW CARB protein bar (OR) 2 scoops Whey Protein Powder in water	
Meal 5 Time: _____	2 Protein Source 0 Active Carbohydrates Free Carbohydrates (as much as you want)	
Bedtime Meal (Optional)	Sugar Free Jell-O 1 cup	

Add fiber supplement in evening, such as Metamucil or other (sugar FREE).
Add spices, pepper, etc. as needed.
Try to eat every two to three hours.
Drink 1¼ gallons of water EVERY DAY!
May have up to 2 diet pops (or) 2 cups a coffee a day.

Active Carbohydrates 2200 Calories

Fruit and Vegetables

APPLE	2.08	3 INCH
APPLESAUCE, MOTT'S	0.76	CUP
APRICOTS (CAN/DEL MONTE LITE)	1.4	CUP
APRICOTS (DRIED)	2.4	OZ
APRICOTS (FRESH 12/LB)	9.9	MEDIUM
ASPARAGUS	45.5	OZ
BANANA	1.6	MEDIUM
BLUEBERRIES (FRESH)	2.05	CUP
BRUSSELS SPROUTS, BOILED	2.8	CUP
CABBAGE, SHREDDED	9.3	CUP
CANTALOUPE	0.9	5 INCH
CARROT (FRESH)	15.2	OZ
CAULIFLOWER	6.5	CUP
CELERY	42	OZ
CHERRIES, FRESH, SWEET W/PIT	1.62	CUP
CHERRIES, DARK (CAN/DEL MONTE)	0.84	CUP
COLLARD GREENS (CAN)	2.8	CUP
COLLARD GREENS (FRESH)	14	CUP
CORN CAKE	4.8	CAKE
CORN (CAN/DEL MONTE NO SODIUM)	12.3	OZ
CUCUMBER, SLICED	12	CUP
EGGPLANT	7.6	CUP
FRUIT, MIXED FROZEN	1.86	CUP
GARLIC, 1 CLOVE	42	CLOVE
GARLIC, TRIMMED	4	OZ
GRAPES	1.48	CUP
GRAPE JUICE/VERY FINE	9	OZ
GRAPEFRUIT	1.83	4 INCH
GREEN BEANS (CAN/DEL MONTE NO SALT)	4.2	CUP
GREEN PEPPER	8.4	MEDIUM
KIWI	11.4	OZ
MUSHROOMS, FRESH	9.4	CUP
ONION, FRESH/CHOPPED	2.81	CUP
ORANGE, NAVAL	2.6	3 INCH

ORANGE, JUICE	12.2	OZ
PAPAYA	1.44	LB.
PAPAYA, PEELED/CUBED	3.1	CUP
PEACH, FRESH, SLICED	2.28	CUP
PEACH (CAN/DEL MONTE EXTRA LITE)	1.4	CUP
PEARS (CAN)	5.6	HALF
PEAS, BLACKEYED (CAN)	0.93	CUP
PEAS (CAN/DEL MONTE NO SODIUM)	12.3	OZ
PEAS, GREEN GIANT FROZEN, SWEET	1.6	CUP
PEAS, EDIBLE-PODDED	2.8	CUP
PINEAPPLE, FRESH/DICED	2.15	CUP
PINEAPPLE, DEL MONTE SNACK CAN (LITE)	2.4	3.5 OZ
PINEAPPLE (CAN/DOLE LITE SYRUP)	9.9	SLICE
PRUNES, DOLE, DRIED	2.4	OZ
PUMPKIN (CAN)	3.35	CUP
RAISINS	0.35	CUP
RED PEPPER	8.4	MEDIUM
STRAWBERRIES (FRESH)	1.75	PINT
STRAWBERRIES (FROZEN)	2.25	CUP
SQUASH, CAN, STOKLEY	1.68	CUP
SQUASH, FRESH BAKED	1.48	CUP
TANGERINE	4.55	2.5 INCH
TOMATO (CAN)	15.7	OZ
TOMATO, FRESH	6.45	3 INCH
TOMATO, JUICE	27	OZ
VEGETABLES, MIXED (FROZEN)	1.87	CUP
WATERMELLON	1.1	1X10 INCH
ZUCCHINI, FRESH, SLICED	9.3	CUP

Yogurts and Desserts

DING DONG	1.05	DING
DREYERS FROZEN FAT FREE YOGURT	0.9	CUP
FRUIT ROLL-UP	2.4	ROLL-UP
POPCORN, WHITE	3.35	TBLSP
TCBY, SOFT SERVE/NONFAT/NO SUGAR	1.05	CUP
YOGURT, FAT FREE, MOUNTAIN HIGH	8	OZ
YOGURT, FAT FREE, DANNON	8	OZ
LUCERN, YOGURT, NONFAT, LITE	8	OZ

YOGURT, YOPLAIT, FAT FREE, LITE	6	OZ
YOGURT,YOPLAIT ORIGINAL/99% FAT FREE	6	OZ
YOGURT, HORIZON, FF / BLUEBERRY	6	OZ
PLANTER DRIED WALNUT PIECES	0.2	CUP
RAW ALMONDS, TOASTED	1	OZ
PECANS, DRIED	0.88	OZ
PEANUTS, DRY ROASTED	0.2	CUP
HOT CHOCOLATE	3	ENVEL.
ALMONDS, SHELLED	1	OZ

Cereals

CEREAL, CHEERIOS	1.53	CUP
CEREAL, COCOA KRISPIES	1.05	CUP
CEREAL, GRAPENUTS	0.42	CUP
CEREAL, HONEY NUT TOASTY O'S	1.53	CUP
CEREAL, WHEATIES	1.53	CUP
CEREAL, KELLOGG'S ALL BRAN	1.05	CUP
CEREAL, KELLOGG'S CORN FLAKES	1.53	CUP
CEREAL, KELLOGG'S RAISIN BRAN	1	CUP
CEREAL, KELLOGG'S CRACKLIN' OAT BRAN	0.64	CUP
CEREAL, NABISCO SHREDDED WHEAT	2.1	PIECE
CEREAL, NAB. SHREDDED WHEAT (SPOON)	0.99	CUP
CEREAL, RICE KRISPIES	1.9	CUP
CEREAL, BENEFIT NUTRITION, PROTEIN +	0.8	CUP
CREAM OF WHEAT	4.2	TBL/DRY
GRANOLA, CW POST HEARTY	0.4	CUP
GRANOLA, KELLOGG'S LOW FAT	2	CUP
OATMEAL (PRE-COOK MEASUREMENT)	0.6	CUP

Breads

BREAD, OROWHEAT LITE	2.95	SLICE
BREAD, SUSAN'S HOMEMADE/18 SLICES	1.31	SLICE
BREAD, SUSAN'S HOMEMADE	0.072	LOAF
BUN, WONDER REDUCED CALORIE LITE	1.48	BUN
CRACKER, ZESTA SALTINES	9.84	CRACKER
TORTILLA (CAROLYN)	0.695	TORT

TORTILLA, TORTILLA'S MEXICO, FLOUR	1.074	TORT
TORTILLA, TORTILLA'S MEXICO, CORN	1.31	TORT
TRISCUITS	1.2	OZ
WAFFLE, EGGO, HOMESTYLE	1.53	WAFFLE
WHOLE GRAIN/WHOLE WHEAT FLOUR	0.412	CUP

Rice/Potatoes/Beans

BLACK BEANS (BOILED)	0.74	CUP
BLACK BEANS (DRY)	0.6	CUP
CHICKPEAS/GARBANZO BEANS	0.22	CUP
KIDNEY BEANS (BOILED)	0.25	CUP
LIMA BEANS (BOILED)	0.81	CUP
NAVY BEANS (BOILED)	0.65	CUP
NAVY BEANS (CAN)	0.7	CUP
PINTO BEANS (BOILED)	0.72	CUP
PINTO BEANS (CAN)	0.88	CUP
PINTO BEANS (DRY)	0.28	CUP
PORK & BEANS (VAN CAMPS)	0.76	CUP
POTATO, SWEET	1.43	5"X2"
POTATO	10	OZ
RICE CAKE	3.35	CAKE
RICE, WHITE, BASMATI	0.7	CUP (C)
RICE, BROWN LONG GRAIN	0.84	CUP (C)
RICE, INSTANT, MINUTE BRAND	0.525	CUP(UC)
RICE, WHITE, LONG GRAIN	0.263	CUP(UC)
SOYBEANS (BOILED)	0.66	CUP
YAM, BOILED OR BAKED	1.06	CUP

Pasta

MACARONI, DAVINI TWIST	0.64	CUP/DRY
MACARONI, HOSPITALITY ELBOW	0.35	CUP/DRY
MACARONI, AM. BEAUTY ELBOW	0.4	CUP/DRY
PASTA, CREAMETTE PLAIN	1.6	OZ
SPAGHETTI, EDEN WHOLE WHEAT	1.6	OZ/UC

Protein Sources 2200 Calories

White Meat

CHICKEN BREAST (HORMEL/CAN)	1.12	CAN
CHICKEN BREAST (SKINLESS)	5.6	OZ
CHICKEN (LEG W/SKIN & BONE)	0.64	
CHICKEN (THIGH W/SKIN & BONE)	1.1	
CHICKEN (LEG & THIGH W/SKIN & BONE)	0.4	
HAM, BAR S, XTRA LEAN, 96% FAT FREE	4.25	OZ
HAM, DAK CAN	5.6	OZ
PORK, SIRLOIN, LEAN W/FAT	1.68	OZ
TURKEY BREAST (SKINLESS)	3.14	OZ
TURKEY BREAST (HORMEL/CAN)	0.96	CAN
TURKEY BRST/OVEN ROAST/SFWY/89% FF	6.7	OZ
VENISON/ANTELOPE	3.75	OZ

Red Meat

HAMBURGER (10% FAT)	3	OZ
HAMBURGER (15% FAT)	2.48	OZ
HAMBURGER (20% FAT)	2.4	OZ
HAMBURGER (27% FAT)	2.04	OZ
LAMB, SHOULDER	1.92	OZ
STEAK, BOTTOM ROUND	2.84	OZ
STEAK, BRISKET (FLAT HALF)	2.68	OZ
STEAK, CHUCK, ARM	2.77	OZ
STEAK, CHUCK, BLADE	2.38	OZ
STEAK, EYE ROUND	3.53	OZ
STEAK, FLANK	2.87	OZ
STEAK, NEW YORK STRIP	3.35	OZ
STEAK, PORTERHOUSE	2.74	OZ
STEAK, RIBEYE	2.65	OZ
STEAK, ROUND TIP	3.22	OZ
STEAK, SHANK (CROSSCUTS)	2.95	OZ
STEAK, T-BONE	2.8	OZ
STEAK, TENDERLOIN	2.83	OZ
STEAK, TOP LOIN	2.88	OZ
STEAK, TOP ROUND	3.3	OZ

STEAK, TOP SIRLOIN	3.06	OZ
STEAK, TYSON SEASONED BEEF STRIPS	3.6	OZ
TACO/BURRITO MEAT/SMART GROUND	0.88	CUP
OSCAR MAYER BACON	5.6	SLICE
LITTLE SIZZLER BROWN/SERVE SAUSAGE	2.2	LINK

Sea Food

BASS, FRESHWATER, DRY HEAT	4.08	OZ
BASS, STRIPED, DRY HEAT	4.8	OZ
COD, ATLANTIC, DRY HEAT	5.65	OZ
CRAB, ALASKA KING, MOIST HEAT	6.15	OZ
CRAB, BLUE, MOIST HEAT	5.8	OZ
FLOUNDER, DRY HEAT	5.1	OZ
HADDOCK, DRY HEAT	5.3	OZ
HALIBUT, DRY HEAT	4.25	OZ
LOBSTER, NORTHERN, MOIST HEAT	6.1	OZ
MAHI MAHI	6.9	OZ
ORANGE ROUGHY, DRY HEAT	6.6	OZ
PERCH, DRY HEAT	5.1	OZ
PERCH, OCEAN/ATLANTIC, DRY HEAT	4.9	OZ
SALMON, ATLANTIC, DRY HEAT	3.25	OZ
SHRIMP, MOIST HEAT	6	OZ
TROUT, DRY HEAT	3.1	OZ
TUNA BURGER, AHI/OMEGA FOODS	6	OZ
TUNA (CAN/LOW SODIUM	0.96	CAN
TUNA, WATER (CAN)	1.12	CAN
TUNA, WHITE (LOW SALT, 5 OZ)	0.96	CAN
TUNA, WHITE (5 OZ)	0.96	CAN
TUNA, FILLET/STEAK	3.8	OZ
WALLEYE, BAKED/BROILED/MICRO	5	OZ

Vegetarian

IVES VEG. COUSINE VEGGY DOG	2.8	DOG
SOY MILK (TRIS)	1.25	CUP
SOY MILK (SYLVIA)	1.15	CUP

Eggs/Dairy

1% COTTAGE CHEESE, NORDICA	1.05	CUP
2% COTTAGE CHEESE (LOW FAT)	0.84	CUP
COTTAGE CHEESE (LUCERNE FAT FREE)	1.05	CUP
COTT CHEESE MARIGOLD/DRY CURD	1.6	CUP
COTT CHEESE MARIGOLD/DRY CURD	25.7	TBLSP
COTT CHEESE BREAKSTONES FAT FREE	1.05	CUP
CHEDDER, SHREDDED, FAT FREE, KHF	0.93	CUP
CHEDDER, SHREDDED, 94% FAT FREE, HC	0.84	CUP
CHEESE, COLBY/MOZZARELLA	1.53	OZ
EGG WHITE	9.9	
EGG, WHOLE	2.25	
EGG BEATERS	1.4	CUP
MOZZARELLA SHREDDED, FAT FREE, KHF	0.84	CUP
SKIM MOZZARELLA STRING CHEESE	2.1	OZ

Free Carbs, Supplements, Fast Foods
2200 calories

Free Carbs

ASPARAGUS
BROCCOLI
CABBAGE
CAULIFLOWER
CELERY
CUCUMBER
GREEN BEANS
GREEN PEPPERS
GREEN SQUASH
LETTUCE, ICEBERG
LETTUCE, LEAF/SHREDDED
MUSHROOMS
ONION
PICKLES (DILL)

RADISH
RED PEPPERS
SPINACH (CAN/NO SALT)
SPINACH (FRESH)
TOMATO (EXCLUDING JUICE)
ZUCCHINI

Supplements/Fast Foods

ATKINS BAR	0.75	BAR
EAS ADVANTEDGE, C&C/LEM/BLUE	0.75	BAR
BAR, ZONE	0.75	BAR
BAR, PURE PROTEIN, 50 G.	0.75	BAR
BAR, W.W. PURE PROTEIN, 78 G.	0.5	BAR
BAR, PROTEIN REVOLUTION, PBJ	0.75	BAR
BAR, FIBAR, PEANUT BUTTER, 1.2 OZ	1	BAR
BAR, PREMIER 1, PROTEIN 8, CHOC/COCO	0.5	BAR
BAR, PREFERRED BAR, CHOC./FUDG/RAS	0.5	BAR
BAR, PREFERRED BAR, CHOC./FUDG/BROW	0.5	BAR
ALIVE, HI CARB POWDER	3	TBLSP
POWERADE	2	SERVING
PROTEIN,GNC P.P. EGG/WHEY	1.25	SERVING
PROTEIN. GNC P.PERF. WHEY	4	SCOOP
OPTIMUM NUTRITION WHEY	1.5	SCOOP
SYNTRAX WHEY PROTEIN	1.75	SCOOP
TRI PROTEIN PLUS POWDER	1	SERVING
HW STRAWBERRY PROT. POWD.	1.5	SCOOP
BIOCHEM WHEY PRO 290	2	SCOOP
HUMAN DEV. TECH. WHEY	1.25	SCOOP
NATURADE 100% SOY PROTEIN	0.5	CUP
SUPER GREEN PRO 96-SOY	0.5	CUP
100% PURE WHEY, PROLAB	1.25	SCOOP
ECLIPSE BULK UP WHEY	1.75	SCOOP
VITAMIN WORLD WHEY 100%	1.25	SCOOP
ULT. NUT. PROSTAR WHEY	1.25	SCOOP
RED WINE	6.5	OZ
MET RX CH.RST.PNT.PRO + BAR	0.5	BAR
MET RX BAV. MINT. PRO + BAR	0.5	BAR
MET AFTER FX BAR	0.5	BAR

MET RX CH. CH. CHIP PRO + BAR	0.5	BAR
MET RX SOURCE ONE BAR	0.55	BAR
MET RX CHOC. GRAHCRK CHIP BAR	0.5	BAR
MET RX PEANUT BUTTER BAR	0.5	BAR
MET RX DRINK MIX, MRP	0.5	SERVING
MET RX PRO 50, ANABOLIC DRIVE	0.5	SERVING
MET RX PRO 60, ANABOLIC DRIVE	0.5	SERVING
MET RX PROTEIN PLUS	2	SCOOP
MET RX KETO PRO	2	SCOOP
NUTRI FORCE DRINK MIX, MRP	0.5	SERVING
EAS MYO. DEL. CH/PB BAR	0.5	BAR
EAS MYOPLEX + DELUXE	0.5	SERVING
EAS MYOPLEX LITE	0.75	SERVING
ADVANT EDGE QUICK STIR PROTEIN DRINK	0.75	SERVING
EAS NEUROGAIN	3.5	SCOOP
EAS PHOSPHAGEN HP	1	SCOOP
EAS PRECISION PROTEIN	1.5	SCOOP
EAS SIMPLY PROTEIN	2.25	SCOOP
EAS WHEY PROTEIN	1.5	SCOOP
EAS SUPPER SHAKE	0.33	SHAKE
VITAMIN WORLD DAILY RX, MRP	0.5	SHAKE
VITAMIN WORLD PROTOPLEX DELUXE, MRP	0.5	SHAKE
VITAMIN WORLD PRE. ENG. WHEY PROT.	1.75	SCOOP
PERFECT RX, MRP, CHOCOLATE	0.5	SHAKE
OPTI PRO	0.5	SHAKE
ARBY'S CHICK. SAND. R.DELX.LITE	0.5	BURGER
ARBY'S SIDE SALAD	1	SALAD
ARBY'S GARDEN SALAD	1	SALAD
ARBY'S RST. CHCK. SALAD	1	SALAD
ARBY'S RED. CAL. ITAL. DRESSING	1	PACKET
ARBY'S RED RANCH DRESSING	1	PACKET
MCD'S VINEG. LITE SALAD DR.	1	PACKET
MCD'S GARDEN SALAD	1	SALAD
MCD'S VINEG. LITE SALAD DR.	1	PACKET
P.HUT. HAND-TOSS CHEESE	0.5	SLICE
P.HUT. HAND-TOSS HAM	0.75	SLICE
P.HUT. HAND-TOSS VEG. LUV.	0.75	SLICE
P.HUT. HAND-TOSS PEPPERON	0.5	SLICE

P.HUT. THIN/CRISP CHEESE	0.75	SLICE
P.HUT. THIN/CRISP HAM	0.75	SLICE
P.HUT. THIN/CRISP VEG. LUV.	0.75	SLICE
P.HUT. THIN/CRISP PEPPERON	0.75	SLICE
SW 6" COLD SUB/VEGG. DELIT	1	SUB
SW 6" COLD SUB/TURK. BRST.	1	SUB
SW 6" COLD SUB/TURK.B/HAM	1	SUB
SW 6" COLD SUB/HAM	1	SUB
SW 6" COLD SUB/ROAST BEEF	1	SUB
SW 6" COLD SUB/SFOOD,CRAB	1	SUB
SW 6" COLD SUB/COLD CUT 3	1	SUB
SW 6" COLD SUB/TUNA	1	SUB
SW 6" HOT SUB/RST.CHICK.BR.	1	SUB
SW 6" HOT SUB/STAK/CHEESE	1	SUB
SW 6" HOT SUB/SUB MELT	1	SUB
SW VEGGIE DELITE SALAD	1	SALAD
SW TURKEY BREAST SALAD	1	SALAD
SW ROAST BEEF SALAD	1	SALAD
SW TURK. BRST/HAM SALAD	1	SALAD
SW RST. CHICK. BR. SALAD	1	SALAD
SW SEAFOOD/CRAB SALAD	0.75	SALAD
SW STEAK/CHEESE SALAD	0.75	SALAD
SW SUBWAY MELT SALAD	0.75	SALAD
SW COLD CUT 3 SALAD	0.75	SALAD
SW FAT FREE ITALIAN DRESS	1	OZ
SW FAT FREE FRENCH DRESS	1	OZ
SW FAT FREE RANCH DRESS	1	OZ
SW DELI STYLE TURKEY BR.	0.5	SNDWCH
SW DELI STYLE HAM	0.5	SNDWCH
SW DELI STYLE ROAST BEEF	0.5	SNDWCH
TB GRILLED STEAK SOFT TACO	0.55	TACO
WAHOO'S CHBROIL FISH TACO	0.75	TACO
WENDI'S SIDE SALAD	1	SALAD
WENDI'S FF FRENCH DRESSING	1	OZ
WENDI'S ITALIAN RED. F/C DRESS	1	OZ
WENDI'S SMALL CHILI	0.75	BOWL
WENDI'S GRILLED CHICK. FILLET	1	MEAT

2300 Calories / Day Eating Plan		
What Does Your Doctor Look Like Naked?		

Name: _____

Date: _____

Exercise: 30 – 40 min in AM Before Food		Write what you eat here:
Meal 1 Time: _____	2 Protein Source 3 Active Carbohydrates	
Meal 2 Time:	2 oz Raw Almonds	
Meal 3 Time: _____	1 Protein Source 2 Active Carbohydrates Free Carbohydrates (as much as you want)	
Meal 4 Time:	1 LOW CARB protein bar	
Meal 5 Time: _____	2 Protein Source 0 Active Carbohydrates Free Carbohydrates (as much as you want)	
Bed Time Meal (Optional)	Sugar Free Jell-O 1 cup	

Add fiber supplement in evening such as Metamucil or other (sugar FREE).
Add spices, pepper, etc. as needed.
Try to eat every two to three hours
Drink 1 ¼ gallons of water EVERY DAY!
May have up to 2 diet pops (or) 2 cups a coffee a day

Active Carbohydrates 2300 Calories

Fruit and Vegetables

APPLE	2.08	3 INCH
APPLESAUCE, MOTT'S	0.76	CUP
APRICOTS (CAN/DEL MONTE LITE)	1.4	CUP
APRICOTS (DRIED)	2.4	OZ
APRICOTS (FRESH 12/LB)	9.9	MEDIUM
ASPARAGUS	45.5	OZ
BANANA	1.6	MEDIUM
BLUEBERRIES (FRESH)	2.05	CUP
BRUSSELS SPROUTS, BOILED	2.8	CUP
CABBAGE, SHREDDED	9.3	CUP
CANTALOUPE	0.9	5 INCH
CARROT (FRESH)	15.2	OZ
CAULIFLOWER	6.5	CUP
CELERY	42	OZ
CHERRIES, FRESH, SWEET W/PIT	1.62	CUP
CHERRIES, DARK, CAN, DEL MONTE	0.84	CUP
COLLARD GREENS (CANNED)	2.8	CUP
COLLARD GREENS (FRESH)	14	CUP
CORN CAKE	4.8	CAKE
CORN, CAN/NO SODIUM, DEL. MONTE	12.3	OZ
CUCUMBER, SLICED	12	CUP
EGGPLANT	7.6	CUP
FRUIT, MIXED FROZEN	1.86	CUP
GARLIC, 1 CLOVE	42	CLOVE
GARLIC, TRIMMED	4	OZ
GRAPES	1.48	CUP
GRAPEJIUCE/VERYFINE	9	OZ
GRAPEFRUIT	1.83	4 INCH
GREEN BEANS, DEL MONTE, CAN NO SALT	4.2	CUP
GREEN PEPPER	8.4	MEDIUM
KIWI	11.4	OZ
MUSHROOMS, FRESH	9.4	CUP
ONION, FRESH/CHOPPED	2.81	CUP
ORANGE, NAVAL	2.6	3 INCH

ORANGE, JUICE	12.2	OZ
PAPAYA	1.44	LB.
PAPAYA, PEELED/CUBED	3.1	CUP
PEACH, FRESH, SLICED	2.28	CUP
PEACH, CAN, DEL MONTE. EXTRA LITE	1.4	CUP
PEARS (CANNED)	5.6	HALF
PEAS, BLACK-EYED (CAN)	0.93	CUP
PEAS, CAN/NO SODIUM, DEL MONTE)	12.3	OZ
PEAS, GREEN GIANT FROZEN, SWEET	1.6	CUP
PEAS, EDIBLE-PODDED	2.8	CUP
PINEAPPLE, FRESH/DICED	2.15	CUP
PINEAPPLE, DEL MONTE SNACK CAN (LITE)	2.4	3.5 OZ
PINEAPPLE, DOLE CAN (LITE SYRUP)	9.9	SLICE
PRUNES, DOLE, DRIED	2.4	OZ
PUMPKIN (CANNED)	3.35	CUP
RAISENS	0.35	CUP
RED PEPPER	8.4	MEDIUM
STRAWBERRIES (FRESH)	1.75	PINT
STRAWBERRIES (FROZEN)	2.25	CUP
SQUASH, CAN, STOKLEY	1.68	CUP
SQUASH, FRESH BAKED	1.48	CUP
TANGERINE	4.55	2.5 INCH
TOMATO, CANNED	15.7	OZ
TOMATO, FRESH	6.45	3 INCH
TOMATO, JUICE	27	OZ
VEGETABLES, MIXED (FROZEN)	1.87	CUP
WATERMELLON	1.1	1X10 INCH
ZUCCHINI, FRESH, SLICED	9.3	CUP

Yogurts and Desserts

DING DONG	1.05	DING
DREYERS FROZEN FAT FREE YOGURT	0.9	CUP
FRUIT ROLL UP	2.4	ROLL UP
POPCORN, WHITE	3.35	TBLSP
TCBY, SOFT SERVE/NON FAT/NO SUGAR	1.05	CUP
YOGURT, FAT FREE, MOUNTAIN HIGH	8	OZ
YOGURT, FAT FREE, DANNON	8	OZ
LUCERN, YOGURT, NONFAT, LITE	8	OZ

YOGURT, YOPLAIT, FAT FREE, LITE	6	OZ
YOGURT, YOPLAIT ORIGINAL/99% FAT FREE	6	OZ
YOGURT, HORIZON, FF / BLUEBERRY	6	OZ
PLANTER DRIED WALNUT PIECES	0.2	CUP
RAW ALMONDS, TOASTED	1	OZ
PECANS, DRIED	0.88	OZ
PEANUTS, DRY ROASTED	0.2	CUP
HOT CHOCOLATE	3	ENVEL.
ALMONDS, SHELLED	1	OZ

Cereals

CEREAL, CHEERIOS	1.53	CUP
CEREAL, COCOA KRISPIES	1.05	CUP
CEREAL, GRAPENUTS	0.42	CUP
CEREAL, HONEY NUT TOASTY O'S	1.53	CUP
CEREAL, WHEATIES	1.53	CUP
CEREAL, KELLOGG'S ALL BRAN	1.05	CUP
CEREAL, KELLOGG'S CORN FLAKES	1.53	CUP
CEREAL, KELLOGG'S RAISEN BRAN	1	CUP
CEREAL, KELLOGG'S CRACKLIN' OAT BRAN	0.64	CUP
CEREAL, NABISCO SHREDDED WHEAT	2.1	PIECE
CEREAL, NAB. SHREDDED WHEAT (SPOON)	0.99	CUP
CEREAL, RICE KRISPIES	1.9	CUP
CEREAL, BENEFIT NUTRITION, PROTEIN +	0.8	CUP
CREAM OF WHEAT	4.2	TBL/DRY
GRANOLA, CW POST HEARTY	0.4	CUP
GRANOLA, KELLOGG'S LOW FAT	2	CUP
OATMEAL (PRE-COOK MEASUREMENT)	0.6	CUP

Breads

BREAD, OROWHEAT LITE	2.95	SLICE
BREAD, SUSAN'S HOMEMADE/18 SLICES	1.31	SLICE
BREAD, SUSAN'S HOMEMADE	0.072	LOAF
BUN, WONDER REDUCED CALORIE LITE	1.48	BUN
CRACKER, ZESTA SALTINES	9.84	CRACKER
TORTILLA, (CAROLYN)	0.695	TORT

TORTILLA, TORTILLA'S MEXICO, FLOUR	1.074	TORT
TORTILLA, TORTILLA'S MEXICO, CORN	1.31	TORT
TRISCUITS	1.2	OZ
WAFFLE, EGGO, HOMESTYLE	1.53	WAFFLE
WHOLE GRAIN/WHOLE WHEAT FLOUR	0.412	CUP

Rice/Potatoes/Beans

BLACK BEANS (BOILED)	0.74	CUP
BLACK BEANS (DRY)	0.6	CUP
CHICKPEAS / GARBANZO BEANS	0.22	CUP
KIDNEY BEANS (BOILED)	0.25	CUP
LIMA BEANS (BOILED)	0.81	CUP
NAVY BEANS (BOILED)	0.65	CUP
NAVY BEANS (CANNED)	0.7	CUP
PINTO BEANS (BOILED)	0.72	CUP
PINTO BEANS (CANNED)	0.88	CUP
PINTO BEANS (DRY)	0.28	CUP
PORK & BEANS / VAN CAMPS	0.76	CUP
POTATO, SWEET	1.43	5"X2"
POTATOE	10	OZ
RICE CAKE	3.35	CAKE
RICE, WHITE, BASMATI	0.7	CUP (C)
RICE, BROWN LONG GRAIN	0.84	CUP (C)
RICE, INSTANT, MINUTE BRAND	0.525	CUP(UC)
RICE, WHITE, LONG GRAIN	0.263	CUP(UC)
SOYBEANS (BOILED)	0.66	CUP
YAM, BOILED OR BAKED	1.06	CUP

Pasta

MACARONI, DAVINI TWIST	0.64	CUP/DRY
MACARONI, HOSPITALITY ELBOW	0.35	CUP/DRY
MACARONI, AM. BEAUTY ELBOW	0.4	CUP/DRY
PASTA, CREAMETTE PLAIN	1.6	OZ
SPAGHETTI, EDEN WHOLE WHEAT	1.6	OZ/UC

Protein Sources 2300 Calories

White Meat

CHICKEN BREAST (HORMEL/CAN)	1.12	CAN
CHICKEN BREAST (SKINLESS)	5.6	OZ
CHICKEN (LEG W/ SKIN & BONE)	0.64	
CHICKEN (THIGH W/ SKIN & BONE)	1.1	
CHICKEN (LEG & THIGH W/ SKIN & BONE)	0.4	
HAM, BAR S, XTRA LEAN, 96% FAT FREE	4.25	OZ
HAM, DAK CANNED	5.6	OZ
PORK, SIRLOIN, LEAN W/ FAT	1.68	OZ
TURKEY BREAST (SKINLESS)	3.14	OZ
TURKEY BREAST (HORMEL/CAN)	0.96	CAN
TURKEY BRST/OVEN ROAST/SFWY/89% FF	6.7	OZ
VENISON / ANTELOPE	3.75	OZ

Red Meat

HAMBURGER, (10 % FAT)	3	OZ
HAMBURGER, (15 % FAT)	2.48	OZ
HAMBURGER, (20 % FAT)	2.4	OZ
HAMBURGER, (27 % FAT)	2.04	OZ
LAMB, SHOULDER	1.92	OZ
STEAK, BOTTOM ROUND	2.84	OZ
STEAK, BRISKET (FLAT HALF)	2.68	OZ
STEAK, CHUCK, ARM	2.77	OZ
STEAK, CHUCK, BLADE	2.38	OZ
STEAK, EYE ROUND	3.53	OZ
STEAK, FLANK	2.87	OZ
STEAK, NEW YORK STRIP	3.35	OZ
STEAK, PORTERHOUSE	2.74	OZ
STEAK, RIB EYE	2.65	OZ
STEAK, ROUND TIP	3.22	OZ
STEAK, SHANK (CROSSCUTS)	2.95	OZ
STEAK, T-BONE	2.8	OZ
STEAK, TENDERLOIN	2.83	OZ
STEAK, TOP LOIN	2.88	OZ
STEAK, TOP ROUND	3.3	OZ

STEAK, TOP SIRLOIN	3.06	OZ
STEAK, TYSON SEASONED BEEF STRIPS	3.6	OZ
TACO/BURRITO MEAT/SMART GROUND	0.88	CUP
OSCAR MAYER BACON	5.6	SLICE
LITTLE SIZZLER BROWN/SERVE SAUSAGE	2.2	LINK

Sea Food

BASS, FRESHWATER, DRY HEAT	4.08	OZ
BASS, STRIPED, DRY HEAT	4.8	OZ
COD, ATLANTIC, DRY HEAT (DRY HEAT)	5.65	OZ
CRAB, ALASKA KING, MOIST HEAT	6.15	OZ
CRAB, BLUE, MOIST HEAT	5.8	OZ
FLOUNDER, DRY HEAT	5.1	OZ
HADDOCK, DRY HEAT	5.3	OZ
HALIBUT, DRY HEAT	4.25	OZ
LOBSTER, NORTHERN, MOIST HEAT	6.1	OZ
MAHI MAHI	6.9	OZ
ORANGE ROUGHY, DRY HEAT	6.6	OZ
PERCH, DRY HEAT	5.1	OZ
PERCH, OCEAN/ATLANTIC, DRY HEAT	4.9	OZ
SALMON, ATLANTIC, DRY HEAT	3.25	OZ
SHRIMP, MOIST HEAT	6	OZ
TROUT, DRY HEAT	3.1	OZ
TUNA BURGER, AHI / OMEGA FOODS	6	OZ
TUNA, LOW SODIUM, CANNED	0.96	CAN
TUNA, WATER, CANNED	1.12	CAN
TUNA, WHITE / LO SALT, CAN (1 CAN / 5 OZ)	0.96	CAN
TUNA, WHITE, CAN (1 CAN / 5 OZ)	0.96	CAN
TUNA, FILLET/STEAK	3.8	OZ
WALLEYE, BAKED/BROILED/MICRO	5	OZ

Vegetarian

IVES VEG. COUSINE VEGGY DOG	2.8	DOG
SOY MILK (TRIS)	1.25	CUP
SOY MILK (SYLVIA)	1.15	CUP

Eggs/Dairy

1 % COTTAGE CHEESE, NORDICA	1.05	CUP
2 % COTTAGE CHEESE (LOW FAT)	0.84	CUP
COTTAGE CHEESE (LUCERNE FAT FREE)	1.05	CUP
COTT CHEESE MARIGOLD/DRY CURD	1.6	CUP
COTT CHEESE MARIGOLD/DRY CURD	25.7	TBLSP
COTT CHEESE BREAKSTONES FAT FREE	1.05	CUP
CHEDDER, SHREDDED, FAT FREE, KHF	0.93	CUP
CHEDDER, SHREDDED, 94% FAT FREE, HC	0.84	CUP
CHEESE, COLBY/MOZZARELLA	1.53	OZ
EGG WHITE	9.9	
EGG, WHOLE	2.25	
EGG BEATERS	1.4	CUP
MOZZARELLA SHREDDED, FAT FREE, KHF	0.84	CUP
SKIM MOZZARELLA STRING CHEESE	2.1	OZ

Free Carbs, Supplements, Fast Foods
2300 calories

Free Carbs
ASPARAGUS
BROCCOLI
CABBAGE
CAULIFLOWER
CELERY
CUCUMBER
GREEN BEANS
GREEN PEPPERS
GREEN SQUASH
LETTUCE, ICEBERG
LETTUCE, LEAF/SHREDDED
MUSHROOMS
ONION
PICKLES (DILL)
RADISH

RED PEPPERS
SPINICH (CAN) NO SALT
SPINICH (FRESH)
TOMATO (EXCLUDING JUICE)
ZUCCHINI

Supplements/Fast Foods

ATKINS BAR	0.75	BAR
EAS ADVANTEDGE, C&C/LEM/BLUE	0.75	BAR
BAR, ZONE	0.75	BAR
BAR, PURE PROTEIN, 50 G.	0.75	BAR
BAR, W.W. PURE PROTEIN, 78 G.	0.5	BAR
BAR, PROTEIN REVOLUTION, PBJ	0.75	BAR
BAR, FIBAR, PEANUT BUTTER, 1.2 OZ	1	BAR
BAR, PREMIER 1, PROTEIN 8, CHOC/COCO	0.5	BAR
BAR, PREFERRED BAR, CHOC./FUDG/RAS	0.5	BAR
BAR, PREFERRED BAR, CHOC./FUDG/BROW	0.5	BAR
ALIVE, HI CARB POWDER	3	TBLSP
POWERADE	2	SERVING
PROTEIN,GNC P.P. EGG/WHEY	1.25	SERVING
PROTEIN. GNC P.PERF. WHEY	4	SCOOP
OPTIMUM NUTRITION WHEY	1.5	SCOOP
SYNTRAX WHEY PROTEIN	1.75	SCOOP
TRI PROTEIN PLUS POWDER	1	SERVING
HW STRAWBERRY PROT. POWD.	1.5	SCOOP
BIOCHEM WHEY PRO 290	2	SCOOP
HUMAN DEV. TECH. WHEY	1.25	SCOOP
NATURADE 100% SOY PROTEIN	0.5	CUP
SUPER GREEN PRO 96 - SOY	0.5	CUP
100% PURE WHEY, PROLAB	1.25	SCOOP
ECLIPSE BULK UP WHEY	1.75	SCOOP
VITAMIN WORLD WHEY 100%	1.25	SCOOP
ULT. NUT. PROSTAR WHEY	1.25	SCOOP
RED WINE	6.5	OZ
MET RX CH.RST.PNT.PRO + BAR	0.5	BAR
MET RX BAV. MINT. PRO + BAR	0.5	BAR
MET AFTER FX BAR	0.5	BAR
MET RX CH. CH. CHIP PRO + BAR	0.5	BAR

MET RX SOURCE ONE BAR	0.55	BAR
MET RX CHOC. GRAHCRK CHIP BAR	0.5	BAR
MET RX PEANUT BUTTER BAR	0.5	BAR
MET RX DRINK MIX, MRP	0.5	SERVING
MET RX PRO 50, ANABOLIC DRIVE	0.5	SERVING
MET RX PRO 60, ANABOLIC DRIVE	0.5	SERVING
MET RX PROTEIN PLUS	2	SCOOP
MET RX KETO PRO	2	SCOOP
NUTRI FORCE DRINK MIX, MRP	0.5	SERVING
EAS MYO. DEL. CH/PB BAR	0.5	BAR
EAS MYOPLEX + DELUXE	0.5	SERVING
EAS MYOPLEX LITE	0.75	SERVING
ADVANT EDGE QUICK STIR PROTEIN DRINK	0.75	SERVING
EAS NEUROGAIN	3.5	SCOOP
EAS PHOSPHAGEN HP	1	SCOOP
EAS PRECISION PROTEIN	1.5	SCOOP
EAS SIMPLY PROTEIN	2.25	SCOOP
EAS WHEY PROTEIN	1.5	SCOOP
EAS SUPPER SHAKE	0.33	SHAKE
VITAMIN WORLD DAILY RX, MRP	0.5	SHAKE
VITAMIN WORLD PROTOPLEX DELUXE, MRP	0.5	SHAKE
VITAMIN WORLD PRE. ENG. WHEY PROT.	1.75	SCOOP
PERFECT RX, MRP, CHOCOLATE	0.5	SHAKE
OPTI PRO	0.5	SHAKE
ARBY'S CHICK. SAND. R.DELX.LITE	0.5	BURGER
ARBY'S SIDE SALAD	1	SALAD
ARBY'S GARDEN SALAD	1	SALAD
ARBY'S RST. CHCK. SALAD	1	SALAD
ARBY'S RED. CAL. ITAL. DRESSING	1	PACKET
ARBY'S RED RANCH DRESSING	1	PACKET
MCD'S VINEG. LITE SALAD DR.	1	PACKET
MCD'S GARDEN SALAD	1	SALAD
MCD'S VINEG. LITE SALAD DR.	1	PACKET
P.HUT. HAND TOSS CHEESE	0.5	SLICE
P.HUT. HAND TOSS HAM	0.75	SLICE
P.HUT. HAND TOSS VEG. LUV.	0.75	SLICE
P.HUT. HAND TOSS PEPPERON	0.5	SLICE
P.HUT. THIN/CRISP CHEESE	0.75	SLICE

P.HUT. THIN/CRISP HAM	0.75	SLICE
P.HUT. THIN/CRISP VEG. LUV.	0.75	SLICE
P.HUT. THIN/CRISP PEPPERON	0.75	SLICE
SW 6" COLD SUB/VEGG. DELIT	1	SUB
SW 6" COLD SUB/TURK. BRST.	1	SUB
SW 6" COLD SUB/TURK.B/HAM	1	SUB
SW 6" COLD SUB/HAM	1	SUB
SW 6" COLD SUB/ROAST BEEF	1	SUB
SW 6" COLD SUB/SFOOD,CRAB	1	SUB
SW 6" COLD SUB/COLD CUT 3	1	SUB
SW 6" COLD SUB/TUNA	1	SUB
SW 6" HOT SUB/RST.CHICK.BR.	1	SUB
SW 6" HOT SUB/STAK/CHEESE	1	SUB
SW 6" HOT SUB/SUB MELT	1	SUB
SW VEGGIE DELITE SALAD	1	SALAD
SW TURKEY BREAST SALAD	1	SALAD
SW ROAST BEEF SALAD	1	SALAD
SW TURK. BRST/HAM SALAD	1	SALAD
SW RST. CHICK. BR. SALAD	1	SALAD
SW SEAFOOD/CRAB SALAD	0.75	SALAD
SW STEAK/CHEESE SALAD	0.75	SALAD
SW SUBWAY MELT SALAD	0.75	SALAD
SW COLD CUT 3 SALAD	0.75	SALAD
SW FAT FREE ITALIAN DRESS	1	OZ
SW FAT FREE FRENCH DRESS	1	OZ
SW FAT FREE RANCH DRESS	1	OZ
SW DELI STYLE TURKEY BR.	0.5	SNDWCH
SW DELI STYLE HAM	0.5	SNDWCH
SW DELI STYLE ROAST BEEF	0.5	SNDWCH
TB GRILLED STEAK SOFT TACO	0.55	TACO
WAHOO'S CHBROIL FISH TACO	0.75	TACO
WENDI'S SIDE SALAD	1	SALAD
WENDI'S FF FRENCH DRESSING	1	OZ
WENDI'S ITALIAN RED. F/C DRESS	1	OZ
WENDI'S SMALL CHILI	0.75	BOWL
WENDI'S GRILLED CHICK. FILLET	1	MEAT

2400 Calories/Day Eating Plan		
What Does Your Doctor Look Like Naked?		
Name: _____ Date: _____		
Exercise: 30-40 min in a.m. before food		Write what you eat here:
Meal 1 Time: _____	2 Protein Source 3 Active Carbohydrates	
Meal 2 Time: _____	2 oz Raw Almonds	
Meal 3 Time: _____	1 Protein Source 2 Active Carbohydrates Free Carbohydrates (as much as you want)	
Meal 4 Time: _____	1 LOW CARB protein bar (OR) 2 scoops Whey Protein Powder in water	
Meal 5 Time: _____	2 Protein Source 0 Active Carbohydrates Free Carbohydrates (as much as you want)	
BEDTIME Meal (Optional)	Sugar Free Jell-O 1 cup	
Add fiber supplement in evening, such as Metamucil or other (sugar FREE). Add spices, pepper, etc. as needed. Try to eat every two to three hours. Drink 1¼ gallons of water EVERY DAY! May have up to 2 diet pops (or) 2 cups a coffee a day.		

Active Carbohydrates 2400 Calories

Fruit and Vegetables

APPLE	2.29	3 INCH
APPLESAUCE, MOTT'S	0.84	CUP
APRICOTS (CAN/DEL MONTE LITE)	1.54	CUP
APRICOTS (DRIED)	2.65	OZ
APRICOTS (FRESH 12/LB)	10.9	MEDIUM
ASPARAGUS	50	OZ
BANANA	1.76	MEDIUM
BLUEBERRIES (FRESH)	2.26	CUP
BRUSSELS SPROUTS, BOILED	3.09	CUP
CABBAGE, SHREDDED	10.3	CUP
CANTALOUPE	0.98	5 INCH
CARROT (FRESH)	16.7	OZ
CAULIFLOWER	7.13	CUP
CELERY	46.3	OZ
CHERRIES, FRESH, SWEET W/PIT	1.78	CUP
CHERRIES, DARK (CAN/DEL MONTE)	0.925	CUP
COLLARD GREENS (CAN)	3.09	CUP
COLLARD GREENS (FRESH)	15.4	CUP
CORN CAKE	5.3	CAKE
CORN (CAN/DEL MONTE NO SODIUM)	13.5	OZ
CUCUMBER, SLICED	13.2	CUP
EGGPLANT	8.4	CUP
FRUIT, MIXED FROZEN	2.06	CUP
GARLIC, 1 CLOVE	46	CLOVE
GARLIC, TRIMMED	4.4	OZ
GRAPES	1.63	CUP
GRAPE JUICE/VERYFINE	9.9	OZ
GRAPEFRUIT	2.01	4 INCH
GREEN BEANS (CAN/DEL MONTE NO SALT)	4.61	CUP
GREEN PEPPER	9.25	MEDIUM
KIWI	12.5	OZ
MUSHROOMS, FRESH	10.3	CUP
ONION, FRESH/CHOPPED	3.09	CUP
ORANGE, NAVAL	2.85	3 INCH

ORANGE, JUICE	13.5	OZ
PAPAYA	1.585	LB.
PAPAYA, PEELED/CUBED	3.44	CUP
PEACH, FRESH, SLICED	2.5	CUP
PEACH (CAN/DEL MONTE EXTRA LITE)	1.54	CUP
PEARS (CAN)	6.15	HALF
PEAS, BLACKEYED (CAN)	1.03	CUP
PEAS (CAN/DEL MONTE NO SODIUM)	13.5	OZ
PEAS, GREEN GIANT FROZEN, SWEET	1.77	CUP
PEAS, EDIBLE-PODDED	3.1	CUP
PINEAPPLE, FRESH/DICED	2.37	CUP
PINEAPPLE, DEL MONTE SNACK CAN (LITE)	2.65	3.5 OZ
PINEAPPLE (CAN/DOLE LITE SYRUP)	10.9	SLICE
PRUNES, DOLE, DRIED	2.65	OZ
PUMPKIN (CAN)	3.7	CUP
RAISINS	0.385	CUP
RED PEPPER	9.25	MEDIUM
STRAWBERRIES (FRESH)	1.9	PINT
STRAWBERRIES (FROZEN)	2.47	CUP
SQUASH, CAN, STOKLEY	1.85	CUP
SQUASH, FRESH BAKED	1.63	CUP
TANGERINE	5	2.5 INCH
TOMATO, CAN	17.2	OZ
TOMATO, FRESH	7.1	3 INCH
TOMATO, JUICE	29.5	OZ
VEGETABLES, MIXED (FROZEN)	2.5	CUP
WATERMELLON	1.22	1X10 INCH
ZUCCHINI, FRESH, SLICED	10.3	CUP

Yogurts and Desserts

DING DONG	1.16	DING
DREYERS FROZEN FAT FREE YOGURT	1.03	CUP
FRUIT ROLL-UP	2.65	ROLL-UP
POPCORN, WHITE	3.7	TBLSP
TCBY, SOFT SERVE/NONFAT/NO SUGAR	1.16	CUP
YOGURT, FAT FREE, MOUNTAIN HIGH	8	OZ
YOGURT, FAT FREE, DANNON	8	OZ
LUCERN, YOGURT, NONFAT, LITE	8	OZ

YOGURT, YOPLAIT, FAT FREE, LITE	6	OZ
YOGURT,YOPLAIT ORIGINAL/99% FAT FREE	6	OZ
YOGURT, HORIZON, FF / BLUEBERRY	6	OZ
PLANTER DRIED WALNUT PIECES	0.2	CUP
RAW ALMONDS, TOASTED	1	OZ
PECANS, DRIED	0.88	OZ
PEANUTS, DRY ROASTED	0.2	CUP
HOT CHOCOLATE	3	ENVEL.
ALMONDS, SHELLED	1	OZ

Cereals

CEREAL, CHEERIOS	1.69	CUP
CEREAL, COCOA KRISPIES	1.16	CUP
CEREAL, GRAPENUTS	0.462	CUP
CEREAL, HONEY NUT TOASTY O'S	1.68	CUP
CEREAL, WHEATIES	1.68	CUP
CEREAL, KELLOGG'S ALL BRAN	1.16	CUP
CEREAL, KELLOGG'S CORN FLAKES	1.68	CUP
CEREAL, KELLOGG'S RAISIN BRAN	1.09	CUP
CEREAL, KELLOGG'S CRACKLIN' OAT BRAN	0.7	CUP
CEREAL, NABISCO SHREDDED WHEAT	2.32	PIECE
CEREAL, NAB. SHREDDED WHEAT (SPOON)	1.09	CUP
CEREAL, RICE KRISPIES	2.1	CUP
CEREAL, BENEFIT NUTRITION, PROTEIN +	0.88	CUP
CREAM OF WHEAT	4.63	TBL/DRY
GRANOLA, CW POST HEARTY	0.44	CUP
GRANOLA, KELLOGG'S LOW FAT	3	CUP
OATMEAL (PRE-COOK MEASUREMENT)	0.66	CUP

Breads

BREAD, OROWHEAT LITE	4.63	SLICE
BREAD, SUSAN'S HOMEMADE/18 SLICES	2.05	SLICE
BREAD, SUSAN'S HOMEMADE	0.113	LOAF
BUN, WONDER REDUCED CALORIE LITE	2.31	BUN
CRACKER, ZESTA SALTINES	5.15	CRACKER
TORTILLA (CAROLYN)	1.09	TORT
TORTILLA, TORTILLA'S MEXICO, FLOUR	1.68	TORT

TORTILLA, TORTILLA'S MEXICO, CORN	2.06	TORT
TRISCUITS	1.32	OZ
WAFFLE, EGGO, HOMESTYLE	1.69	WAFFLE
WHOLE GRAIN/WHOLE WHEAT FLOUR	0.455	CUP

Rice/Potatoes/Beans

BLACK BEANS (BOILED)	0.82	CUP
BLACK BEANS (DRY)	0.66	CUP
CHICKPEAS/GARBANZO BEANS	0.22	CUP
KIDNEY BEANS (BOILED)	0.25	CUP
LIMA BEANS (BOILED)	0.89	CUP
NAVY BEANS (BOILED)	0.72	CUP
NAVY BEANS (CAN)	0.77	CUP
PINTO BEANS (BOILED)	0.79	CUP
PINTO BEANS (CAN)	0.975	CUP
PINTO BEANS (DRY)	0.309	CUP
PORK & BEANS/VAN CAMPS	0.84	CUP
POTATO, SWEET	1.57	5"X2"
POTATO	11	OZ
RICE CAKE	3.7	CAKE
RICE, WHITE, BASMATI	0.772	CUP (C)
RICE, BROWN LONG GRAIN	0.925	CUP (C)
RICE, INSTANT, MINUTE BRAND	0.58	CUP(UC)
RICE, WHITE, LONG GRAIN	0.29	CUP(UC)
SOYBEANS (BOILED)	0.75	CUP
YAM, BOILED OR BAKED	1.17	CUP

Pasta

MACARONI, DAVINI TWIST	0.7	CUP/DRY
MACARONI, HOSPITALITY ELBOW	0.385	CUP/DRY
MACARONI, AM. BEAUTY ELBOW	0.44	CUP/DRY
PASTA, CREAMETTE PLAIN	1.77	OZ
SPAGHETTI, EDEN WHOLE WHEAT	1.76	OZ/UC

Protein Sources 2400 Calories

White Meat

CHICKEN BREAST (HORMEL/CAN)	1.23	CAN
CHICKEN BREAST (SKINLESS)	6.18	OZ
CHICKEN (LEG W/ SKIN & BONE)	0.7	
CHICKEN (THIGH W/ SKIN & BONE)	1.21	
CHICKEN (LEG & THIGH W/ SKIN & BONE)	0.443	
HAM, BAR S, XTRA LEAN, 96% FAT FREE	5.3	OZ
HAM, DAK CAN	6.15	OZ
PORK, SIRLOIN, LEAN W/ FAT	1.85	OZ
TURKEY BREAST (SKINLESS)	3.47	OZ
TURKEY BREAST (HORMEL/CAN)	1.06	CAN
TURKEY BRST/OVEN ROAST/SFWY/89% FF	7.4	OZ
VENISON / ANTELOPE	4.15	OZ

Red Meat

HAMBURGER (10% FAT)	3.3	OZ
HAMBURGER (15% FAT)	2.73	OZ
HAMBURGER (20% FAT)	2.65	OZ
HAMBURGER (27% FAT)	2.24	OZ
LAMB, SHOULDER	2.1	OZ
STEAK, BOTTOM ROUND	3.13	OZ
STEAK, BRISKET (FLAT HALF)	2.95	OZ
STEAK, CHUCK, ARM	3.04	OZ
STEAK, CHUCK, BLADE	2.6	OZ
STEAK, EYE ROUND	3.9	OZ
STEAK, FLANK	3.16	OZ
STEAK, NEW YORK STRIP	3.7	OZ
STEAK, PORTERHOUSE	3	OZ
STEAK, RIBEYE	2.91	OZ
STEAK, ROUND TIP	3.55	OZ
STEAK, SHANK (CROSSCUTS)	3.25	OZ
STEAK, T-BONE	3.05	OZ
STEAK, TENDERLOIN	3.1	OZ
STEAK, TOP LOIN	3.15	OZ
STEAK, TOP ROUND	3.64	OZ

STEAK, TOP SIRLOIN	3.38	OZ
STEAK, TYSON SEASONED BEEF STRIPS	3.95	OZ
TACO/BURRITO MEAT/SMART GROUND	0.96	CUP
OSCAR MAYER BACON	6.15	SLICE
LITTLE SIZZLER BROWN/SERVE SAUSAGE	2.4	LINK

Sea Food

BASS, FRESHWATER, DRY HEAT	4.5	OZ
BASS, STRIPED, DRY HEAT	5.3	OZ
COD, ATLANTIC, DRY HEAT	6.25	OZ
CRAB, ALASKA KING, MOIST HEAT	6.8	OZ
CRAB, BLUE, MOIST HEAT	6.4	OZ
FLOUNDER, DRY HEAT	5.6	OZ
HADDOCK, DRY HEAT	5.85	OZ
HALIBUT, DRY HEAT	4.67	OZ
LOBSTER, NORTHERN, MOIST HEAT	6.7	OZ
MAHI MAHI	7.6	OZ
ORANGE ROUGHY, DRY HEAT	7.33	OZ
PERCH, DRY HEAT	5.6	OZ
PERCH, OCEAN/ATLANTIC, DRY HEAT	5.4	OZ
SALMON, ATLANTIC, DRY HEAT	3.57	OZ
SHRIMP, MOIST HEAT	6.6	OZ
TROUT, DRY HEAT	3.45	OZ
TUNA BURGER, AHI / OMEGA FOODS	6.6	OZ
TUNA, LOW SODIUM, CAN	1.06	CAN
TUNA, WATER, CAN	1.23	CAN
TUNA, WHITE / LOW SALT, CAN (5 OZ)	1.06	CAN
TUNA, WHITE, CAN (5 OZ)	1.06	CAN
TUNA, FILLET/STEAK	4.2	OZ
WALLEYE, BAKED/BROILED/MICRO	5.5	OZ

Vegetarian

IVES VEG. COUSINE VEGGY DOG	3.08	DOG
SOY MILK (TRIS)	2	CUP
SOY MILK (SYLVIA)	1.75	CUP

Eggs/Dairy

1 % COTTAGE CHEESE, NORDICA	1.16	CUP
2 % COTTAGE CHEESE (LOW FAT)	0.925	CUP
COTTAGE CHEESE (LUCERNE FAT FREE)	1.16	CUP
COTT CHEESE MARIGOLD/DRY CURD	1.77	CUP
COTT CHEESE MARIGOLD/DRY CURD	28.3	TBLSP
COTT CHEESE BREAKSTONES FAT FREE	1.16	CUP
CHEDDER, SHREDDED, FAT FREE, KHF	1.03	CUP
CHEDDER, SHREDDED, 94% FAT FREE, HC	0.925	CUP
CHEESE, COLBY/MOZZARELLA	1.69	OZ
EGG WHITE	10.9	
EGG, WHOLE	2.46	
EGG BEATERS	1.54	CUP
MOZZARELLA SHREDDED, FAT FREE, KHF	0.92	CUP
SKIM MOZZARELLA STRING CHEESE	2.32	OZ

Free Carbs, Supplements, Fast Foods
2400 calories

Free Carbs

ASPARAGUS
BROCCOLI
CABBAGE
CAULIFLOWER
CELERY
CUCUMBER
GREEN BEANS
GREEN PEPPERS
GREEN SQUASH
LETTUCE, ICEBERG
LETTUCE, LEAF/SHREDDED
MUSHROOMS
ONION
PICKLES (DILL)
RADISH

RED PEPPERS
SPINACH (CAN/NO SALT)
SPINACH (FRESH)
TOMATO (EXCLUDING JUICE)
ZUCCHINI

Supplements/Fast Foods

ATKINS BAR	0.75	BAR
EAS ADVANTEDGE, C&C/LEM/BLUE	0.75	BAR
BAR, ZONE	0.75	BAR
BAR, PURE PROTEIN, 50 G.	1	BAR
BAR, W.W. PURE PROTEIN, 78 G.	0.5	BAR
BAR, PROTEIN REVOLUTION, PBJ	0.75	BAR
BAR, FIBAR, PEANUT BUTTER, 1.2 OZ	1.25	BAR
BAR, PREMIER 1, PROTEIN 8, CHOC/COCO	0.5	BAR
BAR, PREFERRED BAR, CHOC./FUDG/RAS	0.75	BAR
BAR, PREFERRED BAR, CHOC./FUDG/BROW	0.75	BAR
ALIVE, HI CARB POWDER	1	TBLSP
POWERADE	2	SERVING
PROTEIN,GNC P.P. EGG/WHEY	1.5	SERVING
PROTEIN. GNC P.PERF. WHEY	4	SCOOP
OPTIMUM NUTRITION WHEY	1.5	SCOOP
SYNTRAX WHEY PROTEIN	2	SCOOP
TRI PROTEIN PLUS POWDER	1.25	SERVING
HW STRAWBERRY PROT. POWD.	1.75	SCOOP
BIOCHEM WHEY PRO 290	2.25	SCOOP
HUMAN DEV. TECH. WHEY	1.25	SCOOP
NATURADE 100% SOY PROTEIN	0.5	CUP
SUPER GREEN PRO 96 - SOY	0.5	CUP
100% PURE WHEY, PROLAB	1.25	SCOOP
ECLIPSE BULK UP WHEY	1.75	SCOOP
VITAMIN WORLD WHEY 100%	1.5	SCOOP
ULT. NUT. PROSTAR WHEY	1.5	SCOOP
RED WINE	7	OZ
MET RX CH.RST.PNT.PRO + BAR	0.5	BAR
MET RX BAV. MINT. PRO + BAR	0.75	BAR
MET AFTER FX BAR	0.75	BAR
MET RX CH. CH. CHIP PRO + BAR	0.5	BAR

MET RX SOURCE ONE BAR	0.75	BAR
MET RX CHOC. GRAHCRK CHIP BAR	0.5	BAR
MET RX PEANUT BUTTER BAR	0.5	BAR
MET RX DRINK MIX, MRP	0.75	SERVING
MET RX PRO 50, ANABOLIC DRIVE	0.5	SERVING
MET RX PRO 60, ANABOLIC DRIVE	0.5	SERVING
MET RX PROTEIN PLUS	2.25	SCOOP
MET RX KETO PRO	2.25	SCOOP
NUTRI FORCE DRINK MIX, MRP	0.5	SERVING
EAS MYO. DEL. CH/PB BAR	0.5	BAR
EAS MYOPLEX + DELUXE	0.5	SERVING
EAS MYOPLEX LITE	0.75	SERVING
ADVANT EDGE QUICK STIR PROTEIN DRINK	0.75	SERVING
EAS NEUROGAIN	1	SCOOP
EAS PHOSPHAGEN HP	1.25	SCOOP
EAS PRECISION PROTEIN	1.75	SCOOP
EAS SIMPLY PROTEIN	3	SCOOP
EAS WHEY PROTEIN	1.5	SCOOP
EAS SUPPER SHAKE	0.33	SHAKE
VITAMIN WORLD DAILY RX, MRP	0.5	SHAKE
VITAMIN WORLD PROTOPLEX DELUXE, MRP	0.5	SHAKE
VITAMIN WORLD PRE. ENG. WHEY PROT.	1.75	SCOOP
PERFECT RX, MRP, CHOCOLATE	0.75	SHAKE
OPTI PRO	0.5	SHAKE
ARBY'S CHICK. SAND. R.DELX.LITE	0.5	BURGER
ARBY'S SIDE SALAD	1	SALAD
ARBY'S GARDEN SALAD	1	SALAD
ARBY'S RST. CHCK. SALAD	1	SALAD
ARBY'S RED. CAL. ITAL. DRESSING	1	PACKET
ARBY'S RED RANCH DRESSING	1	PACKET
MCD'S VINEG. LITE SALAD DR.	1	PACKET
MCD'S GARDEN SALAD	1	SALAD
MCD'S VINEG. LITE SALAD DR.	1	PACKET
P.HUT. HAND-TOSS CHEESE	0.5	SLICE
P.HUT. HAND-TOSS HAM	0.75	SLICE
P.HUT. HAND-TOSS VEG. LUV.	0.75	SLICE
P.HUT. HAND-TOSS PEPPERON	0.75	SLICE
P.HUT. THIN/CRISP CHEESE	0.75	SLICE

P.HUT. THIN/CRISP HAM	1	SLICE
P.HUT. THIN/CRISP VEG. LUV.	1	SLICE
P.HUT. THIN/CRISP PEPPERON	0.75	SLICE
SW 6" COLD SUB/VEGG. DELIT	1	SUB
SW 6" COLD SUB/TURK. BRST.	1	SUB
SW 6" COLD SUB/TURK.B/HAM	1	SUB
SW 6" COLD SUB/HAM	1	SUB
SW 6" COLD SUB/ROAST BEEF	1	SUB
SW 6" COLD SUB/SFOOD,CRAB	1	SUB
SW 6" COLD SUB/COLD CUT 3	1	SUB
SW 6" COLD SUB/TUNA	1	SUB
SW 6" HOT SUB/RST.CHICK.BR.	1	SUB
SW 6" HOT SUB/STAK/CHEESE	1	SUB
SW 6" HOT SUB/SUB MELT	1	SUB
SW VEGGIE DELITE SALAD	1	SALAD
SW TURKEY BREAST SALAD	1	SALAD
SW ROAST BEEF SALAD	1	SALAD
SW TURK. BRST/HAM SALAD	1	SALAD
SW RST. CHICK. BR. SALAD	0.75	SALAD
SW SEAFOOD/CRAB SALAD	0.75	SALAD
SW STEAK/CHEESE SALAD	0.75	SALAD
SW SUBWAY MELT SALAD	0.75	SALAD
SW COLD CUT 3 SALAD	0.75	SALAD
SW FAT FREE ITALIAN DRESS	1	OZ
SW FAT FREE FRENCH DRESS	1	OZ
SW FAT FREE RANCH DRESS	1	OZ
SW DELI STYLE TURKEY BR.	0.75	SNDWCH
SW DELI STYLE HAM	0.75	SNDWCH
SW DELI STYLE ROAST BEEF	0.75	SNDWCH
TB GRILLED STEAK SOFT TACO	0.75	TACO
WAHOO'S CHBROIL FISH TACO	0.5	TACO
WENDI'S SIDE SALAD	1	SALAD
WENDI'S FF FRENCH DRESSING	1	OZ
WENDI'S ITALIAN RED. F/C DRESS	1	OZ
WENDI'S SMALL CHILI	0.75	BOWL
WENDI'S GRILLED CHICK. FILLET	1	MEAT

	2500 Calories/Day Eating Plan	
	What Does Your Doctor Look Like Naked?	

Name: _____

Date: _____

Exercise: 30-40 min in a.m. before food		Write what you eat here:
Meal 1 Time: _____	2 Protein Sources 3 Active Carbohydrates	
Meal 2 Time: _____	3 oz Raw Almonds	
Meal 3 Time: _____	1 Protein Source 2 Active Carbohydrates Free Carbohydrates (as much as you want)	
Meal 4 Time: _____	1 LOW CARB protein bar (OR) 2 scoops Whey Protein Powder in water	
Meal 5 Time: _____	2 Protein Source 0 Active Carbohydrates Free Carbohydrates (as much as you want)	
Bedtime Meal (Optional)	Sugar Free Jell-O 1 cup	

Add fiber supplement in evening, such as Metamucil or other (sugar FREE).
Add spices, pepper, etc. as needed.
Try to eat every two to three hours
Drink 1½ gallons of water EVERY DAY!
May have up to 2 diet pops (or) 2 cups a coffee a day

Active Carbohydrates 2500 Calories

Fruit and Vegetables

APPLE	2.2	3 INCH
APPLESAUCE, MOTT'S	0.81	CUP
APRICOTS (CAN/DEL MONTE LITE)	1.49	CUP
APRICOTS (DRIED)	2.55	OZ
APRICOTS (FRESH 12/LB)	10.5	MEDIUM
ASPARAGUS	48	OZ
BANANA	1.7	MEDIUM
BLUEBERRIES (FRESH)	2.18	CUP
BRUSSELS SPROUTS, BOILED	2.97	CUP
CABBAGE, SHREDDED	9.9	CUP
CANTALOUPE	0.95	5 INCH
CARROT (FRESH)	16.1	OZ
CAULIFLOWER	6.85	CUP
CELERY	44.5	OZ
CHERRIES, FRESH, SWEET W/PIT	1.72	CUP
CHERRIES, DARK (CAN/DEL MONTE)	0.89	CUP
COLLARD GREENS (CAN)	2.97	CUP
COLLARD GREENS (FRESH)	14.9	CUP
CORN CAKE	5.1	CAKE
CORN (CAN/DEL MONTE NO SODIUM)	13	OZ
CUCUMBER, SLICED	12.7	CUP
EGGPLANT	8.1	CUP
FRUIT, MIXED FROZEN	1.98	CUP
GARLIC, 1 CLOVE	44.5	CLOVE
GARLIC, TRIMMED	4.25	OZ
GRAPES	1.57	CUP
GRAPE JUICE/VERYFINE	9.5	OZ
GRAPEFRUIT	1.94	4 INCH
GREEN BEANS (CAN/DEL MONTE NO SALT)	4.45	CUP
GREEN PEPPER	8.9	MEDIUM
KIWI	12	OZ
MUSHROOMS, FRESH	9.9	CUP
ONION, FRESH/CHOPPED	2.97	CUP
ORANGE, NAVAL	2.75	3 INCH

ORANGE, JUICE	13	OZ
PAPAYA	1.525	LB.
PAPAYA, PEELED/CUBED	3.3	CUP
PEACH, FRESH, SLICED	2.41	CUP
PEACH (CAN/DEL MONTE EXTRA LITE)	1.49	CUP
PEARS (CAN)	5.9	HALF
PEAS, BLACK-EYED (CAN)	0.99	CUP
PEAS (CAN/DEL MONTE NO SODIUM)	13	OZ
PEAS, GREEN GIANT FROZEN, SWEET	1.7	CUP
PEAS, EDIBLE-PODDED	2.97	CUP
PINEAPPLE, FRESH/DICED	2.29	CUP
PINEAPPLE, DEL MONTE SNACK CAN (LITE)	2.53	3.5 OZ
PINEAPPLE (CAN/DOLE LITE SYRUP)	10.5	SLICE
PRUNES, DOLE, DRIED	2.55	OZ
PUMPKIN (CAN)	3.57	CUP
RAISINS	0.37	CUP
RED PEPPER	8.9	MEDIUM
STRAWBERRIES (FRESH)	1.84	PINT
STRAWBERRIES (FROZEN)	2.38	CUP
SQUASH, CAN, STOKLEY	1.78	CUP
SQUASH, FRESH BAKED	1.57	CUP
TANGERINE	4.83	2.5 INCH
TOMATO, CAN	16.7	OZ
TOMATO, FRESH	6.85	3 INCH
TOMATO, JUICE	28.5	OZ
VEGETABLES, MIXED (FROZEN)	1.98	CUP
WATERMELLON	1.17	1X10 INCH
ZUCCHINI, FRESH, SLICED	9.9	CUP

Yogurts and Desserts

DING DONG	1.11	DING
DREYERS FROZEN FAT FREE YOGURT	0.99	CUP
FRUIT ROLL-UP	2.55	ROLL-UP
POPCORN, WHITE	3.57	TBLSP
TCBY, SOFT SERVE/NONFAT/NO SUGAR	1.11	CUP
YOGURT, FAT FREE, MOUNTAIN HIGH	8	OZ
YOGURT, FAT FREE, DANNON	8	OZ

LUCERN, YOGURT, NONFAT, LITE	8	OZ
YOGURT, YOPLAIT, FAT FREE, LITE	6	OZ
YOGURT,YOPLAIT ORIGINAL/99% FAT FREE	6	OZ
YOGURT, HORIZON, FF / BLUEBERRY	6	OZ
PLANTER DRIED WALNUT PIECES	0.2	CUP
RAW ALMONDS, TOASTED	1	OZ
PECANS, DRIED	0.75	OZ
PEANUTS, DRY ROASTED	0.2	CUP
HOT CHOCOLATE	3.5	ENVEL.
ALMONDS, SHELLED	1	OZ

Cereals

CEREAL, CHEERIOS	1.62	CUP
CEREAL, COCOA KRISPIES	1.11	CUP
CEREAL, GRAPENUTS	0.445	CUP
CEREAL, HONEY NUT TOASTY O'S	1.62	CUP
CEREAL, WHEATIES	1.62	CUP
CEREAL, KELLOGG'S ALL BRAN	1.11	CUP
CEREAL, KELLOGG'S CORN FLAKES	1.62	CUP
CEREAL, KELLOGG'S RAISIN BRAN	1.05	CUP
CEREAL, KELLOGG'S CRACKLIN' OAT BRAN	0.7	CUP
CEREAL, NABISCO SHREDDED WHEAT	2.23	PIECE
CEREAL, NAB. SHREDDED WHEAT (SPOON)	1.05	CUP
CEREAL, RICE KRISPIES	2.03	CUP
CEREAL, BENEFIT NUTRITION, PROTEIN +	0.85	CUP
CREAM OF WHEAT	4.45	TBL/DRY
GRANOLA, CW POST HEARTY	0.425	CUP
GRANOLA, KELLOGG'S LOW FAT	2	CUP
OATMEAL (PRE-COOK MEASUREMENT)	0.636	CUP

Breads

BREAD, OROWHEAT LITE	4.47	SLICE
BREAD, SUSAN'S HOMEMADE/18 SLICES	1.97	SLICE
BREAD, SUSAN'S HOMEMADE	0.11	LOAF
BUN, WONDER REDUCED CALORIE LITE	2.23	BUN
CRACKER, ZESTA SALTINES	14.9	CRACKER

TORTILLA (CAROLYN)	1.05	TORT
TORTILLA, TORTILLA'S MEXICO, FLOUR	1.62	TORT
TORTILLA, TORTILLA'S MEXICO, CORN	1.98	TORT
TRISCUITS	1.27	OZ
WAFFLE, EGGO, HOMESTYLE	1.17	WAFFLE
WHOLE GRAIN/WHOLE WHEAT FLOUR	0.438	CUP

Rice/Potatoes/Beans

BLACK BEANS (BOILED)	0.79	CUP
BLACK BEANS (DRY)	0.636	CUP
CHICKPEAS/GARBANZO BEANS	0.25	CUP
KIDNEY BEANS (BOILED)	0.25	CUP
LIMA BEANS (BOILED)	0.86	CUP
NAVY BEANS (BOILED)	0.69	CUP
NAVY BEANS (CAN)	0.745	CUP
PINTO BEANS (BOILED)	0.76	CUP
PINTO BEANS (CAN)	0.94	CUP
PINTO BEANS (DRY)	0.297	CUP
PORK & BEANS/VAN CAMPS	0.81	CUP
POTATO, SWEET	1.51	5"X2"
POTATO	10.6	OZ
RICE CAKE	3.56	CAKE
RICE, WHITE, BASMATI	0.745	CUP (C)
RICE, BROWN LONG GRAIN	0.89	CUP (C)
RICE, INSTANT, MINUTE BRAND	0.558	CUP(UC)
RICE, WHITE, LONG GRAIN	0.279	CUP(UC)
SOYBEANS (BOILED)	0.5	CUP
YAM, BOILED OR BAKED	1.13	CUP

Pasta

MACARONI, DAVINI TWIST	0.68	CUP/DRY
MACARONI, HOSPITALITY ELBOW	0.37	CUP/DRY
MACARONI, AM. BEAUTY ELBOW	0.425	CUP/DRY
PASTA, CREAMETTE PLAIN	1.7	OZ
SPAGHETTI, EDEN WHOLE WHEAT	1.7	OZ/UC

Protein Sources 2500 Calories

White Meat

CHICKEN BREAST (HORMEL/CAN)	1.19	CAN
CHICKEN BREAST (SKINLESS)	5.95	OZ
CHICKEN (LEG W/ SKIN & BONE)	0.675	
CHICKEN (THIGH W/SKIN & BONE)	1.165	
CHICKEN (LEG & THIGH W/SKIN & BONE)	0.428	
HAM, BAR S, XTRA LEAN, 96% FAT FREE	5.1	OZ
HAM, DAK CAN	5.95	OZ
PORK, SIRLOIN, LEAN W/FAT	1.78	OZ
TURKEY BREAST (SKINLESS)	3.33	OZ
TURKEY BREAST (HORMEL/CAN)	1.02	CAN
TURKEY BRST/OVEN ROAST/SFWY/89% FF	7.1	OZ
VENISON / ANTELOPE	3.98	OZ

Red Meat

HAMBURGER (10% FAT)	3.16	OZ
HAMBURGER (15% FAT)	2.62	OZ
HAMBURGER (20% FAT)	2.55	OZ
HAMBURGER (27% FAT)	2.16	OZ
LAMB, SHOULDER	2.03	OZ
STEAK, BOTTOM ROUND	3.01	OZ
STEAK, BRISKET (FLAT HALF)	2.84	OZ
STEAK, CHUCK, ARM	2.92	OZ
STEAK, CHUCK, BLADE	2.52	OZ
STEAK, EYE ROUND	3.74	OZ
STEAK, FLANK	3.04	OZ
STEAK, NEW YORK STRIP	3.57	OZ
STEAK, PORTERHOUSE	2.9	OZ
STEAK, RIBEYE	2.8	OZ
STEAK, ROUND TIP	3.42	OZ
STEAK, SHANK (CROSSCUTS)	3.14	OZ
STEAK, T-BONE	2.94	OZ
STEAK, TENDERLOIN	2.99	OZ
STEAK, TOP LOIN	3.05	OZ
STEAK, TOP ROUND	3.5	OZ

STEAK, TOP SIRLOIN	3.24	OZ
STEAK, TYSON SEASONED BEEF STRIPS	3.83	OZ
TACO/BURRITO MEAT/SMART GROUND	0.93	CUP
OSCAR MAYER BACON	5.95	SLICE
LITTLE SIZZLER BROWN/SERVE SAUSAGE	2.32	LINK

Sea Food

BASS, FRESHWATER, DRY HEAT	4.33	OZ
BASS, STRIPED, DRY HEAT	5.1	OZ
COD, ATLANTIC, DRY HEAT	6	OZ
CRAB, ALASKA KING, MOIST HEAT	6.53	OZ
CRAB, BLUE, MOIST HEAT	6.15	OZ
FLOUNDER, DRY HEAT	5.4	OZ
HADDOCK, DRY HEAT	5.65	OZ
HALIBUT, DRY HEAT	4.5	OZ
LOBSTER, NORTHERN, MOIST HEAT	6.45	OZ
MAHI MAHI	7.35	OZ
ORANGE ROUGHY, DRY HEAT	7.05	OZ
PERCH, DRY HEAT	5.4	OZ
PERCH, OCEAN/ATLANTIC, DRY HEAT	5.2	OZ
SALMON, ATLANTIC, DRY HEAT	3.44	OZ
SHRIMP, MOIST HEAT	6.36	OZ
TROUT, DRY HEAT	3.33	OZ
TUNA BURGER, AHI / OMEGA FOODS	6.38	OZ
TUNA, LOW SODIUM, CAN	1.02	CAN
TUNA, WATER, CAN	1.19	CAN
TUNA, WHITE/LOW SALT, CAN (5 OZ)	1.02	CAN
TUNA, WHITE, CAN (5 OZ)	1.02	CAN
TUNA, FILLET/STEAK	4.05	OZ
WALLEYE, BAKED/BROILED/MICRO	5.3	OZ

Vegetarian

IVES VEG. COUSINE VEGGY DOG	2.98	DOG
SOY MILK (TRIS)	2	CUP
SOY MILK (SYLVIA)	1.75	CUP

Eggs/Dairy

1% COTTAGE CHEESE, NORDICA	1.12	CUP
2% COTTAGE CHEESE (LOW FAT)	0.89	CUP
COTTAGE CHEESE (LUCERNE FAT FREE)	1.11	CUP
COTT CHEESE MARIGOLD/DRY CURD	1.7	CUP
COTT CHEESE MARIGOLD/DRY CURD	27.2	TBLSP
COTT CHEESE BREAKSTONES FAT FREE	1.11	CUP
CHEDDER, SHREDDED, FAT FREE, KHF	0.99	CUP
CHEDDER, SHREDDED, 94% FAT FREE, HC	0.89	CUP
CHEESE, COLBY/MOZZARELLA	1.62	OZ
EGG WHITE	10.5	
EGG, WHOLE	2.38	
EGG BEATERS	1.49	CUP
MOZZARELLA SHREDDED, FAT FREE, KHF	0.89	CUP
SKIM MOZZARELLA STRING CHEESE	2.23	OZ

Free Carbs, Supplements, Fast Foods
2500 calories

Free Carbs

ASPARAGUS
BROCCOLI
CABBAGE
CAULIFLOWER
CELERY
CUCUMBER
GREEN BEANS
GREEN PEPPERS
GREEN SQUASH
LETTUCE, ICEBERG
LETTUCE, LEAF/SHREDDED
MUSHROOMS
ONION
PICKLES (DILL)
RADISH

RED PEPPERS
SPINACH (CAN/NO SALT)
SPINACH (FRESH)
TOMATO (EXCLUDING JUICE)
ZUCCHINI

Supplements/Fast Foods

ATKINS BAR	0.75	BAR
EAS ADVANTEDGE, C&C/LEM/BLUE	0.75	BAR
BAR, ZONE	0.75	BAR
BAR, PURE PROTEIN, 50 G.	0.75	BAR
BAR, W.W. PURE PROTEIN, 78 G.	0.5	BAR
BAR, PROTEIN REVOLUTION, PBJ	0.75	BAR
BAR, FIBAR, PEANUT BUTTER, 1.2 OZ	1.25	BAR
BAR, PREMIER 1, PROTEIN 8, CHOC/COCO	0.5	BAR
BAR, PREFERRED BAR, CHOC./FUDG/RAS	0.75	BAR
BAR, PREFERRED BAR, CHOC./FUDG/BROW	0.75	BAR
ALIVE, HI CARB POWDER	4	TBLSP
POWERADE	2	SERVING
PROTEIN,GNC P.P. EGG/WHEY	1.25	SERVING
PROTEIN. GNC P.PERF. WHEY	4	SCOOP
OPTIMUM NUTRITION WHEY	1.5	SCOOP
SYNTRAX WHEY PROTEIN	1.75	SCOOP
TRI PROTEIN PLUS POWDER	1.25	SERVING
HW STRAWBERRY PROT. POWD.	1.75	SCOOP
BIOCHEM WHEY PRO 290	2	SCOOP
HUMAN DEV. TECH. WHEY	1.25	SCOOP
NATURADE 100% SOY PROTEIN	0.5	CUP
SUPER GREEN PRO 96 - SOY	0.5	CUP
100% PURE WHEY, PROLAB	1.25	SCOOP
ECLIPSE BULK UP WHEY	1.75	SCOOP
VITAMIN WORLD WHEY 100%	1.5	SCOOP
ULT. NUT. PROSTAR WHEY	1.5	SCOOP
RED WINE	7	OZ
MET RX CH.RST.PNT.PRO + BAR	0.5	BAR
MET RX BAV. MINT. PRO + BAR	0.5	BAR
MET AFTER FX BAR	0.5	BAR
MET RX CH. CH. CHIP PRO + BAR	0.5	BAR

MET RX SOURCE ONE BAR	0.75	BAR
MET RX CHOC. GRAHCRK CHIP BAR	0.5	BAR
MET RX PEANUT BUTTER BAR	0.5	BAR
MET RX DRINK MIX, MRP	0.5	SERVING
MET RX PRO 50, ANABOLIC DRIVE	0.5	SERVING
MET RX PRO 60, ANABOLIC DRIVE	0.5	SERVING
MET RX PROTEIN PLUS	2.5	SCOOP
MET RX KETO PRO	2.25	SCOOP
NUTRI FORCE DRINK MIX, MRP	0.5	SERVING
EAS MYO. DEL. CH/PB BAR	0.5	BAR
EAS MYOPLEX + DELUXE	0.5	SERVING
EAS MYOPLEX LITE	0.75	SERVING
ADVANT EDGE QUICK STIR PROTEIN DRINK	0.75	SERVING
EAS NEUROGAIN	3.5	SCOOP
EAS PHOSPHAGEN HP	1	SCOOP
EAS PRECISION PROTEIN	1.75	SCOOP
EAS SIMPLY PROTEIN	3	SCOOP
EAS WHEY PROTEIN	1.5	SCOOP
EAS SUPPER SHAKE	0.33	SHAKE
VITAMIN WORLD DAILY RX, MRP	0.5	SHAKE
VITAMIN WORLD PROTOPLEX DELUXE, MRP	0.5	SHAKE
VITAMIN WORLD PRE. ENG. WHEY PROT.	2	SCOOP
PERFECT RX, MRP, CHOCOLATE	0.5	SHAKE
OPTI PRO	0.5	SHAKE
ARBY'S CHICK. SAND. R.DELX.LITE	0.5	BURGER
ARBY'S SIDE SALAD	1	SALAD
ARBY'S GARDEN SALAD	1	SALAD
ARBY'S RST. CHCK. SALAD	1	SALAD
ARBY'S RED. CAL. ITAL. DRESSING	1	PACKET
ARBY'S RED RANCH DRESSING	1	PACKET
MCD'S VINEG. LITE SALAD DR.	1	PACKET
MCD'S GARDEN SALAD	1	SALAD
MCD'S VINEG. LITE SALAD DR.	1	PACKET
P.HUT. HAND-TOSS CHEESE	0.75	SLICE
P.HUT. HAND-TOSS HAM	0.75	SLICE
P.HUT. HAND-TOSS VEG. LUV.	0.75	SLICE
P.HUT. HAND-TOSS PEPPERON	0.75	SLICE
P.HUT. THIN/CRISP CHEESE	0.75	SLICE

P.HUT. THIN/CRISP HAM	0.75	SLICE
P.HUT. THIN/CRISP VEG. LUV.	0.75	SLICE
P.HUT. THIN/CRISP PEPPERON	0.75	SLICE
SW 6" COLD SUB/VEGG. DELIT	1	SUB
SW 6" COLD SUB/TURK. BRST.	1	SUB
SW 6" COLD SUB/TURK.B/HAM	1	SUB
SW 6" COLD SUB/HAM	1	SUB
SW 6" COLD SUB/ROAST BEEF	1	SUB
SW 6" COLD SUB/SFOOD,CRAB	1	SUB
SW 6" COLD SUB/COLD CUT 3	1	SUB
SW 6" COLD SUB/TUNA	1	SUB
SW 6" HOT SUB/RST.CHICK.BR.	1	SUB
SW 6" HOT SUB/STAK/CHEESE	1	SUB
SW 6" HOT SUB/SUB MELT	1	SUB
SW VEGGIE DELITE SALAD	1	SALAD
SW TURKEY BREAST SALAD	1	SALAD
SW ROAST BEEF SALAD	1	SALAD
SW TURK. BRST/HAM SALAD	1	SALAD
SW RST. CHICK. BR. SALAD	0.75	SALAD
SW SEAFOOD/CRAB SALAD	0.75	SALAD
SW STEAK/CHEESE SALAD	0.5	SALAD
SW SUBWAY MELT SALAD	0.5	SALAD
SW COLD CUT 3 SALAD	0.5	SALAD
SW FAT FREE ITALIAN DRESS	1	OZ
SW FAT FREE FRENCH DRESS	1	OZ
SW FAT FREE RANCH DRESS	1	OZ
SW DELI STYLE TURKEY BR.	0.5	SNDWCH
SW DELI STYLE HAM	0.5	SNDWCH
SW DELI STYLE ROAST BEEF	0.5	SNDWCH
TB GRILLED STEAK SOFT TACO	0.5	TACO
WAHOO'S CHBROIL FISH TACO	0.5	TACO
WENDI'S SIDE SALAD	1	SALAD
WENDI'S FF FRENCH DRESSING	1	OZ
WENDI'S ITALIAN RED. F/C DRESS	1	OZ
WENDI'S SMALL CHILI	0.75	BOWL
WENDI'S GRILLED CHICK. FILLET	1.5	MEAT

2600 Calories/Day Eating Plan		
What Does Your Doctor Look Like Naked?		
Name: _____ Date: _____		
Exercise: 30-40 min in a.m. before food		Write what you eat here:
Meal 1 Time: _____	2 Protein Sources 3 Active Carbohydrates	
Meal 2 Time: _____	3 oz Raw Almonds	
Meal 3 Time: _____	1 Protein Source 2 Active Carbohydrates Free Carbohydrates (as much as you want)	
Meal 4 Time: _____	1 LOW CARB protein bar (OR) 2.5 scoops Whey Protein Powder in water	
Meal 5 Time: _____	2 Protein Source 0 Active Carbohydrates Free Carbohydrates (as much as you want)	
Bedtime Meal (Optional)	Sugar Free Jell-O 1 cup	
Add fiber supplement in evening , such as Metamucil or other (sugar FREE). Add spices, pepper, etc. as needed. Try to eat every two to three hours. Drink 1⅓ gallons of water EVERY DAY! May have up to 2 diet pops (or) 2 cups a coffee a day		

Active Carbohydrates 2600 Calories

Fruit and Vegetables

APPLE	2.29	3 INCH
APPLESAUCE, MOTT'S	0.84	CUP
APRICOTS (CAN/DEL MONTE LITE)	1.54	CUP
APRICOTS (DRIED)	2.65	OZ
APRICOTS (FRESH 12/LB)	10.9	MEDIUM
ASPARAGUS	50	OZ
BANANA	1.76	MEDIUM
BLUEBERRIES (FRESH)	2.26	CUP
BRUSSELS SPROUTS, BOILED	3.09	CUP
CABBAGE, SHREDDED	10.3	CUP
CANTALOUPE	0.98	5 INCH
CARROT (FRESH)	16.7	OZ
CAULIFLOWER	7.13	CUP
CELERY	46.3	OZ
CHERRIES, FRESH, SWEET W/PIT	1.78	CUP
CHERRIES, DARK (CAN/DEL MONTE)	0.925	CUP
COLLARD GREENS (CAN)	3.09	CUP
COLLARD GREENS (FRESH)	15.4	CUP
CORN CAKE	5.3	CAKE
CORN (CAN/DEL MONTE NO SODIUM)	13.5	OZ
CUCUMBER, SLICED	13.2	CUP
EGGPLANT	8.4	CUP
FRUIT, MIXED FROZEN	2.06	CUP
GARLIC, 1 CLOVE	46	CLOVE
GARLIC, TRIMMED	4.4	OZ
GRAPES	1.63	CUP
GRAPE JUICE/VERYFINE	9.9	OZ
GRAPEFRUIT	2.01	4 INCH
GREEN BEANS (CAN/DEL MONTE NO SALT)	4.61	CUP
GREEN PEPPER	9.25	MEDIUM
KIWI	12.5	OZ
MUSHROOMS, FRESH	10.3	CUP
ONION, FRESH/CHOPPED	3.09	CUP
ORANGE, NAVAL	2.85	3 INCH

ORANGE, JUICE	13.5	OZ
PAPAYA	1.585	LB.
PAPAYA, PEELED/CUBED	3.44	CUP
PEACH, FRESH, SLICED	2.5	CUP
PEACH (CAN/DEL MONTE EXTRA LITE)	1.54	CUP
PEARS (CAN)	6.15	HALF
PEAS, BLACKEYED (CAN)	1.03	CUP
PEAS (CAN/DEL MONTE NO SODIUM)	13.5	OZ
PEAS, GREEN GIANT FROZEN, SWEET	1.77	CUP
PEAS, EDIBLE-PODDED	3.1	CUP
PINEAPPLE, FRESH/DICED	2.37	CUP
PINEAPPLE, DEL MONTE SNACK CAN (LITE)	2.65	3.5 OZ
PINEAPPLE (CAN/DOLE LITE SYRUP)	10.9	SLICE
PRUNES, DOLE, DRIED	2.65	OZ
PUMPKIN (CAN)	3.7	CUP
RAISINS	0.385	CUP
RED PEPPER	9.25	MEDIUM
STRAWBERRIES (FRESH)	1.9	PINT
STRAWBERRIES (FROZEN)	2.47	CUP
SQUASH, CAN, STOKLEY	1.85	CUP
SQUASH, FRESH BAKED	1.63	CUP
TANGERINE	5	2.5 INCH
TOMATO, CAN	17.2	OZ
TOMATO, FRESH	7.1	3 INCH
TOMATO, JUICE	29.5	OZ
VEGETABLES, MIXED (FROZEN)	2.5	CUP
WATERMELLON	1.22	1X10 INCH
ZUCCHINI, FRESH, SLICED	10.3	CUP

Yogurts and Desserts

DING DONG	1.16	DING
DREYERS FROZEN FAT FREE YOGURT	1.03	CUP
FRUIT ROLL-UP	2.65	ROLL-UP
POPCORN, WHITE	3.7	TBLSP
TCBY, SOFT SERVE/NONFAT/NO SUGAR	1.16	CUP
YOGURT, FAT FREE, MOUNTAIN HIGH	8	OZ
YOGURT, FAT FREE, DANNON	8	OZ
LUCERN, YOGURT, NONFAT, LITE	8	OZ

YOGURT, YOPLAIT, FAT FREE, LITE	6	OZ
YOGURT, YOPLAIT ORIGINAL/99% FAT FREE	6	OZ
YOGURT, HORIZON, FF/BLUEBERRY	6	OZ
PLANTER DRIED WALNUT PIECES	0.2	CUP
RAW ALMONDS, TOASTED	1	OZ
PECANS, DRIED	0.88	OZ
PEANUTS, DRY ROASTED	0.2	CUP
HOT CHOCOLATE	3	ENVEL.
ALMONDS, SHELLED	1	OZ

Cereals

CEREAL, CHEERIOS	1.69	CUP
CEREAL, COCOA KRISPIES	1.16	CUP
CEREAL, GRAPENUTS	0.462	CUP
CEREAL, HONEY NUT TOASTY O'S	1.68	CUP
CEREAL, WHEATIES	1.68	CUP
CEREAL, KELLOGG'S ALL BRAN	1.16	CUP
CEREAL, KELLOGG'S CORN FLAKES	1.68	CUP
CEREAL, KELLOGG'S RAISIN BRAN	1.09	CUP
CEREAL, KELLOGG'S CRACKLIN' OAT BRAN	0.7	CUP
CEREAL, NABISCO SHREDDED WHEAT	2.32	PIECE
CEREAL, NAB. SHREDDED WHEAT (SPOON)	1.09	CUP
CEREAL, RICE KRISPIES	2.1	CUP
CEREAL, BENEFIT NUTRITION, PROTEIN +	0.88	CUP
CREAM OF WHEAT	4.63	TBL/DRY
GRANOLA, CW POST HEARTY	0.44	CUP
GRANOLA, KELLOGG'S LOW FAT	3	CUP
OATMEAL (PRE-COOK MEASUREMENT)	0.66	CUP

Breads

BREAD, OROWHEAT LITE	4.63	SLICE
BREAD, SUSAN'S HOMEMADE/18 SLICES	2.05	SLICE
BREAD, SUSAN'S HOMEMADE	0.113	LOAF
BUN, WONDER REDUCED CALORIE LITE	2.31	BUN
CRACKER, ZESTA SALTINES	5.15	CRACKER
TORTILLA (CAROLYN)	1.09	TORT
TORTILLA, TORTILLA'S MEXICO, FLOUR	1.68	TORT

TORTILLA, TORTILLA'S MEXICO, CORN	2.06	TORT
TRISCUITS	1.32	OZ
WAFFLE, EGGO, HOMESTYLE	1.69	WAFFLE
WHOLE GRAIN/WHOLE WHEAT FLOUR	0.455	CUP

Rice/Potatoes/Beans

BLACK BEANS (BOILED)	0.82	CUP
BLACK BEANS (DRY)	0.66	CUP
CHICKPEAS/GARBANZO BEANS	0.22	CUP
KIDNEY BEANS (BOILED)	0.25	CUP
LIMA BEANS (BOILED)	0.89	CUP
NAVY BEANS (BOILED)	0.72	CUP
NAVY BEANS (CAN)	0.77	CUP
PINTO BEANS (BOILED)	0.79	CUP
PINTO BEANS (CAN)	0.975	CUP
PINTO BEANS (DRY)	0.309	CUP
PORK & BEANS/VAN CAMPS	0.84	CUP
POTATO, SWEET	1.57	5"X2"
POTATO	11	OZ
RICE CAKE	3.7	CAKE
RICE, WHITE, BASMATI	0.772	CUP (C)
RICE, BROWN LONG GRAIN	0.925	CUP (C)
RICE, INSTANT, MINUTE BRAND	0.58	CUP(UC)
RICE, WHITE, LONG GRAIN	0.29	CUP(UC)
SOYBEANS (BOILED)	0.75	CUP
YAM, BOILED OR BAKED	1.17	CUP

Pasta

MACARONI, DAVINI TWIST	0.7	CUP/DRY
MACARONI, HOSPITALITY ELBOW	0.385	CUP/DRY
MACARONI, AM. BEAUTY ELBOW	0.44	CUP/DRY
PASTA, CREAMETTE PLAIN	1.77	OZ
SPAGHETTI, EDEN WHOLE WHEAT	1.76	OZ/UC

Protein Sources 2600 Calories

White Meat

CHICKEN BREAST (HORMEL/CAN)	1.23	CAN
CHICKEN BREAST (SKINLESS)	6.18	OZ
CHICKEN (LEG W/SKIN & BONE)	0.7	
CHICKEN (THIGH W/SKIN & BONE)	1.21	
CHICKEN (LEG & THIGH W/SKIN & BONE)	0.443	
HAM, BAR S, XTRA LEAN, 96% FAT FREE	5.3	OZ
HAM, DAK CAN	6.15	OZ
PORK, SIRLOIN, LEAN W/FAT	1.85	OZ
TURKEY BREAST (SKINLESS)	3.47	OZ
TURKEY BREAST (HORMEL/CAN)	1.06	CAN
TURKEY BRST/OVEN ROAST/SFWY/89% FF	7.4	OZ
VENISON/ANTELOPE	4.15	OZ

Red Meat

HAMBURGER (10% FAT)	3.3	OZ
HAMBURGER (15% FAT)	2.73	OZ
HAMBURGER (20% FAT)	2.65	OZ
HAMBURGER (27% FAT)	2.24	OZ
LAMB, SHOULDER	2.1	OZ
STEAK, BOTTOM ROUND	3.13	OZ
STEAK, BRISKET (FLAT HALF)	2.95	OZ
STEAK, CHUCK, ARM	3.04	OZ
STEAK, CHUCK, BLADE	2.6	OZ
STEAK, EYE ROUND	3.9	OZ
STEAK, FLANK	3.16	OZ
STEAK, NEW YORK STRIP	3.7	OZ
STEAK, PORTERHOUSE	3	OZ
STEAK, RIBEYE	2.91	OZ
STEAK, ROUND TIP	3.55	OZ
STEAK, SHANK (CROSSCUTS)	3.25	OZ
STEAK, T-BONE	3.05	OZ
STEAK, TENDERLOIN	3.1	OZ
STEAK, TOP LOIN	3.15	OZ
STEAK, TOP ROUND	3.64	OZ

STEAK, TOP SIRLOIN	3.38	OZ
STEAK, TYSON SEASONED BEEF STRIPS	3.95	OZ
TACO/BURRITO MEAT/SMART GROUND	0.96	CUP
OSCAR MAYER BACON	6.15	SLICE
LITTLE SIZZLER BROWN/SERVE SAUSAGE	2.4	LINK

Sea Food

BASS, FRESHWATER, DRY HEAT	4.5	OZ
BASS, STRIPED, DRY HEAT	5.3	OZ
COD, ATLANTIC, DRY HEAT	6.25	OZ
CRAB, ALASKA KING, MOIST HEAT	6.8	OZ
CRAB, BLUE, MOIST HEAT	6.4	OZ
FLOUNDER, DRY HEAT	5.6	OZ
HADDOCK, DRY HEAT	5.85	OZ
HALIBUT, DRY HEAT	4.67	OZ
LOBSTER, NORTHERN, MOIST HEAT	6.7	OZ
MAHI MAHI	7.6	OZ
ORANGE ROUGHY, DRY HEAT	7.33	OZ
PERCH, DRY HEAT	5.6	OZ
PERCH, OCEAN/ATLANTIC, DRY HEAT	5.4	OZ
SALMON, ATLANTIC, DRY HEAT	3.57	OZ
SHRIMP, MOIST HEAT	6.6	OZ
TROUT, DRY HEAT	3.45	OZ
TUNA BURGER, AHI / OMEGA FOODS	6.6	OZ
TUNA, LOW SODIUM, CAN	1.06	CAN
TUNA, WATER, CAN	1.23	CAN
TUNA, WHITE/LOW SALT, CAN (5 OZ)	1.06	CAN
TUNA, WHITE, CAN (5 OZ)	1.06	CAN
TUNA, FILLET/STEAK	4.2	OZ
WALLEYE, BAKED/BROILED/MICRO	5.5	OZ

Vegetarian

IVES VEG. COUSINE VEGGY DOG	3.08	DOG
SOY MILK (TRIS)	2	CUP
SOY MILK (SYLVIA)	1.75	CUP

Eggs/Dairy

1 % COTTAGE CHEESE, NORDICA	1.16	CUP
2 % COTTAGE CHEESE (LOW FAT)	0.925	CUP
COTTAGE CHEESE (LUCERNE FAT FREE)	1.16	CUP
COTT CHEESE MARIGOLD/DRY CURD	1.77	CUP
COTT CHEESE MARIGOLD/DRY CURD	28.3	TBLSP
COTT CHEESE BREAKSTONES FAT FREE	1.16	CUP
CHEDDER, SHREDDED, FAT FREE, KHF	1.03	CUP
CHEDDER, SHREDDED, 94% FAT FREE, HC	0.925	CUP
CHEESE, COLBY/MOZZARELLA	1.69	OZ
EGG WHITE	10.9	
EGG, WHOLE	2.46	
EGG BEATERS	1.54	CUP
MOZZARELLA SHREDDED, FAT FREE, KHF	0.92	CUP
SKIM MOZZARELLA STRING CHEESE	2.32	OZ

Free Carbs, Supplements, Fast Foods
2600 calories

Free Carbs

ASPARAGUS
BROCCOLI
CABBAGE
CAULIFLOWER
CELERY
CUCUMBER
GREEN BEANS
GREEN PEPPERS
GREEN SQUASH
LETTUCE, ICEBERG
LETTUCE, LEAF/SHREDDED
MUSHROOMS
ONION
PICKLES (DILL)
RADISH

RED PEPPERS
SPINACH (CAN/NO SALT)
SPINACH (FRESH)
TOMATO (EXCLUDING JUICE)
ZUCCHINI

Supplements/Fast Foods

ATKINS BAR	0.75	BAR
EAS ADVANTEDGE, C&C/LEM/BLUE	0.75	BAR
BAR, ZONE	0.75	BAR
BAR, PURE PROTEIN, 50 G.	1	BAR
BAR, W.W. PURE PROTEIN, 78 G.	0.5	BAR
BAR, PROTEIN REVOLUTION, PBJ	0.75	BAR
BAR, FIBAR, PEANUT BUTTER, 1.2 OZ	1.25	BAR
BAR, PREMIER 1, PROTEIN 8, CHOC/COCO	0.5	BAR
BAR, PREFERRED BAR, CHOC./FUDG/RAS	0.75	BAR
BAR, PREFERRED BAR, CHOC./FUDG/BROW	0.75	BAR
ALIVE, HI CARB POWDER	1	TBLSP
POWERADE	2	SERVING
PROTEIN,GNC P.P. EGG/WHEY	1.5	SERVING
PROTEIN. GNC P.PERF. WHEY	4	SCOOP
OPTIMUM NUTRITION WHEY	1.5	SCOOP
SYNTRAX WHEY PROTEIN	2	SCOOP
TRI PROTEIN PLUS POWDER	1.25	SERVING
HW STRAWBERRY PROT. POWD.	1.75	SCOOP
BIOCHEM WHEY PRO 290	2.25	SCOOP
HUMAN DEV. TECH. WHEY	1.25	SCOOP
NATURADE 100% SOY PROTEIN	0.5	CUP
SUPER GREEN PRO 96 - SOY	0.5	CUP
100% PURE WHEY, PROLAB	1.25	SCOOP
ECLIPSE BULK UP WHEY	1.75	SCOOP
VITAMIN WORLD WHEY 100%	1.5	SCOOP
ULT. NUT. PROSTAR WHEY	1.5	SCOOP
RED WINE	7	OZ
MET RX CH.RST.PNT.PRO + BAR	0.5	BAR
MET RX BAV. MINT. PRO + BAR	0.75	BAR
MET AFTER FX BAR	0.75	BAR
MET RX CH. CH. CHIP PRO + BAR	0.5	BAR

MET RX SOURCE ONE BAR	0.75	BAR
MET RX CHOC. GRAHCRK CHIP BAR	0.5	BAR
MET RX PEANUT BUTTER BAR	0.5	BAR
MET RX DRINK MIX, MRP	0.75	SERVING
MET RX PRO 50, ANABOLIC DRIVE	0.5	SERVING
MET RX PRO 60, ANABOLIC DRIVE	0.5	SERVING
MET RX PROTEIN PLUS	2.25	SCOOP
MET RX KETO PRO	2.25	SCOOP
NUTRI FORCE DRINK MIX, MRP	0.5	SERVING
EAS MYO. DEL. CH/PB BAR	0.5	BAR
EAS MYOPLEX + DELUXE	0.5	SERVING
EAS MYOPLEX LITE	0.75	SERVING
ADVANT EDGE QUICK STIR PROTEIN DRINK	0.75	SERVING
EAS NEUROGAIN	1	SCOOP
EAS PHOSPHAGEN HP	1.25	SCOOP
EAS PRECISION PROTEIN	1.75	SCOOP
EAS SIMPLY PROTEIN	3	SCOOP
EAS WHEY PROTEIN	1.5	SCOOP
EAS SUPPER SHAKE	0.33	SHAKE
VITAMIN WORLD DAILY RX, MRP	0.5	SHAKE
VITAMIN WORLD PROTOPLEX DELUXE, MRP	0.5	SHAKE
VITAMIN WORLD PRE. ENG. WHEY PROT.	1.75	SCOOP
PERFECT RX, MRP, CHOCOLATE	0.75	SHAKE
OPTI PRO	0.5	SHAKE
ARBY'S CHICK. SAND. R.DELX.LITE	0.5	BURGER
ARBY'S SIDE SALAD	1	SALAD
ARBY'S GARDEN SALAD	1	SALAD
ARBY'S RST. CHCK. SALAD	1	SALAD
ARBY'S RED. CAL. ITAL. DRESSING	1	PACKET
ARBY'S RED RANCH DRESSING	1	PACKET
MCD'S VINEG. LITE SALAD DR.	1	PACKET
MCD'S GARDEN SALAD	1	SALAD
MCD'S VINEG. LITE SALAD DR.	1	PACKET
P.HUT. HAND-TOSS CHEESE	0.5	SLICE
P.HUT. HAND-TOSS HAM	0.75	SLICE
P.HUT. HAND-TOSS VEG. LUV.	0.75	SLICE
P.HUT. HAND-TOSS PEPPERON	0.75	SLICE
P.HUT. THIN/CRISP CHEESE	0.75	SLICE

P.HUT. THIN/CRISP HAM	1	SLICE
P.HUT. THIN/CRISP VEG. LUV.	1	SLICE
P.HUT. THIN/CRISP PEPPERON	0.75	SLICE
SW 6" COLD SUB/VEGG. DELIT	1	SUB
SW 6" COLD SUB/TURK. BRST.	1	SUB
SW 6" COLD SUB/TURK.B/HAM	1	SUB
SW 6" COLD SUB/HAM	1	SUB
SW 6" COLD SUB/ROAST BEEF	1	SUB
SW 6" COLD SUB/SFOOD,CRAB	1	SUB
SW 6" COLD SUB/COLD CUT 3	1	SUB
SW 6" COLD SUB/TUNA	1	SUB
SW 6" HOT SUB/RST.CHICK.BR.	1	SUB
SW 6" HOT SUB/STAK/CHEESE	1	SUB
SW 6" HOT SUB/SUB MELT	1	SUB
SW VEGGIE DELITE SALAD	1	SALAD
SW TURKEY BREAST SALAD	1	SALAD
SW ROAST BEEF SALAD	1	SALAD
SW TURK. BRST/HAM SALAD	1	SALAD
SW RST. CHICK. BR. SALAD	0.75	SALAD
SW SEAFOOD/CRAB SALAD	0.75	SALAD
SW STEAK/CHEESE SALAD	0.75	SALAD
SW SUBWAY MELT SALAD	0.75	SALAD
SW COLD CUT 3 SALAD	0.75	SALAD
SW FAT FREE ITALIAN DRESS	1	OZ
SW FAT FREE FRENCH DRESS	1	OZ
SW FAT FREE RANCH DRESS	1	OZ
SW DELI STYLE TURKEY BR.	0.75	SNDWCH
SW DELI STYLE HAM	0.75	SNDWCH
SW DELI STYLE ROAST BEEF	0.75	SNDWCH
TB GRILLED STEAK SOFT TACO	0.75	TACO
WAHOO'S CHBROIL FISH TACO	0.5	TACO
WENDI'S SIDE SALAD	1	SALAD
WENDI'S FF FRENCH DRESSING	1	OZ
WENDI'S ITALIAN RED. F/C DRESS	1	OZ
WENDI'S SMALL CHILI	0.75	BOWL
WENDI'S GRILLED CHICK. FILLET	1	MEAT

2700 Calories/Day Eating Plan		
What Does Your Doctor Look Like Naked?		
Name: _____		
Date: _____		
Exercise: 30-40 min in a.m. before food		Write what you eat here:
Meal 1 Time: _____	2 Protein Sources 3 Active Carbohydrates	
Meal 2 Time: _____	3 oz Raw Almonds	
Meal 3 Time: _____	1 Protein Source 2 Active Carbohydrates Free Carbohydrates (as much as you want)	
Meal 4 Time: _____	1 LOW CARB protein bar(OR) 2.5 scoops Whey Protein Powder in water AND 1 oz String Cheese	
Meal 5 Time: _____	2 Protein Source 0 Active Carbohydrates Free Carbohydrates (as much as you want)	
Bedtime Meal (Optional)	Sugar Free Jell-O 1 cup	
Add fiber supplement in evening, such as Metamucil or other (sugar FREE). Add spices, pepper, etc. as needed. Try to eat every two to three hours. Drink 1⅓ gallons of water EVERY DAY! May have up to 2 diet pops (or) 2 cups a coffee a day.		

Active Carbohydrates 2700 Calories

Fruit and Vegetables

APPLE	2.29	3 INCH
APPLESAUCE, MOTT'S	0.84	CUP
APRICOTS (CAN/DEL MONTE LITE)	1.54	CUP
APRICOTS (DRIED)	2.65	OZ
APRICOTS (FRESH 12/LB)	10.9	MEDIUM
ASPARAGUS	50	OZ
BANANA	1.76	MEDIUM
BLUEBERRIES (FRESH)	2.26	CUP
BRUSSELS SPROUTS, BOILED	3.09	CUP
CABBAGE, SHREDDED	10.3	CUP
CANTALOUPE	0.98	5 INCH
CARROT (FRESH)	16.7	OZ
CAULIFLOWER	7.13	CUP
CELERY	46.3	OZ
CHERRIES, FRESH, SWEET W/PIT	1.78	CUP
CHERRIES, DARK (CAN/DEL MONTE)	0.925	CUP
COLLARD GREENS (CAN)	3.09	CUP
COLLARD GREENS (FRESH)	15.4	CUP
CORN CAKE	5.3	CAKE
CORN (CAN/DEL MONTE NO SODIUM)	13.5	OZ
CUCUMBER, SLICED	13.2	CUP
EGGPLANT	8.4	CUP
FRUIT, MIXED FROZEN	2.06	CUP
GARLIC, 1 CLOVE	46	CLOVE
GARLIC, TRIMMED	4.4	OZ
GRAPES	1.63	CUP
GRAPE JUICE/VERYFINE	9.9	OZ
GRAPEFRUIT	2.01	4 INCH
GREEN BEANS (CAN/DEL MONTE NO SALT)	4.61	CUP
GREEN PEPPER	9.25	MEDIUM
KIWI	12.5	OZ
MUSHROOMS, FRESH	10.3	CUP
ONION, FRESH/CHOPPED	3.09	CUP
ORANGE, NAVAL	2.85	3 INCH

ORANGE, JUICE	13.5	OZ
PAPAYA	1.585	LB.
PAPAYA, PEELED/CUBED	3.44	CUP
PEACH, FRESH, SLICED	2.5	CUP
PEACH (CAN/DEL MONTE EXTRA LITE)	1.54	CUP
PEARS (CAN)	6.15	HALF
PEAS, BLACKEYED (CAN)	1.03	CUP
PEAS (CAN/DEL MONTE NO SODIUM)	13.5	OZ
PEAS, GREEN GIANT FROZEN, SWEET	1.77	CUP
PEAS, EDIBLE-PODDED	3.1	CUP
PINEAPPLE, FRESH/DICED	2.37	CUP
PINEAPPLE, DEL MONTE SNACK CAN (LITE)	2.65	3.5 OZ
PINEAPPLE (CAN/DOLE LITE SYRUP)	10.9	SLICE
PRUNES, DOLE, DRIED	2.65	OZ
PUMPKIN (CAN)	3.7	CUP
RAISINS	0.385	CUP
RED PEPPER	9.25	MEDIUM
STRAWBERRIES (FRESH)	1.9	PINT
STRAWBERRIES (FROZEN)	2.47	CUP
SQUASH, CAN, STOKLEY	1.85	CUP
SQUASH, FRESH BAKED	1.63	CUP
TANGERINE	5	2.5 INCH
TOMATO, CAN	17.2	OZ
TOMATO, FRESH	7.1	3 INCH
TOMATO, JUICE	29.5	OZ
VEGETABLES, MIXED (FROZEN)	2.5	CUP
WATERMELLON	1.22	1X10 INCH
ZUCCHINI, FRESH, SLICED	10.3	CUP

Yogurts and Desserts

DING DONG	1.16	DING
DREYERS FROZEN FAT FREE YOGURT	1.03	CUP
FRUIT ROLL-UP	2.65	ROLL-UP
POPCORN, WHITE	3.7	TBLSP
TCBY, SOFT SERVE/NONFAT/NO SUGAR	1.16	CUP
YOGURT, FAT FREE, MOUNTAIN HIGH	8	OZ
YOGURT, FAT FREE, DANNON	8	OZ
LUCERN, YOGURT, NONFAT, LITE	8	OZ

YOGURT, YOPLAIT, FAT FREE, LITE	6	OZ
YOGURT,YOPLAIT ORIGINAL/99% FAT FREE	6	OZ
YOGURT, HORIZON, FF / BLUEBERRY	6	OZ
PLANTER DRIED WALNUT PIECES	0.2	CUP
RAW ALMONDS, TOASTED	1	OZ
PECANS, DRIED	0.88	OZ
PEANUTS, DRY ROASTED	0.2	CUP
HOT CHOCOLATE	3	ENVEL.
ALMONDS, SHELLED	1	OZ

Cereals

CEREAL, CHEERIOS	1.69	CUP
CEREAL, COCOA KRISPIES	1.16	CUP
CEREAL, GRAPENUTS	0.462	CUP
CEREAL, HONEY NUT TOASTY O'S	1.68	CUP
CEREAL, WHEATIES	1.68	CUP
CEREAL, KELLOGG'S ALL BRAN	1.16	CUP
CEREAL, KELLOGG'S CORN FLAKES	1.68	CUP
CEREAL, KELLOGG'S RAISIN BRAN	1.09	CUP
CEREAL, KELLOGG'S CRACKLIN' OAT BRAN	0.7	CUP
CEREAL, NABISCO SHREDDED WHEAT	2.32	PIECE
CEREAL, NAB. SHREDDED WHEAT (SPOON)	1.09	CUP
CEREAL, RICE KRISPIES	2.1	CUP
CEREAL, BENEFIT NUTRITION, PROTEIN +	0.88	CUP
CREAM OF WHEAT	4.63	TBL/DRY
GRANOLA, CW POST HEARTY	0.44	CUP
GRANOLA, KELLOGG'S LOW FAT	3	CUP
OATMEAL (PRE-COOK MEASUREMENT)	0.66	CUP

Breads

BREAD, OROWHEAT LITE	4.63	SLICE
BREAD, SUSAN'S HOMEMADE/18 SLICES	2.05	SLICE
BREAD, SUSAN'S HOMEMADE	0.113	LOAF
BUN, WONDER REDUCED CALORIE LITE	2.31	BUN
CRACKER, ZESTA SALTINES	5.15	CRACKER
TORTILLA (CAROLYN)	1.09	TORT
TORTILLA, TORTILLA'S MEXICO, FLOUR	1.68	TORT

TORTILLA, TORTILLA'S MEXICO, CORN	2.06	TORT
TRISCUITS	1.32	OZ
WAFFLE, EGGO, HOMESTYLE	1.69	WAFFLE
WHOLE GRAIN/WHOLE WHEAT FLOUR	0.455	CUP

Rice/Potatoes/Beans

BLACK BEANS (BOILED)	0.82	CUP
BLACK BEANS (DRY)	0.66	CUP
CHICKPEAS/GARBANZO BEANS	0.22	CUP
KIDNEY BEANS (BOILED)	0.25	CUP
LIMA BEANS (BOILED)	0.89	CUP
NAVY BEANS (BOILED)	0.72	CUP
NAVY BEANS (CAN)	0.77	CUP
PINTO BEANS (BOILED)	0.79	CUP
PINTO BEANS (CAN)	0.975	CUP
PINTO BEANS (DRY)	0.309	CUP
PORK & BEANS/VAN CAMPS	0.84	CUP
POTATO, SWEET	1.57	5"X2"
POTATO	11	OZ
RICE CAKE	3.7	CAKE
RICE, WHITE, BASMATI	0.772	CUP (C)
RICE, BROWN LONG GRAIN	0.925	CUP (C)
RICE, INSTANT, MINUTE BRAND	0.58	CUP(UC)
RICE, WHITE, LONG GRAIN	0.29	CUP(UC)
SOYBEANS (BOILED)	0.75	CUP
YAM, BOILED OR BAKED	1.17	CUP

Pasta

MACARONI, DAVINI TWIST	0.7	CUP/DRY
MACARONI, HOSPITALITY ELBOW	0.385	CUP/DRY
MACARONI, AM. BEAUTY ELBOW	0.44	CUP/DRY
PASTA, CREAMETTE PLAIN	1.77	OZ
SPAGHETTI, EDEN WHOLE WHEAT	1.76	OZ/UC

Protein Sources 2700 Calories

White Meat

CHICKEN BREAST (HORMEL/CAN)	1.23	CAN
CHICKEN BREAST (SKINLESS)	6.18	OZ
CHICKEN (LEG W/SKIN & BONE)	0.7	
CHICKEN (THIGH W/SKIN & BONE)	1.21	
CHICKEN (LEG & THIGH W/SKIN & BONE)	0.443	
HAM, BAR S, XTRA LEAN, 96% FAT FREE	5.3	OZ
HAM, DAK CAN	6.15	OZ
PORK, SIRLOIN, LEAN W/FAT	1.85	OZ
TURKEY BREAST (SKINLESS)	3.47	OZ
TURKEY BREAST (HORMEL/CAN)	1.06	CAN
TURKEY BRST/OVEN ROAST/SFWY/89% FF	7.4	OZ
VENISON/ANTELOPE	4.15	OZ

Red Meat

HAMBURGER (10% FAT)	3.3	OZ
HAMBURGER (15% FAT)	2.73	OZ
HAMBURGER (20% FAT)	2.65	OZ
HAMBURGER (27% FAT)	2.24	OZ
LAMB, SHOULDER	2.1	OZ
STEAK, BOTTOM ROUND	3.13	OZ
STEAK, BRISKET (FLAT HALF)	2.95	OZ
STEAK, CHUCK, ARM	3.04	OZ
STEAK, CHUCK, BLADE	2.6	OZ
STEAK, EYE ROUND	3.9	OZ
STEAK, FLANK	3.16	OZ
STEAK, NEW YORK STRIP	3.7	OZ
STEAK, PORTERHOUSE	3	OZ
STEAK, RIBEYE	2.91	OZ
STEAK, ROUND TIP	3.55	OZ
STEAK, SHANK (CROSSCUTS)	3.25	OZ
STEAK, T-BONE	3.05	OZ
STEAK, TENDERLOIN	3.1	OZ
STEAK, TOP LOIN	3.15	OZ
STEAK, TOP ROUND	3.64	OZ

STEAK, TOP SIRLOIN	3.38	OZ
STEAK, TYSON SEASONED BEEF STRIPS	3.95	OZ
TACO/BURRITO MEAT/SMART GROUND	0.96	CUP
OSCAR MAYER BACON	6.15	SLICE
LITTLE SIZZLER BROWN/SERVE SAUSAGE	2.4	LINK

Sea Food

BASS, FRESHWATER, DRY HEAT	4.5	OZ
BASS, STRIPED, DRY HEAT	5.3	OZ
COD, ATLANTIC, DRY HEAT	6.25	OZ
CRAB, ALASKA KING, MOIST HEAT	6.8	OZ
CRAB, BLUE, MOIST HEAT	6.4	OZ
FLOUNDER, DRY HEAT	5.6	OZ
HADDOCK, DRY HEAT	5.85	OZ
HALIBUT, DRY HEAT	4.67	OZ
LOBSTER, NORTHERN, MOIST HEAT	6.7	OZ
MAHI MAHI	7.6	OZ
ORANGE ROUGHY, DRY HEAT	7.33	OZ
PERCH, DRY HEAT	5.6	OZ
PERCH, OCEAN/ATLANTIC, DRY HEAT	5.4	OZ
SALMON, ATLANTIC, DRY HEAT	3.57	OZ
SHRIMP, MOIST HEAT	6.6	OZ
TROUT, DRY HEAT	3.45	OZ
TUNA BURGER, AHI/OMEGA FOODS	6.6	OZ
TUNA, LOW SODIUM, CAN	1.06	CAN
TUNA, WATER, CAN	1.23	CAN
TUNA, WHITE/LOW SALT, CAN (5 OZ)	1.06	CAN
TUNA, WHITE, CAN (5 OZ)	1.06	CAN
TUNA, FILLET/STEAK	4.2	OZ
WALLEYE, BAKED/BROILED/MICRO	5.5	OZ

Vegetarian

IVES VEG. COUSINE VEGGY DOG	3.08	DOG
SOY MILK (TRIS)	2	CUP
SOY MILK (SYLVIA)	1.75	CUP

Eggs/Dairy

1% COTTAGE CHEESE, NORDICA	1.16	CUP
2% COTTAGE CHEESE (LOW FAT)	0.925	CUP
COTTAGE CHEESE (LUCERNE FAT FREE)	1.16	CUP
COTT CHEESE MARIGOLD/DRY CURD	1.77	CUP
COTT CHEESE MARIGOLD/DRY CURD	28.3	TBLSP
COTT CHEESE BREAKSTONES FAT FREE	1.16	CUP
CHEDDER, SHREDDED, FAT FREE, KHF	1.03	CUP
CHEDDER, SHREDDED, 94% FAT FREE, HC	0.925	CUP
CHEESE, COLBY/MOZZARELLA	1.69	OZ
EGG WHITE	10.9	
EGG, WHOLE	2.46	
EGG BEATERS	1.54	CUP
MOZZARELLA SHREDDED, FAT FREE, KHF	0.92	CUP
SKIM MOZZARELLA STRING CHEESE	2.32	OZ

Free Carbs, Supplements, Fast Foods
2700 calories

Free Carbs

ASPARAGUS
BROCCOLI
CABBAGE
CAULIFLOWER
CELERY
CUCUMBER
GREEN BEANS
GREEN PEPPERS
GREEN SQUASH
LETTUCE, ICEBERG
LETTUCE, LEAF/SHREDDED
MUSHROOMS
ONION
PICKLES (DILL)
RADISH

RED PEPPERS
SPINACH (CAN/NO SALT)
SPINACH (FRESH)
TOMATO (EXCLUDING JUICE)
ZUCCHINI

Supplements/Fast Foods

ATKINS BAR	0.75	BAR
EAS ADVANTEDGE, C&C/LEM/BLUE	0.75	BAR
BAR, ZONE	0.75	BAR
BAR, PURE PROTEIN, 50 G.	1	BAR
BAR, W.W. PURE PROTEIN, 78 G.	0.5	BAR
BAR, PROTEIN REVOLUTION, PBJ	0.75	BAR
BAR, FIBAR, PEANUT BUTTER, 1.2 OZ	1.25	BAR
BAR, PREMIER 1, PROTEIN 8, CHOC/COCO	0.5	BAR
BAR, PREFERRED BAR, CHOC./FUDG/RAS	0.75	BAR
BAR, PREFERRED BAR, CHOC./FUDG/BROW	0.75	BAR
ALIVE, HI CARB POWDER	1	TBLSP
POWERADE	2	SERVING
PROTEIN,GNC P.P. EGG/WHEY	1.5	SERVING
PROTEIN. GNC P.PERF. WHEY	4	SCOOP
OPTIMUM NUTRITION WHEY	1.5	SCOOP
SYNTRAX WHEY PROTEIN	2	SCOOP
TRI PROTEIN PLUS POWDER	1.25	SERVING
HW STRAWBERRY PROT. POWD.	1.75	SCOOP
BIOCHEM WHEY PRO 290	2.25	SCOOP
HUMAN DEV. TECH. WHEY	1.25	SCOOP
NATURADE 100% SOY PROTEIN	0.5	CUP
SUPER GREEN PRO 96 - SOY	0.5	CUP
100% PURE WHEY, PROLAB	1.25	SCOOP
ECLIPSE BULK UP WHEY	1.75	SCOOP
VITAMIN WORLD WHEY 100%	1.5	SCOOP
ULT. NUT. PROSTAR WHEY	1.5	SCOOP
RED WINE	7	OZ
MET RX CH.RST.PNT.PRO + BAR	0.5	BAR
MET RX BAV. MINT. PRO + BAR	0.75	BAR
MET AFTER FX BAR	0.75	BAR
MET RX CH. CH. CHIP PRO + BAR	0.5	BAR

MET RX SOURCE ONE BAR	0.75	BAR
MET RX CHOC. GRAHCRK CHIP BAR	0.5	BAR
MET RX PEANUT BUTTER BAR	0.5	BAR
MET RX DRINK MIX, MRP	0.75	SERVING
MET RX PRO 50, ANABOLIC DRIVE	0.5	SERVING
MET RX PRO 60, ANABOLIC DRIVE	0.5	SERVING
MET RX PROTEIN PLUS	2.25	SCOOP
MET RX KETO PRO	2.25	SCOOP
NUTRI FORCE DRINK MIX, MRP	0.5	SERVING
EAS MYO. DEL. CH/PB BAR	0.5	BAR
EAS MYOPLEX + DELUXE	0.5	SERVING
EAS MYOPLEX LITE	0.75	SERVING
ADVANT EDGE QUICK STIR PROTEIN DRINK	0.75	SERVING
EAS NEUROGAIN	1	SCOOP
EAS PHOSPHAGEN HP	1.25	SCOOP
EAS PRECISION PROTEIN	1.75	SCOOP
EAS SIMPLY PROTEIN	3	SCOOP
EAS WHEY PROTEIN	1.5	SCOOP
EAS SUPPER SHAKE	0.33	SHAKE
VITAMIN WORLD DAILY RX, MRP	0.5	SHAKE
VITAMIN WORLD PROTOPLEX DELUXE, MRP	0.5	SHAKE
VITAMIN WORLD PRE. ENG. WHEY PROT.	1.75	SCOOP
PERFECT RX, MRP, CHOCOLATE	0.75	SHAKE
OPTI PRO	0.5	SHAKE
ARBY'S CHICK. SAND. R.DELX.LITE	0.5	BURGER
ARBY'S SIDE SALAD	1	SALAD
ARBY'S GARDEN SALAD	1	SALAD
ARBY'S RST. CHCK. SALAD	1	SALAD
ARBY'S RED. CAL. ITAL. DRESSING	1	PACKET
ARBY'S RED RANCH DRESSING	1	PACKET
MCD'S VINEG. LITE SALAD DR.	1	PACKET
MCD'S GARDEN SALAD	1	SALAD
MCD'S VINEG. LITE SALAD DR.	1	PACKET
P.HUT. HAND-TOSS CHEESE	0.5	SLICE
P.HUT. HAND-TOSS HAM	0.75	SLICE
P.HUT. HAND-TOSS VEG. LUV.	0.75	SLICE
P.HUT. HAND-TOSS PEPPERON	0.75	SLICE
P.HUT. THIN/CRISP CHEESE	0.75	SLICE

P.HUT. THIN/CRISP HAM	1	SLICE
P.HUT. THIN/CRISP VEG. LUV.	1	SLICE
P.HUT. THIN/CRISP PEPPERON	0.75	SLICE
SW 6" COLD SUB/VEGG. DELIT	1	SUB
SW 6" COLD SUB/TURK. BRST.	1	SUB
SW 6" COLD SUB/TURK.B/HAM	1	SUB
SW 6" COLD SUB/HAM	1	SUB
SW 6" COLD SUB/ROAST BEEF	1	SUB
SW 6" COLD SUB/SFOOD,CRAB	1	SUB
SW 6" COLD SUB/COLD CUT 3	1	SUB
SW 6" COLD SUB/TUNA	1	SUB
SW 6" HOT SUB/RST.CHICK.BR.	1	SUB
SW 6" HOT SUB/STAK/CHEESE	1	SUB
SW 6" HOT SUB/SUB MELT	1	SUB
SW VEGGIE DELITE SALAD	1	SALAD
SW TURKEY BREAST SALAD	1	SALAD
SW ROAST BEEF SALAD	1	SALAD
SW TURK. BRST/HAM SALAD	1	SALAD
SW RST. CHICK. BR. SALAD	0.75	SALAD
SW SEAFOOD/CRAB SALAD	0.75	SALAD
SW STEAK/CHEESE SALAD	0.75	SALAD
SW SUBWAY MELT SALAD	0.75	SALAD
SW COLD CUT 3 SALAD	0.75	SALAD
SW FAT FREE ITALIAN DRESS	1	OZ
SW FAT FREE FRENCH DRESS	1	OZ
SW FAT FREE RANCH DRESS	1	OZ
SW DELI STYLE TURKEY BR.	0.75	SNDWCH
SW DELI STYLE HAM	0.75	SNDWCH
SW DELI STYLE ROAST BEEF	0.75	SNDWCH
TB GRILLED STEAK SOFT TACO	0.75	TACO
WAHOO'S CHBROIL FISH TACO	0.5	TACO
WENDI'S SIDE SALAD	1	SALAD
WENDI'S FF FRENCH DRESSING	1	OZ
WENDI'S ITALIAN RED. F/C DRESS	1	OZ
WENDI'S SMALL CHILI	0.75	BOWL
WENDI'S GRILLED CHICK. FILLET	1	MEAT

2800 Calories/Day Eating Plan		
What Does Your Doctor Look Like Naked?		

Name: _____

Date: _____

Exercise: 30-40 min in a.m. before food		
		Write what you eat here:
Meal 1 Time: _____	2 Protein Sources 3 Active Carbohydrates	
Meal 2 Time: _____	3 oz Raw Almonds	
Meal 3 Time: _____	1 Protein Source 2 Active Carbohydrates Free Carbohydrates (as much as you want)	
Meal 4 Time: _____	1 LOW CARB protein bar (OR) 2.5 scoops Whey Protein Powder in water AND 1 oz String Cheese	
Meal 5 Time: _____	2 Protein Source 0 Active Carbohydrates Free Carbohydrates (as much as you want)	
Bedtime Meal (Optional)	Sugar Free Jell-O 1 cup	

Add fiber supplement in evening, such as Metamucil or other (sugar FREE).
Add spices, pepper, etc. as needed.
Try to eat every two to three hours.
Drink 1⅓ gallons of water EVERY DAY!
May have up to 2 diet pops (or) 2 cups a coffee a day.

Active Carbohydrates 2800 Calories

Fruit and Vegetables

APPLE	2.49	3 INCH
APPLESAUCE, MOTT'S	0.91	CUP
APRICOTS (CAN/DEL MONTE LITE)	1.68	CUP
APRICOTS (DRIED)	2.88	OZ
APRICOTS (FRESH 12/LB)	11.8	MEDIUM
ASPARAGUS	54.4	OZ
BANANA	1.92	MEDIUM
BLUEBERRIES (FRESH)	2.46	CUP
BRUSSELS SPROUTS, BOILED	3.35	CUP
CABBAGE, SHREDDED	11.2	CUP
CANTALOUPE	1.07	5 INCH
CARROT (FRESH)	18.1	OZ
CAULIFLOWER	7.75	CUP
CELERY	50	OZ
CHERRIES, FRESH, SWEET W/PIT	1.94	CUP
CHERRIES, DARK (CAN/DEL MONTE)	1	CUP
COLLARD GREENS (CAN)	3.36	CUP
COLLARD GREENS (FRESH)	16.8	CUP
CORN CAKE	5.75	CAKE
CORN (CAN/DEL MONTE NO SODIUM)	14.7	OZ
CUCUMBER, SLICED	14.4	CUP
EGGPLANT	9.1	CUP
FRUIT, MIXED FROZEN	2.24	CUP
GARLIC, 1 CLOVE	50	CLOVE
GARLIC, TRIMMED	4.8	OZ
GRAPES	1.77	CUP
GRAPE JUICE/VERYFINE	10.7	OZ
GRAPEFRUIT	2.19	4 INCH
GREEN BEANS (CAN/DEL MONTE NO SALT)	5	CUP
GREEN PEPPER	10	MEDIUM
KIWI	13.5	OZ
MUSHROOMS, FRESH	11.2	CUP
ONION, FRESH/CHOPPED	3.36	CUP
ORANGE, NAVAL	3.1	3 INCH

ORANGE, JUICE	14.6	OZ
PAPAYA	1.72	LB.
PAPAYA, PEELED/CUBED	3.74	CUP
PEACH, FRESH, SLICED	2.72	CUP
PEACH (CAN/DEL MONTE EXTRA LITE)	1.68	CUP
PEARS (CAN)	6.7	HALF
PEAS, BLACKEYED (CAN)	1.12	CUP
PEAS (CAN/DEL MONTE NO SODIUM)	14.7	OZ
PEAS, GREEN GIANT FROZEN, SWEET	1.92	CUP
PEAS, EDIBLE-PODDED	3.35	CUP
PINEAPPLE, FRESH/DICED	2.58	CUP
PINEAPPLE, DEL MONTE SNACK CAN (LITE)	2.88	3.5 OZ
PINEAPPLE (CAN/DOLE LITE SYRUP)	11.88	SLICE
PRUNES, DOLE, DRIED	2.88	OZ
PUMPKIN (CAN)	4	CUP
RAISINS	0.42	CUP
RED PEPPER	10	MEDIUM
STRAWBERRIES (FRESH)	2.08	PINT
STRAWBERRIES (FROZEN)	2.69	CUP
SQUASH, CAN, STOKLEY	2	CUP
SQUASH, FRESH BAKED	1.77	CUP
TANGERINE	5.45	2.5 INCH
TOMATO, CAN	18.8	OZ
TOMATO, FRESH	7.7	3 INCH
TOMATO, JUICE	32	OZ
VEGETABLES, MIXED (FROZEN)	2.24	CUP
WATERMELLON	1.32	1X10 INCH
ZUCCHINI, FRESH, SLICED	11.2	CUP

Yogurts and Desserts

DING DONG	1.26	DING
DREYERS FROZEN FAT FREE YOGURT	1.12	CUP
FRUIT ROLL-UP	2.88	ROLL-UP
POPCORN, WHITE	4	TBLSP
TCBY, SOFT SERVE/NONFAT/NO SUGAR	1.26	CUP
YOGURT, FAT FREE, MOUNTAIN HIGH	8	OZ
YOGURT, FAT FREE, DANNON	8	OZ
LUCERN, YOGURT, NONFAT, LITE	8	OZ

YOGURT, YOPLAIT, FAT FREE, LITE	6	OZ
YOGURT, YOPLAIT ORIGINAL/99% FAT FREE	6	OZ
YOGURT, HORIZON, FF / BLUEBERRY	6	OZ
PLANTER DRIED WALNUT PIECES	0.25	CUP
RAW ALMONDS, TOASTED	1.19	OZ
PECANS, DRIED	1	OZ
PEANUTS, DRY ROASTED	0.2	CUP
HOT CHOCOLATE	4	ENVEL.
ALMONDS, SHELLED	1	OZ

Cereals

CEREAL, CHEERIOS	1.83	CUP
CEREAL, COCOA KRISPIES	1.26	CUP
CEREAL, GRAPENUTS	0.5	CUP
CEREAL, HONEY NUT TOASTY O'S	1.83	CUP
CEREAL, WHEATIES	1.83	CUP
CEREAL, KELLOGG'S ALL BRAN	1.26	CUP
CEREAL, KELLOGG'S CORN FLAKES	1.83	CUP
CEREAL, KELLOGG'S RAISIN BRAN	1.18	CUP
CEREAL, KELLOGG'S CRACKLIN' OAT BRAN	0.76	CUP
CEREAL, NABISCO SHREDDED WHEAT	2.5	PIECE
CEREAL, NAB. SHREDDED WHEAT (SPOON)	1.18	CUP
CEREAL, RICE KRISPIES	2.29	CUP
CEREAL, BENEFIT NUTRITION, PROTEIN +	0.96	CUP
CREAM OF WHEAT	5	TBL/DRY
GRANOLA, CW POST HEARTY	0.48	CUP
GRANOLA, KELLOGG'S LOW FAT	4	CUP
OATMEAL (PRE-COOK MEASUREMENT)	0.72	CUP

Breads

BREAD, OROWHEAT LITE	5	SLICE
BREAD, SUSAN'S HOMEMADE/18 SLICES	2.22	SLICE
BREAD, SUSAN'S HOMEMADE	0.123	LOAF
BUN, WONDER REDUCED CALORIE LITE	2.5	BUN
CRACKER, ZESTA SALTINES	16.8	CRACKER
TORTILLA (CAROLYN)	1.18	TORT
TORTILLA, TORTILLA'S MEXICO, FLOUR	1.83	TORT

TORTILLA, TORTILLA'S MEXICO, CORN	2.24	TORT
TRISCUITS	1.44	OZ
WAFFLE, EGGO, HOMESTYLE	1.83	WAFFLE
WHOLE GRAIN/WHOLE WHEAT FLOUR	0.495	CUP

Rice/Potatoes/Beans

BLACK BEANS (BOILED)	0.89	CUP
BLACK BEANS (DRY)	0.72	CUP
CHICKPEAS/GARBANZO BEANS	0.25	CUP
KIDNEY BEANS (BOILED)	0.25	CUP
LIMA BEANS (BOILED)	0.568	CUP
NAVY BEANS (BOILED)	0.78	CUP
NAVY BEANS (CAN)	0.838	CUP
PINTO BEANS (BOILED)	0.86	CUP
PINTO BEANS (CAN)	1.06	CUP
PINTO BEANS (DRY)	0.335	CUP
PORK & BEANS/VAN CAMPS	0.91	CUP
POTATO, SWEET	1.71	5"X2"
POTATO	12	OZ
RICE CAKE	4	CAKE
RICE, WHITE, BASMATI	0.84	CUP (C)
RICE, BROWN LONG GRAIN	1	CUP (C)
RICE, INSTANT, MINUTE BRAND	0.63	CUP(UC)
RICE, WHITE, LONG GRAIN	0.315	CUP(UC)
SOYBEANS (BOILED)	0.75	CUP
YAM, BOILED OR BAKED	1.27	CUP

Pasta

MACARONI, DAVINI TWIST	0.765	CUP/DRY
MACARONI, HOSPITALITY ELBOW	0.42	CUP/DRY
MACARONI, AM. BEAUTY ELBOW	0.48	CUP/DRY
PASTA, CREAMETTE PLAIN	1.92	OZ
SPAGHETTI, EDEN WHOLE WHEAT	1.92	OZ/UC

Protein Sources 2800 Calories

White Meat

CHICKEN BREAST (HORMEL/CAN)	1.34	CAN
CHICKEN BREAST (SKINLESS)	6.7	OZ
CHICKEN (LEG W/SKIN & BONE)	0.76	
CHICKEN (THIGH W/SKIN & BONE)	1.32	
CHICKEN (LEG & THIGH W/SKIN & BONE)	0.48	
HAM, BAR S, XTRA LEAN, 96% FAT FREE	5.75	OZ
HAM, DAK CAN	6.7	OZ
PORK, SIRLOIN, LEAN W/FAT	2	OZ
TURKEY BREAST (SKINLESS)	3.76	OZ
TURKEY BREAST (HORMEL/CAN)	1.15	CAN
TURKEY BRST/OVEN ROAST/SFWY/89% FF	8	OZ
VENISON/ANTELOPE	4.5	OZ

Red Meat

HAMBURGER (10% FAT)	3.58	OZ
HAMBURGER (15% FAT)	2.96	OZ
HAMBURGER (20% FAT)	2.88	OZ
HAMBURGER (27% FAT)	2.44	OZ
LAMB, SHOULDER	2.29	OZ
STEAK, BOTTOM ROUND	3.4	OZ
STEAK, BRISKET (FLAT HALF)	3.2	OZ
STEAK, CHUCK, ARM	3.3	OZ
STEAK, CHUCK, BLADE	2.84	OZ
STEAK, EYE ROUND	4.22	OZ
STEAK, FLANK	3.44	OZ
STEAK, NEW YORK STRIP	4	OZ
STEAK, PORTERHOUSE	3.27	OZ
STEAK, RIBEYE	3.16	OZ
STEAK, ROUND TIP	3.85	OZ
STEAK, SHANK (CROSSCUTS)	3.53	OZ
STEAK, T-BONE	3.32	OZ
STEAK, TENDERLOIN	3.38	OZ
STEAK, TOP LOIN	3.44	OZ
STEAK, TOP ROUND	3.95	OZ

STEAK, TOP SIRLOIN	3.67	OZ
STEAK, TYSON SEASONED BEEF STRIPS	4.3	OZ
TACO/BURRITO MEAT/SMART GROUND	1.05	CUP
OSCAR MAYER BACON	6.7	SLICE
LITTLE SIZZLER BROWN/SERVE SAUSAGE	2.62	LINK

Sea Food

BASS, FRESHWATER, DRY HEAT	4.9	OZ
BASS, STRIPED, DRY HEAT	5.75	OZ
COD, ATLANTIC, DRY HEAT	6.8	OZ
CRAB, ALASKA KING, MOIST HEAT	7.38	OZ
CRAB, BLUE, MOIST HEAT	6.95	OZ
FLOUNDER, DRY HEAT	6.1	OZ
HADDOCK, DRY HEAT	6.35	OZ
HALIBUT, DRY HEAT	5.08	OZ
LOBSTER, NORTHERN, MOIST HEAT	7.3	OZ
MAHI MAHI	8.3	OZ
ORANGE ROUGHY, DRY HEAT	7.9	OZ
PERCH, DRY HEAT	6.1	OZ
PERCH, OCEAN/ATLANTIC, DRY HEAT	5.86	OZ
SALMON, ATLANTIC, DRY HEAT	3.87	OZ
SHRIMP, MOIST HEAT	7.2	OZ
TROUT, DRY HEAT	3.75	OZ
TUNA BURGER, AHI / OMEGA FOODS	7.2	OZ
TUNA, LOW SODIUM, CAN	1.15	CAN
TUNA, WATER, CAN	1.34	CAN
TUNA, WHITE / LOW SALT, CAN (5 OZ)	1.15	CAN
TUNA, WHITE, CAN (5 OZ)	1.15	CAN
TUNA, FILLET/STEAK	4.57	OZ
WALLEYE, BAKED/BROILED/MICRO	5.97	OZ

Vegetarian

IVES VEG. COUSINE VEGGY DOG	3.35	DOG
SOY MILK (TRIS)	2.25	CUP
SOY MILK (SYLVIA)	2	CUP

Eggs/Dairy

1% COTTAGE CHEESE, NORDICA	1.26	CUP
2% COTTAGE CHEESE (LOW FAT)	1	CUP
COTTAGE CHEESE (LUCERNE FAT FREE)	1.26	CUP
COTT CHEESE MARIGOLD/DRY CURD	1.92	CUP
COTT CHEESE MARIGOLD/DRY CURD	30.5	TBLSP
COTT CHEESE BREAKSTONES FAT FREE	1.26	CUP
CHEDDER, SHREDDED, FAT FREE, KHF	1.12	CUP
CHEDDER, SHREDDED, 94% FAT FREE, HC	1	CUP
CHEESE, COLBY/MOZZARELLA	1.83	OZ
EGG WHITE	11.8	
EGG, WHOLE	2.69	
EGG BEATERS	1.68	CUP
MOZZARELLA SHREDDED, FAT FREE, KHF	1	CUP
SKIM MOZZARELLA STRING CHEESE	2.5	OZ

Free Carbs, Supplements, Fast Foods
2800 calories

Free Carbs

ASPARAGUS
BROCCOLI
CABBAGE
CAULIFLOWER
CELERY
CUCUMBER
GREEN BEANS
GREEN PEPPERS
GREEN SQUASH
LETTUCE, ICEBERG
LETTUCE, LEAF/SHREDDED
MUSHROOMS
ONION
PICKLES (DILL)
RADISH

RED PEPPERS
SPINACH (CAN/NO SALT)
SPINACH (FRESH)
TOMATO (EXCLUDING JUICE)
ZUCCHINI

Supplements/Fast Foods

ATKINS BAR	0.75	BAR
EAS ADVANTEDGE, C&C/LEM/BLUE	0.75	BAR
BAR, ZONE	0.88	BAR
BAR, PURE PROTEIN, 50 G.	1	BAR
BAR, W.W. PURE PROTEIN, 78 G.	0.5	BAR
BAR, PROTEIN REVOLUTION, PBJ	0.88	BAR
BAR, FIBAR, PEANUT BUTTER, 1.2 OZ	1.33	BAR
BAR, PREMIER 1, PROTEIN 8, CHOC/COCO	0.75	BAR
BAR, PREFERRED BAR, CHOC./FUDG/RAS	0.88	BAR
BAR, PREFERRED BAR, CHOC./FUDG/BROW	0.88	BAR
ALIVE, HI CARB POWDER	5	TBLSP
POWERADE	2	SERVING
PROTEIN,GNC P.P. EGG/WHEY	1.5	SERVING
PROTEIN. GNC P.PERF. WHEY	4	SCOOP
OPTIMUM NUTRITION WHEY	1.75	SCOOP
SYNTRAX WHEY PROTEIN	2.25	SCOOP
TRI PROTEIN PLUS POWDER	1.5	SERVING
HW STRAWBERRY PROT. POWD.	2	SCOOP
BIOCHEM WHEY PRO 290	2.5	SCOOP
HUMAN DEV. TECH. WHEY	1.5	SCOOP
NATURADE 100% SOY PROTEIN	0.5	CUP
SUPER GREEN PRO 96 - SOY	0.5	CUP
100% PURE WHEY, PROLAB	0.75	SCOOP
ECLIPSE BULK UP WHEY	2	SCOOP
VITAMIN WORLD WHEY 100%	1.75	SCOOP
ULT. NUT. PROSTAR WHEY	1.75	SCOOP
RED WINE	8	OZ
MET RX CH.RST.PNT.PRO + BAR	0.5	BAR
MET RX BAV. MINT. PRO + BAR	0.75	BAR
MET AFTER FX BAR	0.75	BAR
MET RX CH. CH. CHIP PRO + BAR	0.75	BAR

MET RX SOURCE ONE BAR	0.75	BAR
MET RX CHOC. GRAHCRK CHIP BAR	0.5	BAR
MET RX PEANUT BUTTER BAR	0.5	BAR
MET RX DRINK MIX, MRP	0.75	SERVING
MET RX PRO 50, ANABOLIC DRIVE	0.75	SERVING
MET RX PRO 60, ANABOLIC DRIVE	0.5	SERVING
MET RX PROTEIN PLUS	2.5	SCOOP
MET RX KETO PRO	2.5	SCOOP
NUTRI FORCE DRINK MIX, MRP	0.75	SERVING
EAS MYO. DEL. CH/PB BAR	0.5	BAR
EAS MYOPLEX + DELUXE	0.5	SERVING
EAS MYOPLEX LITE	0.75	SERVING
ADVANT EDGE QUICK STIR PROTEIN DRINK	0.75	SERVING
EAS NEUROGAIN	4	SCOOP
EAS PHOSPHAGEN HP	1	SCOOP
EAS PRECISION PROTEIN	1.75	SCOOP
EAS SIMPLY PROTEIN	3	SCOOP
EAS WHEY PROTEIN	1.75	SCOOP
EAS SUPPER SHAKE	0.33	SHAKE
VITAMIN WORLD DAILY RX, MRP	0.75	SHAKE
VITAMIN WORLD PROTOPLEX DELUXE, MRP	0.5	SHAKE
VITAMIN WORLD PRE. ENG. WHEY PROT.	2	SCOOP
PERFECT RX, MRP, CHOCOLATE	0.75	SHAKE
OPTI PRO	0.75	SHAKE
ARBY'S CHICK. SAND. R.DELX.LITE	0.5	BURGER
ARBY'S SIDE SALAD	1	SALAD
ARBY'S GARDEN SALAD	1	SALAD
ARBY'S RST. CHCK. SALAD	1	SALAD
ARBY'S RED. CAL. ITAL. DRESSING	1	PACKET
ARBY'S RED RANCH DRESSING	1	PACKET
MCD'S VINEG. LITE SALAD DR.	1	PACKET
MCD'S GARDEN SALAD	1	SALAD
MCD'S VINEG. LITE SALAD DR.	1	PACKET
P.HUT. HAND-TOSS CHEESE	0.75	SLICE
P.HUT. HAND-TOSS HAM	0.75	SLICE
P.HUT. HAND-TOSS VEG. LUV.	0.75	SLICE
P.HUT. HAND-TOSS PEPPERON	0.75	SLICE
P.HUT. THIN/CRISP CHEESE	1	SLICE

P.HUT. THIN/CRISP HAM	1	SLICE
P.HUT. THIN/CRISP VEG. LUV.	1	SLICE
P.HUT. THIN/CRISP PEPPERON	0.75	SLICE
SW 6" COLD SUB/VEGG. DELIT	1	SUB
SW 6" COLD SUB/TURK. BRST.	1	SUB
SW 6" COLD SUB/TURK.B/HAM	1	SUB
SW 6" COLD SUB/HAM	1	SUB
SW 6" COLD SUB/ROAST BEEF	1	SUB
SW 6" COLD SUB/SFOOD,CRAB	1	SUB
SW 6" COLD SUB/COLD CUT 3	1	SUB
SW 6" COLD SUB/TUNA	1	SUB
SW 6" HOT SUB/RST.CHICK.BR.	1	SUB
SW 6" HOT SUB/STAK/CHEESE	1	SUB
SW 6" HOT SUB/SUB MELT	1	SUB
SW VEGGIE DELITE SALAD	1	SALAD
SW TURKEY BREAST SALAD	1	SALAD
SW ROAST BEEF SALAD	1	SALAD
SW TURK. BRST/HAM SALAD	1	SALAD
SW RST. CHICK. BR. SALAD	1	SALAD
SW SEAFOOD/CRAB SALAD	1	SALAD
SW STEAK/CHEESE SALAD	0.75	SALAD
SW SUBWAY MELT SALAD	1	SALAD
SW COLD CUT 3 SALAD	1	SALAD
SW FAT FREE ITALIAN DRESS	1	OZ
SW FAT FREE FRENCH DRESS	1	OZ
SW FAT FREE RANCH DRESS	1	OZ
SW DELI STYLE TURKEY BR.	0.75	SNDWCH
SW DELI STYLE HAM	0.75	SNDWCH
SW DELI STYLE ROAST BEEF	0.75	SNDWCH
TB GRILLED STEAK SOFT TACO	0.75	TACO
WAHOO'S CHBROIL FISH TACO	1	TACO
WENDI'S SIDE SALAD	1	SALAD
WENDI'S FF FRENCH DRESSING	1	OZ
WENDI'S ITALIAN RED. F/C DRESS	1	OZ
WENDI'S SMALL CHILI	1	BOWL
WENDI'S GRILLED CHICK. FILLET	1.5	MEAT

	2900 Calories/Day Eating Plan	
	What Does Your Doctor Look Like Naked?	

Name: _____

Date: _____

Exercise: 30-40 min in a.m. before food		Write what you eat here:
Meal 1 Time: _____	2 Protein Sources 3 Active Carbohydrates	
Meal 2 Time:	3 oz Raw Almonds	
Meal 3 Time: _____	1 Protein Source 2 Active Carbohydrates Free Carbohydrates (as much as you want)	
Meal 4 Time: _____	1 LOW CARB protein bar (OR) 2.5 scoops Whey Protein Powder in water AND 1 oz String Cheese	
Meal 5 Time:	2 Protein Source 0 Active Carbohydrates Free Carbohydrates (as much as you want)	
BEDTIME Meal (Optional)	Sugar Free Jell-O 1 cup	

Add fiber supplement in evening, such as Metamucil or other (sugar FREE).
Add spices, pepper, etc. as needed.
Try to eat every two to three hours.
Drink 1⅓ gallons of water EVERY DAY!
May have up to 2 diet pops (or) 2 cups a coffee a day.

Active Carbohydrates 2900 Calories

Fruit and Vegetables

APPLE	2.56	3 INCH
APPLESAUCE, MOTT'S	0.945	CUP
APRICOTS (CAN/DEL MONTE LITE)	1.73	CUP
APRICOTS (DRIED)	2.96	OZ
APRICOTS (FRESH 12/LB)	12.2	MEDIUM
ASPARAGUS	56	OZ
BANANA	1.98	MEDIUM
BLUEBERRIES (FRESH)	2.53	CUP
BRUSSELS SPROUTS, BOILED	3.45	CUP
CABBAGE, SHREDDED	11.5	CUP
CANTALOUPE	1.1	5 INCH
CARROT (FRESH)	18.7	OZ
CAULIFLOWER	7.97	CUP
CELERY	51.8	OZ
CHERRIES, FRESH, SWEET W/PIT	1.99	CUP
CHERRIES, DARK (CAN/DEL MONTE)	1.035	CUP
COLLARD GREENS (CAN)	3.45	CUP
COLLARD GREENS (FRESH)	17.3	CUP
CORN CAKE	5.94	CAKE
CORN (CAN/DEL MONTE NO SODIUM)	15.15	OZ
CUCUMBER, SLICED	14.8	CUP
EGGPLANT	14.8	CUP
FRUIT, MIXED FROZEN	2.3	CUP
GARLIC, 1 CLOVE	51.8	CLOVE
GARLIC, TRIMMED	4.95	OZ
GRAPES	1.82	CUP
GRAPE JUICE/VERYFINE	11.05	OZ
GRAPEFRUIT	2.25	4 INCH
GREEN BEANS (CAN/DEL MONTE NO SALT)	5.18	CUP
GREEN PEPPER	10.35	MEDIUM
KIWI	13.95	OZ
MUSHROOMS, FRESH	11.5	CUP
ONION, FRESH/CHOPPED	3.45	CUP
ORANGE, NAVAL	3.19	3 INCH

ORANGE, JUICE	15.1	OZ
PAPAYA	3.85	LB.
PAPAYA, PEELED/CUBED	1.98	CUP
PEACH, FRESH, SLICED	2.8	CUP
PEACH (CAN/DEL MONTE EXTRA LITE)	1.73	CUP
PEARS (CAN)	6.9	HALF
PEAS, BLACKEYED (CAN)	1.15	CUP
PEAS (CAN/DEL MONTE NO SODIUM)	15.15	OZ
PEAS, GREEN GIANT FROZEN, SWEET	1.98	CUP
PEAS, EDIBLE-PODDED	3.45	CUP
PINEAPPLE, FRESH/DICED	2.66	CUP
PINEAPPLE, DEL MONTE SNACK CAN (LITE)	2.96	3.5 OZ
PINEAPPLE (CAN/DOLE LITE SYRUP)	12.2	SLICE
PRUNES, DOLE, DRIED	2.96	OZ
PUMPKIN (CAN)	4.14	CUP
RAISINS	0.433	CUP
RED PEPPER	10.35	MEDIUM
STRAWBERRIES (FRESH)	2.14	PINT
STRAWBERRIES (FROZEN)	2.76	CUP
SQUASH, CAN, STOKLEY	2.07	CUP
SQUASH, FRESH BAKED	1.82	CUP
TANGERINE	5.6	2.5 INCH
TOMATO, CAN	19.4	OZ
TOMATO, FRESH	8	3 INCH
TOMATO, JUICE	33	OZ
VEGETABLES, MIXED (FROZEN)	2.3	CUP
WATERMELLON	1.36	1X10 INCH
ZUCCHINI, FRESH, SLICED	11.5	CUP

Yogurts and Desserts

DING DONG	1.29	DING
DREYERS FROZEN FAT FREE YOGURT	1.15	CUP
FRUIT ROLL-UP	2.96	ROLL-UP
POPCORN, WHITE	4.15	TBLSP
TCBY, SOFT SERVE/NONFAT/NO SUGAR	1.29	CUP
YOGURT, FAT FREE, MOUNTAIN HIGH	8	OZ
YOGURT, FAT FREE, DANNON	8	OZ
LUCERN, YOGURT, NONFAT, LITE	8	OZ

YOGURT, YOPLAIT, FAT FREE, LITE	6	OZ
YOGURT, YOPLAIT ORIGINAL/99% FAT FREE	6	OZ
YOGURT, HORIZON, FF/BLUEBERRY	6	OZ
PLANTER DRIED WALNUT PIECES	0.25	CUP
RAW ALMONDS, TOASTED	1.25	OZ
PECANS, DRIED	1	OZ
PEANUTS, DRY ROASTED	0.25	CUP
HOT CHOCOLATE	4	ENVEL.
ALMONDS, SHELLED	1.25	OZ

Cereals

CEREAL, CHEERIOS	1.89	CUP
CEREAL, COCOA KRISPIES	1.295	CUP
CEREAL, GRAPENUTS	0.518	CUP
CEREAL, HONEY NUT TOASTY O'S	1.89	CUP
CEREAL, WHEATIES	1.89	CUP
CEREAL, KELLOGG'S ALL BRAN	1.295	CUP
CEREAL, KELLOGG'S CORN FLAKES	1.89	CUP
CEREAL, KELLOGG'S RAISIN BRAN	1.22	CUP
CEREAL, KELLOGG'S CRACKLIN' OAT BRAN	0.785	CUP
CEREAL, NABISCO SHREDDED WHEAT	2.59	PIECE
CEREAL, NAB. SHREDDED WHEAT (SPOON)	1.22	CUP
CEREAL, RICE KRISPIES	2.36	CUP
CEREAL, BENEFIT NUTRITION, PROTEIN +	0.99	CUP
CREAM OF WHEAT	5.18	TBL/DRY
GRANOLA, CW POST HEARTY	0.495	CUP
GRANOLA, KELLOGG'S LOW FAT	4	CUP
OATMEAL (PRE-COOK MEASUREMENT)	0.74	CUP

Breads

BREAD, OROWHEAT LITE	5.18	SLICE
BREAD, SUSAN'S HOMEMADE/18 SLICES	2.29	SLICE
BREAD, SUSAN'S HOMEMADE	0.127	LOAF
BUN, WONDER REDUCED CALORIE LITE	2.59	BUN
CRACKER, ZESTA SALTINES	17.3	CRACKER
TORTILLA (CAROLYN)	1.22	TORT
TORTILLA, TORTILLA'S MEXICO, FLOUR	1.89	TORT

TORTILLA, TORTILLA'S MEXICO, CORN	2.3	TORT
TRISCUITS	1.48	OZ
WAFFLE, EGGO, HOMESTYLE	1.89	WAFFLE
WHOLE GRAIN/WHOLE WHEAT FLOUR	0.51	CUP

Rice/Potatoes/Beans

BLACK BEANS (BOILED)	0.92	CUP
BLACK BEANS (DRY)	0.74	CUP
CHICKPEAS/GARBANZO BEANS	0.25	CUP
KIDNEY BEANS (BOILED)	0.33	CUP
LIMA BEANS (BOILED)	1	CUP
NAVY BEANS (BOILED)	0.8	CUP
NAVY BEANS (CAN)	0.865	CUP
PINTO BEANS (BOILED)	0.886	CUP
PINTO BEANS (CAN)	1.09	CUP
PINTO BEANS (DRY)	0.345	CUP
PORK & BEANS/VAN CAMPS	0.945	CUP
POTATO, SWEET	1.76	5"X2"
POTATO	12.3	OZ
RICE CAKE	4.14	CAKE
RICE, WHITE, BASMATI	0.865	CUP (C)
RICE, BROWN LONG GRAIN	1.035	CUP (C)
RICE, INSTANT, MINUTE BRAND	0.645	CUP(UC)
RICE, WHITE, LONG GRAIN	0.324	CUP(UC)
SOYBEANS (BOILED)	0.75	CUP
YAM, BOILED OR BAKED	1.31	CUP

Pasta

MACARONI, DAVINI TWIST	0.79	CUP/DRY
MACARONI, HOSPITALITY ELBOW	0.433	CUP/DRY
MACARONI, AM. BEAUTY ELBOW	0.495	CUP/DRY
PASTA, CREAMETTE PLAIN	1.98	OZ
SPAGHETTI, EDEN WHOLE WHEAT	1.98	OZ/UC

Protein Sources 2900 Calories

White Meat

CHICKEN BREAST (HORMEL/CAN)	1.38	CAN
CHICKEN BREAST (SKINLESS)	6.9	OZ
CHICKEN (LEG W/ SKIN & BONE)	0.78	
CHICKEN (THIGH W/ SKIN & BONE)	1.355	
CHICKEN (LEG & THIGH W/ SKIN & BONE)	0.496	
HAM, BAR S, XTRA LEAN, 96% FAT FREE	5.93	OZ
HAM, DAK CAN	6.9	OZ
PORK, SIRLOIN, LEAN W/FAT	2.07	OZ
TURKEY BREAST (SKINLESS)	3.87	OZ
TURKEY BREAST (HORMEL/CAN)	1.185	CAN
TURKEY BRST/OVEN ROAST/SFWY/89% FF	8.3	OZ
VENISON / ANTELOPE	4.64	OZ

Red Meat

HAMBURGER (10% FAT)	3.68	OZ
HAMBURGER (15% FAT)	3.05	OZ
HAMBURGER (20% FAT)	2.96	OZ
HAMBURGER (27% FAT)	2.51	OZ
LAMB, SHOULDER	2.36	OZ
STEAK, BOTTOM ROUND	3.5	OZ
STEAK, BRISKET (FLAT HALF)	3.3	OZ
STEAK, CHUCK, ARM	3.4	OZ
STEAK, CHUCK, BLADE	2.92	OZ
STEAK, EYE ROUND	4.35	OZ
STEAK, FLANK	3.54	OZ
STEAK, NEW YORK STRIP	4.14	OZ
STEAK, PORTERHOUSE	3.36	OZ
STEAK, RIBEYE	3.26	OZ
STEAK, ROUND TIP	3.97	OZ
STEAK, SHANK (CROSSCUTS)	3.64	OZ
STEAK, T-BONE	3.42	OZ
STEAK, TENDERLOIN	3.48	OZ
STEAK, TOP LOIN	3.54	OZ
STEAK, TOP ROUND	4.07	OZ

STEAK, TOP SIRLOIN	3.78	OZ
STEAK, TYSON SEASONED BEEF STRIPS	4.45	OZ
TACO/BURRITO MEAT/SMART GROUND	1.08	CUP
OSCAR MAYER BACON	6.9	SLICE
LITTLE SIZZLER BROWN/SERVE SAUSAGE	2.7	LINK

Sea Food

BASS, FRESHWATER, DRY HEAT	5	OZ
BASS, STRIPED, DRY HEAT	5.93	OZ
COD, ATLANTIC, DRY HEAT	7	OZ
CRAB, ALASKA KING, MOIST HEAT	7.6	OZ
CRAB, BLUE, MOIST HEAT	7.15	OZ
FLOUNDER, DRY HEAT	6.3	OZ
HADDOCK, DRY HEAT	6.56	OZ
HALIBUT, DRY HEAT	5.23	OZ
LOBSTER, NORTHERN, MOIST HEAT	7.5	OZ
MAHI MAHI	8.55	OZ
ORANGE ROUGHY, DRY HEAT	8.2	OZ
PERCH, DRY HEAT	6.3	OZ
PERCH, OCEAN/ATLANTIC, DRY HEAT	6.04	OZ
SALMON, ATLANTIC, DRY HEAT	3.99	OZ
SHRIMP, MOIST HEAT	7.4	OZ
TROUT, DRY HEAT	3.86	OZ
TUNA BURGER, AHI/OMEGA FOODS	7.4	OZ
TUNA, LOW SODIUM, CAN	1.185	CAN
TUNA, WATER, CAN	1.38	CAN
TUNA, WHITE/LOW SALT, CAN (5 OZ)	1.18	CAN
TUNA, WHITE, CAN (5 OZ)	1.18	CAN
TUNA, FILLET/STEAK	4.72	OZ
WALLEYE, BAKED/BROILED/MICRO	6.15	OZ

Vegetarian

IVES VEG. COUSINE VEGGY DOG	3.45	DOG
SOY MILK (TRIS)	2.25	CUP
SOY MILK (SYLVIA)	2	CUP

Eggs/Dairy

1% COTTAGE CHEESE, NORDICA	1.295	CUP
2% COTTAGE CHEESE (LOW FAT)	1.035	CUP
COTTAGE CHEESE (LUCERNE FAT FREE)	1.29	CUP
COTT CHEESE MARIGOLD/DRY CURD	1.98	CUP
COTT CHEESE MARIGOLD/DRY CURD	31.6	TBLSP
COTT CHEESE BREAKSTONES FAT FREE	1.295	CUP
CHEDDER, SHREDDED, FAT FREE, KHF	1.15	CUP
CHEDDER, SHREDDED, 94% FAT FREE, HC	1.035	CUP
CHEESE, COLBY/MOZZARELLA	1.89	OZ
EGG WHITE	12.2	
EGG, WHOLE	2.76	
EGG BEATERS	1.73	CUP
MOZZARELLA SHREDDED, FAT FREE, KHF	1.03	CUP
SKIM MOZZARELLA STRING CHEESE	2.59	OZ

Free Carbs, Supplements, Fast Foods
2900 calories

Free Carbs

ASPARAGUS
BROCCOLI
CABBAGE
CAULIFLOWER
CELERY
CUCUMBER
GREEN BEANS
GREEN PEPPERS
GREEN SQUASH
LETTUCE, ICEBERG
LETTUCE, LEAF/SHREDDED
MUSHROOMS
ONION
PICKLES (DILL)
RADISH

RED PEPPERS
SPINACH (CAN/NO SALT)
SPINACH (FRESH)
TOMATO (EXCLUDING JUICE)
ZUCCHINI

Supplements/Fast Foods

ATKINS BAR	1	BAR
EAS ADVANTEDGE, C&C/LEM/BLUE	1	BAR
BAR, ZONE	1	BAR
BAR, PURE PROTEIN, 50 G.	1	BAR
BAR, W.W. PURE PROTEIN, 78 G.	0.5	BAR
BAR, PROTEIN REVOLUTION, PBJ	0.88	BAR
BAR, FIBAR, PEANUT BUTTER, 1.2 OZ	1.5	BAR
BAR, PREMIER 1, PROTEIN 8, CHOC/COCO	0.75	BAR
BAR, PREFERRED BAR, CHOC./FUDG/RAS	1	BAR
BAR, PREFERRED BAR, CHOC./FUDG/BROW	1	BAR
ALIVE, HI CARB POWDER	5	TBLSP
POWERADE	2.5	SERVING
PROTEIN,GNC P.P. EGG/WHEY	1.75	SERVING
PROTEIN. GNC P.PERF. WHEY	5	SCOOP
OPTIMUM NUTRITION WHEY	1.75	SCOOP
SYNTRAX WHEY PROTEIN	2.33	SCOOP
TRI PROTEIN PLUS POWDER	1.5	SERVING
HW STRAWBERRY PROT. POWD.	2.25	SCOOP
BIOCHEM WHEY PRO 290	2.5	SCOOP
HUMAN DEV. TECH. WHEY	1.5	SCOOP
NATURADE 100% SOY PROTEIN	0.5	CUP
SUPER GREEN PRO 96 - SOY	0.5	CUP
100% PURE WHEY, PROLAB	1.5	SCOOP
ECLIPSE BULK UP WHEY	2	SCOOP
VITAMIN WORLD WHEY 100%	1.88	SCOOP
ULT. NUT. PROSTAR WHEY	1.88	SCOOP
RED WINE	8	OZ
MET RX CH.RST.PNT.PRO + BAR	0.5	BAR
MET RX BAV. MINT. PRO + BAR	0.75	BAR
MET AFTER FX BAR	0.75	BAR
MET RX CH. CH. CHIP PRO + BAR	0.75	BAR

MET RX SOURCE ONE BAR	1	BAR
MET RX CHOC. GRAHCRK CHIP BAR	0.5	BAR
MET RX PEANUT BUTTER BAR	0.5	BAR
MET RX DRINK MIX, MRP	0.75	SERVING
MET RX PRO 50, ANABOLIC DRIVE	0.75	SERVING
MET RX PRO 60, ANABOLIC DRIVE	0.5	SERVING
MET RX PROTEIN PLUS	3	SCOOP
MET RX KETO PRO	2.75	SCOOP
NUTRI FORCE DRINK MIX, MRP	0.75	SERVING
EAS MYO. DEL. CH/PB BAR	0.5	BAR
EAS MYOPLEX + DELUXE	0.5	SERVING
EAS MYOPLEX LITE	0.5	SERVING
ADVANT EDGE QUICK STIR PROTEIN DRINK	0.88	SERVING
EAS NEUROGAIN	4.5	SCOOP
EAS PHOSPHAGEN HP	1.5	SCOOP
EAS PRECISION PROTEIN	2	SCOOP
EAS SIMPLY PROTEIN	3.5	SCOOP
EAS WHEY PROTEIN	1.75	SCOOP
EAS SUPPER SHAKE	0.33	SHAKE
VITAMIN WORLD DAILY RX, MRP	0.75	SHAKE
VITAMIN WORLD PROTOPLEX DELUXE, MRP	0.5	SHAKE
VITAMIN WORLD PRE. ENG. WHEY PROT.	2.5	SCOOP
PERFECT RX, MRP, CHOCOLATE	0.75	SHAKE
OPTI PRO	0.75	SHAKE
ARBY'S CHICK. SAND. R.DELX.LITE	0.75	BURGER
ARBY'S SIDE SALAD	1	SALAD
ARBY'S GARDEN SALAD	1	SALAD
ARBY'S RST. CHCK. SALAD	1	SALAD
ARBY'S RED. CAL. ITAL. DRESSING	1	PACKET
ARBY'S RED RANCH DRESSING	1	PACKET
MCD'S VINEG. LITE SALAD DR.	1	PACKET
MCD'S GARDEN SALAD	1	SALAD
MCD'S VINEG. LITE SALAD DR.	1	PACKET
P.HUT. HAND-TOSS CHEESE	0.88	SLICE
P.HUT. HAND-TOSS HAM	1	SLICE
P.HUT. HAND-TOSS VEG. LUV.	0.88	SLICE
P.HUT. HAND-TOSS PEPPERON	0.75	SLICE
P.HUT. THIN/CRISP CHEESE	1	SLICE

P.HUT. THIN/CRISP HAM	1	SLICE
P.HUT. THIN/CRISP VEG. LUV.	1	SLICE
P.HUT. THIN/CRISP PEPPERON	1	SLICE
SW 6" COLD SUB/VEGG. DELIT	1	SUB
SW 6" COLD SUB/TURK. BRST.	1	SUB
SW 6" COLD SUB/TURK.B/HAM	1	SUB
SW 6" COLD SUB/HAM	1	SUB
SW 6" COLD SUB/ROAST BEEF	1	SUB
SW 6" COLD SUB/SFOOD,CRAB	1	SUB
SW 6" COLD SUB/COLD CUT 3	1	SUB
SW 6" COLD SUB/TUNA	1	SUB
SW 6" HOT SUB/RST.CHICK.BR.	1	SUB
SW 6" HOT SUB/STAK/CHEESE	1	SUB
SW 6" HOT SUB/SUB MELT	1	SUB
SW VEGGIE DELITE SALAD	1	SALAD
SW TURKEY BREAST SALAD	1	SALAD
SW ROAST BEEF SALAD	1	SALAD
SW TURK. BRST/HAM SALAD	1	SALAD
SW RST. CHICK. BR. SALAD	1	SALAD
SW SEAFOOD/CRAB SALAD	1	SALAD
SW STEAK/CHEESE SALAD	1	SALAD
SW SUBWAY MELT SALAD	1	SALAD
SW COLD CUT 3 SALAD	1	SALAD
SW FAT FREE ITALIAN DRESS	1	OZ
SW FAT FREE FRENCH DRESS	1	OZ
SW FAT FREE RANCH DRESS	1	OZ
SW DELI STYLE TURKEY BR.	0.88	SNDWCH
SW DELI STYLE HAM	0.88	SNDWCH
SW DELI STYLE ROAST BEEF	0.75	SNDWCH
TB GRILLED STEAK SOFT TACO	0.88	TACO
WAHOO'S CHBROIL FISH TACO	1	TACO
WENDI'S SIDE SALAD	1	SALAD
WENDI'S FF FRENCH DRESSING	1	OZ
WENDI'S ITALIAN RED. F/C DRESS	1	OZ
WENDI'S SMALL CHILI	1	BOWL
WENDI'S GRILLED CHICK. FILLET	1	MEAT

3000 Calories/Day Eating Plan		
What Does Your Doctor Look Like Naked?		
Name: _____		
Date: _____		
Exercise: 30-40 min in a.m. before food		Write what you eat here:
Meal 1 Time: _____	2 Protein Sources 4 Active Carbohydrates	
Meal 2 Time: _____	3 oz Raw Almonds	
Meal 3 Time: _____	2 Protein Source 2 Active Carbohydrates Free Carbohydrates (as much as you want)	
Meal 4 Time: _____	1 LOW CARB protein bar (OR) 2 scoops Whey Protein Powder in water AND 1 oz String Cheese 1 oz Raw Almonds	
Meal 5 Time: _____	2 Protein Source 0 Active Carbohydrates Free Carbohydrates (as much as you want)	
Bedtime Meal (Optional)	Sugar Free Jell-O 1 cup	
Add fiber supplement in evening, such as Metamucil or other (sugar FREE). Add spices, pepper, etc. as needed. Try to eat every two to three hours. Drink 1⅓ gallons of water EVERY DAY! May have up to 2 diet pops (or) 2 cups a coffee a day.		

Active Carbohydrates 3000 Calories

Fruit and Vegetables

APPLE	2.08	3 INCH
APPLESAUCE, MOTT'S	0.76	CUP
APRICOTS (CAN/DEL MONTE LITE)	1.4	CUP
APRICOTS (DRIED)	2.4	OZ
APRICOTS (FRESH 12/LB)	9.9	MEDIUM
ASPARAGUS	45.5	OZ
BANANA	1.6	MEDIUM
BLUEBERRIES (FRESH)	2.05	CUP
BRUSSELS SPROUTS, BOILED	2.8	CUP
CABBAGE, SHREDDED	9.3	CUP
CANTALOUPE	0.9	5 INCH
CARROT (FRESH)	15.2	OZ
CAULIFLOWER	6.5	CUP
CELERY	42	OZ
CHERRIES, FRESH, SWEET W/PIT	1.62	CUP
CHERRIES, DARK (CAN/DEL MONTE)	0.84	CUP
COLLARD GREENS (CAN)	2.8	CUP
COLLARD GREENS (FRESH)	14	CUP
CORN CAKE	4.8	CAKE
CORN (CAN/DEL MONTE NO SODIUM)	12.3	OZ
CUCUMBER, SLICED	12	CUP
EGGPLANT	7.6	CUP
FRUIT, MIXED FROZEN	1.86	CUP
GARLIC, 1 CLOVE	42	CLOVE
GARLIC, TRIMMED	4	OZ
GRAPES	1.48	CUP
GRAPE JUICE/VERYFINE	9	OZ
GRAPEFRUIT	1.83	4 INCH
GREEN BEANS (CAN/DEL MONTE NO SALT)	4.2	CUP
GREEN PEPPER	8.4	MEDIUM
KIWI	11.4	OZ
MUSHROOMS, FRESH	2.81	CUP
ONION, FRESH/CHOPPED	1.968	CUP
ORANGE, NAVAL	2.6	3 INCH

ORANGE, JUICE	12.2	OZ
PAPAYA	1.44	LB.
PAPAYA, PEELED/CUBED	3.1	CUP
PEACH, FRESH, SLICED	2.28	CUP
PEACH (CAN/DEL MONTE EXTRA LITE)	1.4	CUP
PEARS (CAN)	5.6	HALF
PEAS, BLACKEYED (CAN)	0.93	CUP
PEAS (CAN/DEL MONTE NO SODIUM)	12.3	OZ
PEAS, GREEN GIANT FROZEN, SWEET	1.6	CUP
PEAS, EDIBLE-PODDED	2.8	CUP
PINEAPPLE, FRESH/DICED	2.15	CUP
PINEAPPLE, DEL MONTE SNACK CAN (LITE)	2.4	3.5 OZ
PINEAPPLE (CAN/DOLE LITE SYRUP)	9.9	SLICE
PRUNES, DOLE, DRIED	2.4	OZ
PUMPKIN (CAN)	3.35	CUP
RAISINS	0.35	CUP
RED PEPPER	8.4	MEDIUM
STRAWBERRIES (FRESH)	1.75	PINT
STRAWBERRIES (FROZEN)	2.25	CUP
SQUASH, CAN, STOKLEY	1.68	CUP
SQUASH, FRESH BAKED	1.48	CUP
TANGERINE	4.55	2.5 INCH
TOMATO, CAN	15.7	OZ
TOMATO, FRESH	6.45	3 INCH
TOMATO, JUICE	27	OZ
VEGETABLES, MIXED (FROZEN)	1.87	CUP
WATERMELLON	1.1	1X10 INCH
ZUCCHINI, FRESH, SLICED	9.3	CUP

Yogurts and Desserts

DING DONG	1.05	DING
DREYERS FROZEN FAT FREE YOGURT	0.9	CUP
FRUIT ROLL-UP	2.4	ROLL-UP
POPCORN, WHITE	3.35	TBLSP
TCBY, SOFT SERVE/NONFAT/NO SUGAR	1.05	CUP
YOGURT, FAT FREE, MOUNTAIN HIGH	8	OZ
YOGURT, FAT FREE, DANNON	8	OZ
LUCERN, YOGURT, NONFAT, LITE	8	OZ

YOGURT, YOPLAIT, FAT FREE, LITE	6	OZ
YOGURT,YOPLAIT ORIGINAL/99% FAT FREE	6	OZ
YOGURT, HORIZON, FF/BLUEBERRY	6	OZ
PLANTER DRIED WALNUT PIECES	0.2	CUP
RAW ALMONDS, TOASTED	1	OZ
PECANS, DRIED	0.88	OZ
PEANUTS, DRY ROASTED	0.2	CUP
HOT CHOCOLATE	3	ENVEL.
ALMONDS, SHELLED	1	OZ

Cereals

CEREAL, CHEERIOS	1.53	CUP
CEREAL, COCOA KRISPIES	1.05	CUP
CEREAL, GRAPENUTS	0.42	CUP
CEREAL, HONEY NUT TOASTY O'S	1.53	CUP
CEREAL, WHEATIES	1.53	CUP
CEREAL, KELLOGG'S ALL BRAN	1.05	CUP
CEREAL, KELLOGG'S CORN FLAKES	1.53	CUP
CEREAL, KELLOGG'S RAISIN BRAN	1	CUP
CEREAL, KELLOGG'S CRACKLIN' OAT BRAN	0.64	CUP
CEREAL, NABISCO SHREDDED WHEAT	2.1	PIECE
CEREAL, NAB. SHREDDED WHEAT (SPOON)	0.99	CUP
CEREAL, RICE KRISPIES	1.9	CUP
CEREAL, BENEFIT NUTRITION, PROTEIN +	0.8	CUP
CREAM OF WHEAT	4.2	TBL/DRY
GRANOLA, CW POST HEARTY	0.4	CUP
GRANOLA, KELLOGG'S LOW FAT	2	CUP
OATMEAL (PRE-COOK MEASUREMENT)	0.6	CUP

Breads

BREAD, OROWHEAT LITE	4.2	SLICE
BREAD, SUSAN'S HOMEMADE/18 SLICES	1.86	SLICE
BREAD, SUSAN'S HOMEMADE	0.103	LOAF
BUN, WONDER REDUCED CALORIE LITE	2.1	BUN
CRACKER, ZESTA SALTINES	14	CRACKER
TORTILLA (CAROLYN)	0.99	TORT
TORTILLA, TORTILLA'S MEXICO, FLOUR	1.53	TORT

TORTILLA, TORTILLA'S MEXICO, CORN	1.87	TORT
TRISCUITS	1.2	OZ
WAFFLE, EGGO, HOMESTYLE	1.53	WAFFLE
WHOLE GRAIN/WHOLE WHEAT FLOUR	0.412	CUP

Rice/Potatoes/Beans

BLACK BEANS (BOILED)	0.74	CUP
BLACK BEANS (DRY)	0.6	CUP
CHICKPEAS/GARBANZO BEANS	0.2	CUP
KIDNEY BEANS (BOILED)	0.25	CUP
LIMA BEANS (BOILED)	0.81	CUP
NAVY BEANS (BOILED)	0.65	CUP
NAVY BEANS (CAN)	0.7	CUP
PINTO BEANS (BOILED)	0.72	CUP
PINTO BEANS (CAN)	0.88	CUP
PINTO BEANS (DRY)	0.28	CUP
PORK & BEANS/VAN CAMPS	0.76	CUP
POTATO, SWEET	1.43	5"X2"
POTATO	10	OZ
RICE CAKE	3.35	CAKE
RICE, WHITE, BASMATI	0.7	CUP (C)
RICE, BROWN LONG GRAIN	0.84	CUP (C)
RICE, INSTANT, MINUTE BRAND	0.525	CUP(UC)
RICE, WHITE, LONG GRAIN	0.263	CUP(UC)
SOYBEANS (BOILED)	0.66	CUP
YAM, BOILED OR BAKED	1.06	CUP

Pasta

MACARONI, DAVINI TWIST	0.64	CUP/DRY
MACARONI, HOSPITALITY ELBOW	0.35	CUP/DRY
MACARONI, AM. BEAUTY ELBOW	0.4	CUP/DRY
PASTA, CREAMETTE PLAIN	1.6	OZ
SPAGHETTI, EDEN WHOLE WHEAT	1.6	OZ/UC

Protein Sources 3000 Calories

White Meat

CHICKEN BREAST (HORMEL/CAN)	1.12	CAN
CHICKEN BREAST (SKINLESS)	5.6	OZ
CHICKEN (LEG W/SKIN & BONE)	0.64	
CHICKEN (THIGH W/SKIN & BONE)	1.1	
CHICKEN (LEG & THIGH W/SKIN & BONE)	0.4	
HAM, BAR S, XTRA LEAN, 96% FAT FREE	4.25	OZ
HAM, DAK CAN	5.6	OZ
PORK, SIRLOIN, LEAN W/FAT	1.68	OZ
TURKEY BREAST (SKINLESS)	3.14	OZ
TURKEY BREAST (HORMEL/CAN)	0.96	CAN
TURKEY BRST/OVEN ROAST/SFWY/89% FF	6.7	OZ
VENISON/ANTELOPE	3.75	OZ

Red Meat

HAMBURGER (10% FAT)	3	OZ
HAMBURGER (15% FAT)	2.48	OZ
HAMBURGER (20% FAT)	2.4	OZ
HAMBURGER (27% FAT)	2.04	OZ
LAMB, SHOULDER	1.92	OZ
STEAK, BOTTOM ROUND	2.84	OZ
STEAK, BRISKET (FLAT HALF)	2.68	OZ
STEAK, CHUCK, ARM	2.77	OZ
STEAK, CHUCK, BLADE	2.38	OZ
STEAK, EYE ROUND	3.53	OZ
STEAK, FLANK	2.87	OZ
STEAK, NEW YORK STRIP	3.35	OZ
STEAK, PORTERHOUSE	2.74	OZ
STEAK, RIBYE	2.65	OZ
STEAK, ROUND TIP	3.22	OZ
STEAK, SHANK (CROSSCUTS)	2.95	OZ
STEAK, T-BONE	2.8	OZ
STEAK, TENDERLOIN	2.83	OZ
STEAK, TOP LOIN	2.88	OZ
STEAK, TOP ROUND	3.3	OZ

STEAK, TOP SIRLOIN	3.06	OZ
STEAK, TYSON SEASONED BEEF STRIPS	3.6	OZ
TACO/BURRITO MEAT/SMART GROUND	0.88	CUP
OSCAR MAYER BACON	5.6	SLICE
LITTLE SIZZLER BROWN/SERVE SAUSAGE	2.2	LINK

Sea Food

BASS, FRESHWATER, DRY HEAT	4.08	OZ
BASS, STRIPED, DRY HEAT	4.8	OZ
COD, ATLANTIC, DRY HEAT	5.65	OZ
CRAB, ALASKA KING, MOIST HEAT	6.15	OZ
CRAB, BLUE, MOIST HEAT	5.8	OZ
FLOUNDER, DRY HEAT	5.1	OZ
HADDOCK, DRY HEAT	5.3	OZ
HALIBUT, DRY HEAT	4.25	OZ
LOBSTER, NORTHERN, MOIST HEAT	6.1	OZ
MAHI MAHI	6.9	OZ
ORANGE ROUGHY, DRY HEAT	6.6	OZ
PERCH, DRY HEAT	5.1	OZ
PERCH, OCEAN/ATLANTIC, DRY HEAT	4.9	OZ
SALMON, ATLANTIC, DRY HEAT	1.68	OZ
SHRIMP, MOIST HEAT	3.25	OZ
TROUT, DRY HEAT	3.1	OZ
TUNA BURGER, AHI / OMEGA FOODS	6	OZ
TUNA, LOW SODIUM, CAN	0.96	CAN
TUNA, WATER, CAN	1.12	CAN
TUNA, WHITE/LOW SALT, CAN (5 OZ)	0.96	CAN
TUNA, WHITE, CAN (5 OZ)	0.96	CAN
TUNA, FILLET/STEAK	3.8	OZ
WALLEYE, BAKED/BROILED/MICRO	5	OZ

Vegetarian

IVES VEG. COUSINE VEGGY DOG	2.8	DOG
SOY MILK (TRIS)	1.87	CUP
SOY MILK (SYLVIA)	1.5	CUP

Eggs/Dairy

1% COTTAGE CHEESE, NORDICA	1.05	CUP
2% COTTAGE CHEESE (LOW FAT)	0.84	CUP
COTTAGE CHEESE (LUCERNE FAT FREE)	1.05	CUP
COTT CHEESE MARIGOLD/DRY CURD	1.6	CUP
COTT CHEESE MARIGOLD/DRY CURD	25.7	TBLSP
COTT CHEESE BREAKSTONES FAT FREE	1.05	CUP
CHEDDER, SHREDDED, FAT FREE, KHF	0.93	CUP
CHEDDER, SHREDDED, 94% FAT FREE, HC	0.84	CUP
CHEESE, COLBY/MOZZARELLA	1.53	OZ
EGG WHITE	9.9	
EGG, WHOLE	2.25	
EGG BEATERS	1.4	CUP
MOZZARELLA SHREDDED, FAT FREE, KHF	0.84	CUP
SKIM MOZZARELLA STRING CHEESE	2.1	OZ

Free Carbs, Supplements, Fast Foods
3000 calories

Free Carbs

ASPARAGUS
BROCCOLI
CABBAGE
CAULIFLOWER
CELERY
CUCUMBER
GREEN BEANS
GREEN PEPPERS
GREEN SQUASH
LETTUCE, ICEBERG
LETTUCE, LEAF/SHREDDED
MUSHROOMS
ONION
PICKLES (DILL)
RADISH

RED PEPPERS
SPINACH (CAN/NO SALT)
SPINACH (FRESH)
TOMATO (EXCLUDING JUICE)
ZUCCHINI

Supplements/Fast Foods

ATKINS BAR	0.75	BAR
EAS ADVANTEDGE, C&C/LEM/BLUE	0.75	BAR
BAR, ZONE	0.75	BAR
BAR, PURE PROTEIN, 50 G.	0.75	BAR
BAR, W.W. PURE PROTEIN, 78 G.	0.5	BAR
BAR, PROTEIN REVOLUTION, PBJ	0.5	BAR
BAR, FIBAR, PEANUT BUTTER, 1.2 OZ	1	BAR
BAR, PREMIER 1, PROTEIN 8, CHOC/COCO	0.5	BAR
BAR, PREFERRED BAR, CHOC./FUDG/RAS	0.5	BAR
BAR, PREFERRED BAR, CHOC./FUDG/BROW	0.5	BAR
ALIVE, HI CARB POWDER	3	TBLSP
POWERADE	2	SERVING
PROTEIN,GNC P.P. EGG/WHEY	1.25	SERVING
PROTEIN. GNC P.PERF. WHEY	4	SCOOP
OPTIMUM NUTRITION WHEY	1.5	SCOOP
SYNTRAX WHEY PROTEIN	1.75	SCOOP
TRI PROTEIN PLUS POWDER	1	SERVING
HW STRAWBERRY PROT. POWD.	1.5	SCOOP
BIOCHEM WHEY PRO 290	2	SCOOP
HUMAN DEV. TECH. WHEY	1.25	SCOOP
NATURADE 100% SOY PROTEIN	0.5	CUP
SUPER GREEN PRO 96 - SOY	0.5	CUP
100% PURE WHEY, PROLAB	1.25	SCOOP
ECLIPSE BULK UP WHEY	1.25	SCOOP
VITAMIN WORLD WHEY 100%	1.25	SCOOP
ULT. NUT. PROSTAR WHEY	1.25	SCOOP
RED WINE	4	OZ
MET RX CH.RST.PNT.PRO + BAR	0.5	BAR
MET RX BAV. MINT. PRO + BAR	0.5	BAR
MET AFTER FX BAR	0.5	BAR
MET RX CH. CH. CHIP PRO + BAR	0.5	BAR

MET RX SOURCE ONE BAR	0.55	BAR
MET RX CHOC. GRAHCRK CHIP BAR	0.5	BAR
MET RX PEANUT BUTTER BAR	0.5	BAR
MET RX DRINK MIX, MRP	0.5	SERVING
MET RX PRO 50, ANABOLIC DRIVE	0.5	SERVING
MET RX PRO 60, ANABOLIC DRIVE	0.5	SERVING
MET RX PROTEIN PLUS	2	SCOOP
MET RX KETO PRO	2	SCOOP
NUTRI FORCE DRINK MIX, MRP	0.5	SERVING
EAS MYO. DEL. CH/PB BAR	0.5	BAR
EAS MYOPLEX + DELUXE	0.5	SERVING
EAS MYOPLEX LITE	0.75	SERVING
ADVANT EDGE QUICK STIR PROTEIN DRINK	0.75	SERVING
EAS NEUROGAIN	3.5	SCOOP
EAS PHOSPHAGEN HP	1	SCOOP
EAS PRECISION PROTEIN	1.5	SCOOP
EAS SIMPLY PROTEIN	2.75	SCOOP
EAS WHEY PROTEIN	1.5	SCOOP
EAS SUPPER SHAKE	0.33	SHAKE
VITAMIN WORLD DAILY RX, MRP	0.5	SHAKE
VITAMIN WORLD PROTOPLEX DELUXE, MRP	0.5	SHAKE
VITAMIN WORLD PRE. ENG. WHEY PROT.	1.75	SCOOP
PERFECT RX, MRP, CHOCOLATE	0.5	SHAKE
OPTI PRO	0.5	SHAKE
ARBY'S CHICK. SAND. R.DELX.LITE	0.5	BURGER
ARBY'S SIDE SALAD	1	SALAD
ARBY'S GARDEN SALAD	1	SALAD
ARBY'S RST. CHCK. SALAD	1	SALAD
ARBY'S RED. CAL. ITAL. DRESSING	1	PACKET
ARBY'S RED RANCH DRESSING	1	PACKET
MCD'S VINEG. LITE SALAD DR.	1	PACKET
MCD'S GARDEN SALAD	1	SALAD
MCD'S VINEG. LITE SALAD DR.	1	PACKET
P.HUT. HAND-TOSS CHEESE	0.5	SLICE
P.HUT. HAND-TOSS HAM	0.75	SLICE
P.HUT. HAND-TOSS VEG. LUV.	0.75	SLICE
P.HUT. HAND-TOSS PEPPERON	0.5	SLICE
P.HUT. THIN/CRISP CHEESE	0.75	SLICE

P.HUT. THIN/CRISP HAM	0.75	SLICE
P.HUT. THIN/CRISP VEG. LUV.	0.75	SLICE
P.HUT. THIN/CRISP PEPPERON	0.75	SLICE
SW 6" COLD SUB/VEGG. DELIT	1	SUB
SW 6" COLD SUB/TURK. BRST.	1	SUB
SW 6" COLD SUB/TURK.B/HAM	1	SUB
SW 6" COLD SUB/HAM	1	SUB
SW 6" COLD SUB/ROAST BEEF	1	SUB
SW 6" COLD SUB/SFOOD,CRAB	1	SUB
SW 6" COLD SUB/COLD CUT 3	1	SUB
SW 6" COLD SUB/TUNA	1	SUB
SW 6" HOT SUB/RST.CHICK.BR.	1	SUB
SW 6" HOT SUB/STAK/CHEESE	1	SUB
SW 6" HOT SUB/SUB MELT	1	SUB
SW VEGGIE DELITE SALAD	1	SALAD
SW TURKEY BREAST SALAD	1	SALAD
SW ROAST BEEF SALAD	1	SALAD
SW TURK. BRST/HAM SALAD	1	SALAD
SW RST. CHICK. BR. SALAD	0.75	SALAD
SW SEAFOOD/CRAB SALAD	0.75	SALAD
SW STEAK/CHEESE SALAD	0.75	SALAD
SW SUBWAY MELT SALAD	0.75	SALAD
SW COLD CUT 3 SALAD	0.75	SALAD
SW FAT FREE ITALIAN DRESS	1	OZ
SW FAT FREE FRENCH DRESS	1	OZ
SW FAT FREE RANCH DRESS	1	OZ
SW DELI STYLE TURKEY BR.	0.5	SNDWCH
SW DELI STYLE HAM	0.5	SNDWCH
SW DELI STYLE ROAST BEEF	0.5	SNDWCH
TB GRILLED STEAK SOFT TACO	0.55	TACO
WAHOO'S CHBROIL FISH TACO	0.75	TACO
WENDI'S SIDE SALAD	1	SALAD
WENDI'S FF FRENCH DRESSING	1	OZ
WENDI'S ITALIAN RED. F/C DRESS	1	OZ
WENDI'S SMALL CHILI	0.75	BOWL
WENDI'S GRILLED CHICK. FILLET	1	MEAT

3100 Calories/Day Eating Plan		
What Does Your Doctor Look Like Naked?		
Name: _____		
Date: _____		
Exercise: 30-40 min in a.m. before food		Write what you eat here:
Meal 1 Time: _____	2 Protein Sources 4 Active Carbohydrates	
Meal 2 Time: _____	3 oz Raw Almonds	
Meal 3 Time: _____	2 Protein Source 2 Active Carbohydrates Free Carbohydrates (as much as you want)	
Meal 4 Time: _____	1 LOW CARB protein bar (OR) 2 scoops Whey Protein Powder in water AND 1 oz String Cheese 1 oz Raw Almonds	
Meal 5 Time: _____	2 Protein Source 0 Active Carbohydrates Free Carbohydrates (as much as you want)	
Bedtime Meal (Optional)	Sugar Free Jell-O 1 cup	

Add fiber supplement in evening, such as Metamucil or other (sugar FREE).
Add spices, pepper, etc. as needed.
Try to eat every two to three hours.
Drink 1½ gallons of water EVERY DAY!
May have up to 2 diet pops (or) 2 cups a coffee a day.

Active Carbohydrates 3100 Calories

Fruit and Vegetables

APPLE	2.2	3 INCH
APPLESAUCE, MOTT'S	0.81	CUP
APRICOTS (CAN/DEL MONTE LITE)	1.49	CUP
APRICOTS (DRIED)	2.55	OZ
APRICOTS (FRESH 12/LB)	10.5	MEDIUM
ASPARAGUS	48	OZ
BANANA	1.7	MEDIUM
BLUEBERRIES (FRESH)	2.18	CUP
BRUSSELS SPROUTS, BOILED	2.97	CUP
CABBAGE, SHREDDED	9.9	CUP
CANTALOUPE	0.95	5 INCH
CARROT (FRESH)	16.1	OZ
CAULIFLOWER	6.85	CUP
CELERY	44.5	OZ
CHERRIES, FRESH, SWEET W/PIT	1.72	CUP
CHERRIES, DARK (CAN/DEL MONTE)	0.89	CUP
COLLARD GREENS (CAN)	2.97	CUP
COLLARD GREENS (FRESH)	14.9	CUP
CORN CAKE	5.1	CAKE
CORN (CAN/DEL MONTE NO SODIUM)	13	OZ
CUCUMBER, SLICED	12.7	CUP
EGGPLANT	8.1	CUP
FRUIT, MIXED FROZEN	1.98	CUP
GARLIC, 1 CLOVE	44.5	CLOVE
GARLIC, TRIMMED	4.25	OZ
GRAPES	1.57	CUP
GRAPE JUICE/VERYFINE	9.5	OZ
GRAPEFRUIT	1.94	4 INCH
GREEN BEANS (CAN/DEL MONTE NO SALT)	4.45	CUP
GREEN PEPPER	8.9	MEDIUM
KIWI	12	OZ
MUSHROOMS, FRESH	9.9	CUP
ONION, FRESH/CHOPPED	2.97	CUP

ORANGE, NAVAL	2.75	3 INCH
ORANGE, JUICE	13	OZ
PAPAYA	1.525	LB.
PAPAYA, PEELED/CUBED	3.3	CUP
PEACH, FRESH, SLICED	2.41	CUP
PEACH (CAN/DEL MONTE EXTRA LITE)	1.49	CUP
PEARS (CAN)	5.9	HALF
PEAS, BLACKEYED (CAN)	0.99	CUP
PEAS (CAN/DEL MONTE NO SODIUM)	13	OZ
PEAS, GREEN GIANT FROZEN, SWEET	1.7	CUP
PEAS, EDIBLE-PODDED	2.97	CUP
PINEAPPLE, FRESH/DICED	2.29	CUP
PINEAPPLE, DEL MONTE SNACK CAN (LITE)	2.55	3.5 OZ
PINEAPPLE (CAN/DOLE LITE SYRUP)	10.5	SLICE
PRUNES, DOLE, DRIED	2.55	OZ
PUMPKIN (CAN)	3.57	CUP
RAISINS	0.37	CUP
RED PEPPER	8.9	MEDIUM
STRAWBERRIES (FRESH)	1.84	PINT
STRAWBERRIES (FROZEN)	2.38	CUP
SQUASH, CAN, STOKLEY	1.78	CUP
SQUASH, FRESH BAKED	1.57	CUP
TANGERINE	4.83	2.5 INCH
TOMATO, CAN	16.7	OZ
TOMATO, FRESH	6.85	3 INCH
TOMATO, JUICE	28.5	OZ
VEGETABLES, MIXED (FROZEN)	1.98	CUP
WATERMELLON	1.17	1X10 INCH
ZUCCHINI, FRESH, SLICED	9.9	CUP

Yogurts and Desserts

DING DONG	1.11	DING
DREYERS FROZEN FAT FREE YOGURT	0.99	CUP
FRUIT ROLL-UP	2.55	ROLL-UP
POPCORN, WHITE	3.57	TBLSP
TCBY, SOFT SERVE/NONFAT/NO SUGAR	1.11	CUP
YOGURT, FAT FREE, MOUNTAIN HIGH	8	OZ
YOGURT, FAT FREE, DANNON	8	OZ

LUCERN, YOGURT, NONFAT, LITE	8	OZ
YOGURT, YOPLAIT, FAT FREE, LITE	6	OZ
YOGURT,YOPLAIT ORIGINAL/99% FAT FREE	6	OZ
YOGURT, HORIZON, FF/BLUEBERRY	6	OZ
PLANTER DRIED WALNUT PIECES	0.2	CUP
RAW ALMONDS, TOASTED	1	OZ
PECANS, DRIED	0.75	OZ
PEANUTS, DRY ROASTED	0.2	CUP
HOT CHOCOLATE	3.5	ENVEL.
ALMONDS, SHELLED	1	OZ

Cereals

CEREAL, CHEERIOS	1.62	CUP
CEREAL, COCOA KRISPIES	1.11	CUP
CEREAL, GRAPENUTS	0.445	CUP
CEREAL, HONEY NUT TOASTY O'S	1.62	CUP
CEREAL, WHEATIES	1.62	CUP
CEREAL, KELLOGG'S ALL BRAN	1.11	CUP
CEREAL, KELLOGG'S CORN FLAKES	1.62	CUP
CEREAL, KELLOGG'S RAISIN BRAN	1.05	CUP
CEREAL, KELLOGG'S CRACKLIN' OAT BRAN	0.7	CUP
CEREAL, NABISCO SHREDDED WHEAT	2.23	PIECE
CEREAL, NAB. SHREDDED WHEAT (SPOON)	1.05	CUP
CEREAL, RICE KRISPIES	2.03	CUP
CEREAL, BENEFIT NUTRITION, PROTEIN +	0.85	CUP
CREAM OF WHEAT	4.45	TBL/DRY
GRANOLA, CW POST HEARTY	0.425	CUP
GRANOLA, KELLOGG'S LOW FAT	2	CUP
OATMEAL (PRE-COOK MEASUREMENT)	0.636	CUP

Breads

BREAD, OROWHEAT LITE	4.47	SLICE
BREAD, SUSAN'S HOMEMADE/18 SLICES	0.11	SLICE
BREAD, SUSAN'S HOMEMADE	2.97	LOAF
BUN, WONDER REDUCED CALORIE LITE	2.23	BUN
CRACKER, ZESTA SALTINES	14.9	CRACKER
TORTILLA (CAROLYN)	1.05	TORT

TORTILLA, TORTILLA'S MEXICO, FLOUR	1.62	TORT
TORTILLA, TORTILLA'S MEXICO, CORN	1.98	TORT
TRISCUITS	1.27	OZ
WAFFLE, EGGO, HOMESTYLE	1.62	WAFFLE
WHOLE GRAIN/WHOLE WHEAT FLOUR	0.438	CUP

Rice/Potatoes/Beans

BLACK BEANS (BOILED)	0.79	CUP
BLACK BEANS (DRY)	0.636	CUP
CHICKPEAS/GARBANZO BEANS	0.25	CUP
KIDNEY BEANS (BOILED)	0.8	CUP
LIMA BEANS (BOILED)	0.86	CUP
NAVY BEANS (BOILED)	0.69	CUP
NAVY BEANS (CAN)	0.745	CUP
PINTO BEANS (BOILED)	0.76	CUP
PINTO BEANS (CAN)	0.94	CUP
PINTO BEANS (DRY)	0.297	CUP
PORK & BEANS/VAN CAMPS	0.81	CUP
POTATO, SWEET	1.51	5"X2"
POTATO	10.6	OZ
RICE CAKE	3.56	CAKE
RICE, WHITE, BASMATI	0.745	CUP (C)
RICE, BROWN LONG GRAIN	0.89	CUP (C)
RICE, INSTANT, MINUTE BRAND	0.558	CUP(UC)
RICE, WHITE, LONG GRAIN	0.279	CUP(UC)
SOYBEANS (BOILED)	0.5	CUP
YAM, BOILED OR BAKED	1.13	CUP

Pasta

MACARONI, DAVINI TWIST	0.68	CUP/DRY
MACARONI, HOSPITALITY ELBOW	0.37	CUP/DRY
MACARONI, AM. BEAUTY ELBOW	0.425	CUP/DRY
PASTA, CREAMETTE PLAIN	1.7	OZ
SPAGHETTI, EDEN WHOLE WHEAT	1.7	OZ/UC

Protein Sources 3100 Calories

White Meat

CHICKEN BREAST (HORMEL/CAN)	1.19	CAN
CHICKEN BREAST (SKINLESS)	5.95	OZ
CHICKEN (LEG W/ SKIN & BONE)	0.675	
CHICKEN (THIGH W/ SKIN & BONE)	1.165	
CHICKEN (LEG & THIGH W/ SKIN & BONE)	0.428	
HAM, BAR S, XTRA LEAN, 96% FAT FREE	5.1	OZ
HAM, DAK CAN	5.95	OZ
PORK, SIRLOIN, LEAN W/ FAT	1.78	OZ
TURKEY BREAST (SKINLESS)	3.33	OZ
TURKEY BREAST (HORMEL/CAN)	1.02	CAN
TURKEY BRST/OVEN ROAST/SFWY/89% FF	7.1	OZ
VENISON / ANTELOPE	3.98	OZ

Red Meat

HAMBURGER (10% FAT)	3.16	OZ
HAMBURGER (15% FAT)	2.62	OZ
HAMBURGER (20% FAT)	2.55	OZ
HAMBURGER (27% FAT)	2.16	OZ
LAMB, SHOULDER	2	OZ
STEAK, BOTTOM ROUND	2.03	OZ
STEAK, BRISKET (FLAT HALF)	2.84	OZ
STEAK, CHUCK, ARM	2.92	OZ
STEAK, CHUCK, BLADE	2.52	OZ
STEAK, EYE ROUND	3.74	OZ
STEAK, FLANK	3.04	OZ
STEAK, NEW YORK STRIP	3.57	OZ
STEAK, PORTERHOUSE	2.9	OZ
STEAK, RIBEYE	2.8	OZ
STEAK, ROUND TIP	3.42	OZ
STEAK, SHANK (CROSSCUTS)	3.14	OZ
STEAK, T-BONE	2.94	OZ
STEAK, TENDERLOIN	2.99	OZ
STEAK, TOP LOIN	3.05	OZ
STEAK, TOP ROUND	3.5	OZ

STEAK, TOP SIRLOIN	3.24	OZ
STEAK, TYSON SEASONED BEEF STRIPS	3.83	OZ
TACO/BURRITO MEAT/SMART GROUND	0.93	CUP
OSCAR MAYER BACON	5.95	SLICE
LITTLE SIZZLER BROWN/SERVE SAUSAGE	2.32	LINK

Sea Food

BASS, FRESHWATER, DRY HEAT	4.33	OZ
BASS, STRIPED, DRY HEAT	5.1	OZ
COD, ATLANTIC, DRY HEAT	6	OZ
CRAB, ALASKA KING, MOIST HEAT	6.53	OZ
CRAB, BLUE, MOIST HEAT	6.15	OZ
FLOUNDER, DRY HEAT	5.4	OZ
HADDOCK, DRY HEAT	5.65	OZ
HALIBUT, DRY HEAT	4.5	OZ
LOBSTER, NORTHERN, MOIST HEAT	6.45	OZ
MAHI MAHI	7.35	OZ
ORANGE ROUGHY, DRY HEAT	7.05	OZ
PERCH, DRY HEAT	5.4	OZ
PERCH, OCEAN/ATLANTIC, DRY HEAT	5.2	OZ
SALMON, ATLANTIC, DRY HEAT	3.44	OZ
SHRIMP, MOIST HEAT	6.36	OZ
TROUT, DRY HEAT	3.33	OZ
TUNA BURGER, AHI / OMEGA FOODS	6.38	OZ
TUNA, LOW SODIUM, CAN	1.02	CAN
TUNA, WATER, CAN	1.19	CAN
TUNA, WHITE/LOW SALT, CAN (5 OZ)	1.02	CAN
TUNA, WHITE, CAN (5 OZ)	1.02	CAN
TUNA, FILLET/STEAK	4.05	OZ
WALLEYE, BAKED/BROILED/MICRO	5.3	OZ

Vegetarian

IVES VEG. COUSINE VEGGY DOG	2.98	DOG
SOY MILK (TRIS)	2	CUP
SOY MILK (SYLVIA)	1.75	CUP

Eggs/Dairy

1% COTTAGE CHEESE, NORDICA	1.12	CUP
2% COTTAGE CHEESE (LOW FAT)	0.89	CUP
COTTAGE CHEESE (LUCERNE FAT FREE)	1.11	CUP
COTT CHEESE MARIGOLD/DRY CURD	1.7	CUP
COTT CHEESE MARIGOLD/DRY CURD	27.2	TBLSP
COTT CHEESE BREAKSTONES FAT FREE	1.11	CUP
CHEDDER, SHREDDED, FAT FREE, KHF	0.99	CUP
CHEDDER, SHREDDED, 94% FAT FREE, HC	0.89	CUP
CHEESE, COLBY/MOZZARELLA	1.62	OZ
EGG WHITE	10.5	
EGG, WHOLE	2.38	
EGG BEATERS	1.49	CUP
MOZZARELLA SHREDDED, FAT FREE, KHF	0.89	CUP
SKIM MOZZARELLA STRING CHEESE	2.23	OZ

Free Carbs, Supplements, Fast Foods
3100 calories

Free Carbs
ASPARAGUS
BROCCOLI
CABBAGE
CAULIFLOWER
CELERY
CUCUMBER
GREEN BEANS
GREEN PEPPERS
GREEN SQUASH
LETTUCE, ICEBERG
LETTUCE, LEAF/SHREDDED
MUSHROOMS
ONION
PICKLES (DILL)
RADISH

RED PEPPERS
SPINACH (CAN/NO SALT)
SPINACH (FRESH)
TOMATO (EXCLUDING JUICE)
ZUCCHINI

Supplements/Fast Foods

ATKINS BAR	75%	BAR
EAS ADVANTEDGE, C&C/LEM/BLUE	0.75	BAR
BAR, ZONE	0.75	BAR
BAR, PURE PROTEIN, 50 G.	0.75	BAR
BAR, W.W. PURE PROTEIN, 78 G.	0.5	BAR
BAR, PROTEIN REVOLUTION, PBJ	0.75	BAR
BAR, FIBAR, PEANUT BUTTER, 1.2 OZ	1.25	BAR
BAR, PREMIER 1, PROTEIN 8, CHOC/COCO	0.5	BAR
BAR, PREFERRED BAR, CHOC./FUDG/RAS	0.75	BAR
BAR, PREFERRED BAR, CHOC./FUDG/BROW	0.75	BAR
ALIVE, HI CARB POWDER	4	TBLSP
POWERADE	2	SERVING
PROTEIN,GNC P.P. EGG/WHEY	1.25	SERVING
PROTEIN. GNC P.PERF. WHEY	4	SCOOP
OPTIMUM NUTRITION WHEY	1.5	SCOOP
SYNTRAX WHEY PROTEIN	1.75	SCOOP
TRI PROTEIN PLUS POWDER	1.25	SERVING
HW STRAWBERRY PROT. POWD.	1.75	SCOOP
BIOCHEM WHEY PRO 290	2	SCOOP
HUMAN DEV. TECH. WHEY	1.25	SCOOP
NATURADE 100% SOY PROTEIN	0.5	CUP
SUPER GREEN PRO 96 - SOY	0.5	CUP
100% PURE WHEY, PROLAB	1.25	SCOOP
ECLIPSE BULK UP WHEY	1.75	SCOOP
VITAMIN WORLD WHEY 100%	1.5	SCOOP
ULT. NUT. PROSTAR WHEY	1.5	SCOOP
RED WINE	7	OZ
MET RX CH.RST.PNT.PRO + BAR	0.5	BAR
MET RX BAV. MINT. PRO + BAR	0.5	BAR
MET AFTER FX BAR	0.5	BAR
MET RX CH. CH. CHIP PRO + BAR	0.5	BAR

MET RX SOURCE ONE BAR	0.75	BAR
MET RX CHOC. GRAHCRK CHIP BAR	0.5	BAR
MET RX PEANUT BUTTER BAR	0.5	BAR
MET RX DRINK MIX, MRP	0.5	SERVING
MET RX PRO 50, ANABOLIC DRIVE	0.5	SERVING
MET RX PRO 60, ANABOLIC DRIVE	0.5	SERVING
MET RX PROTEIN PLUS	2.5	SCOOP
MET RX KETO PRO	2.25	SCOOP
NUTRI FORCE DRINK MIX, MRP	0.5	SERVING
EAS MYO. DEL. CH/PB BAR	0.5	BAR
EAS MYOPLEX + DELUXE	0.5	SERVING
EAS MYOPLEX LITE	0.75	SERVING
ADVANT EDGE QUICK STIR PROTEIN DRINK	0.75	SERVING
EAS NEUROGAIN	3.5	SCOOP
EAS PHOSPHAGEN HP	1	SCOOP
EAS PRECISION PROTEIN	1.75	SCOOP
EAS SIMPLY PROTEIN	3	SCOOP
EAS WHEY PROTEIN	1.5	SCOOP
EAS SUPPER SHAKE	0.33	SHAKE
VITAMIN WORLD DAILY RX, MRP	0.5	SHAKE
VITAMIN WORLD PROTOPLEX DELUXE, MRP	0.5	SHAKE
VITAMIN WORLD PRE. ENG. WHEY PROT.	2	SCOOP
PERFECT RX, MRP, CHOCOLATE	0.5	SHAKE
OPTI PRO	0.5	SHAKE
ARBY'S CHICK. SAND. R.DELX.LITE	0.5	BURGER
ARBY'S SIDE SALAD	1	SALAD
ARBY'S GARDEN SALAD	1	SALAD
ARBY'S RST. CHCK. SALAD	1	SALAD
ARBY'S RED. CAL. ITAL. DRESSING	1	PACKET
ARBY'S RED RANCH DRESSING	1	PACKET
MCD'S VINEG. LITE SALAD DR.	1	PACKET
MCD'S GARDEN SALAD	1	SALAD
MCD'S VINEG. LITE SALAD DR.	1	PACKET
P.HUT. HAND-TOSS CHEESE	0.75	SLICE
P.HUT. HAND-TOSS HAM	0.75	SLICE
P.HUT. HAND-TOSS VEG. LUV.	0.75	SLICE
P.HUT. HAND-TOSS PEPPERON	0.75	SLICE
P.HUT. THIN/CRISP CHEESE	0.75	SLICE

P.HUT. THIN/CRISP HAM	0.75	SLICE
P.HUT. THIN/CRISP VEG. LUV.	0.75	SLICE
P.HUT. THIN/CRISP PEPPERON	0.75	SLICE
SW 6" COLD SUB/VEGG. DELIT	1	SUB
SW 6" COLD SUB/TURK. BRST.	1	SUB
SW 6" COLD SUB/TURK.B/HAM	1	SUB
SW 6" COLD SUB/HAM	1	SUB
SW 6" COLD SUB/ROAST BEEF	1	SUB
SW 6" COLD SUB/SFOOD,CRAB	1	SUB
SW 6" COLD SUB/COLD CUT 3	1	SUB
SW 6" COLD SUB/TUNA	1	SUB
SW 6" HOT SUB/RST.CHICK.BR.	1	SUB
SW 6" HOT SUB/STAK/CHEESE	1	SUB
SW 6" HOT SUB/SUB MELT	1	SUB
SW VEGGIE DELITE SALAD	1	SALAD
SW TURKEY BREAST SALAD	1	SALAD
SW ROAST BEEF SALAD	1	SALAD
SW TURK. BRST/HAM SALAD	1	SALAD
SW RST. CHICK. BR. SALAD	1	SALAD
SW SEAFOOD/CRAB SALAD	1	SALAD
SW STEAK/CHEESE SALAD	0.75	SALAD
SW SUBWAY MELT SALAD	0.75	SALAD
SW COLD CUT 3 SALAD	0.75	SALAD
SW FAT FREE ITALIAN DRESS	1	OZ
SW FAT FREE FRENCH DRESS	1	OZ
SW FAT FREE RANCH DRESS	1	OZ
SW DELI STYLE TURKEY BR.	0.75	SNDWCH
SW DELI STYLE HAM	0.75	SNDWCH
SW DELI STYLE ROAST BEEF	0.5	SNDWCH
TB GRILLED STEAK SOFT TACO	0.5	TACO
WAHOO'S CHBROIL FISH TACO	1	TACO
WENDI'S SIDE SALAD	1	SALAD
WENDI'S FF FRENCH DRESSING	1	OZ
WENDI'S ITALIAN RED. F/C DRESS	1	OZ
WENDI'S SMALL CHILI	0.75	BOWL
WENDI'S GRILLED CHICK. FILLET	1.5	MEAT

3200 Calories/Day Eating Plan		
What Does Your Doctor Look Like Naked?		

Name: _____

Date: _____

Exercise: 30-40 min in a.m. before food		
		Write what you eat here:
Meal 1 Time: _____	2 Protein Sources 4 Active Carbohydrates	
Meal 2 Time: _____	3 oz Raw Almonds	
Meal 3 Time: _____	2 Protein Source 2 Active Carbohydrates Free Carbohydrates (as much as you want)	
Meal 4 Time: _____	1 LOW CARB protein bar (OR) 2 scoops Whey Protein Powder in water AND 1 oz String Cheese 1 oz Raw Almonds	
Meal 5 Time: _____	2 Protein Source 0 Active Carbohydrates Free Carbohydrates (as much as you want)	
Bedtime Meal (Optional)	Sugar Free Jell-O 1 cup	
Add fiber supplement in evening, such as Metamucil or other (sugar FREE). Add spices, pepper, etc. as needed. Try to eat every two to three hours. Drink 1 ½ gallons of water EVERY DAY! May have up to 2 diet pops (or) 2 cups a coffee a day.		

Active Carbohydrates 3200 Calories

Fruit and Vegetables

APPLE	2.29	3 INCH
APPLESAUCE, MOTT'S	0.84	CUP
APRICOTS (CAN/DEL MONTE LITE)	1.54	CUP
APRICOTS (DRIED)	2.65	OZ
APRICOTS (FRESH)(12/LB)	10.9	MEDIUM
ASPARAGUS	50	OZ
BANANA	1.76	MEDIUM
BLUEBERRIES (FRESH)	2.26	CUP
BRUSSELS SPROUTS, BOILED	3.09	CUP
CABBAGE, SHREDDED	10.3	CUP
CANTALOUPE	0.98	5 INCH
CARROT (FRESH)	16.7	OZ
CAULIFLOWER	7.13	CUP
CELERY	46.3	OZ
CHERRIES, FRESH, SWEET W/PIT	1.78	CUP
CHERRIES, DARK (CAN/DEL MONTE)	0.925	CUP
COLLARD GREENS (CAN)	3.09	CUP
COLLARD GREENS (FRESH)	15.4	CUP
CORN CAKE	5.3	CAKE
CORN (CAN/DEL MONTE NO SODIUM)	13.5	OZ
CUCUMBER, SLICED	13.2	CUP
EGGPLANT	8.4	CUP
FRUIT, MIXED FROZEN	2.06	CUP
GARLIC, 1 CLOVE	46	CLOVE
GARLIC, TRIMMED	4.4	OZ
GRAPES	1.63	CUP
GRAPE JUICE/VERYFINE	9.9	OZ
GRAPEFRUIT	2.01	4 INCH
GREEN BEANS (CAN/DEL MONTE NO SALT)	4.61	CUP
GREEN PEPPER	9.25	MEDIUM
KIWI	12.5	OZ
MUSHROOMS, FRESH	10.3	CUP
ONION, FRESH/CHOPPED	3.09	CUP
ORANGE, NAVAL	2.85	3 INCH

ORANGE, JUICE	13.5	OZ
PAPAYA	1.585	LB.
PAPAYA, PEELED/CUBED	3.44	CUP
PEACH, FRESH, SLICED	2.5	CUP
PEACH (CAN/DEL MONTE EXTRA LITE)	1.54	CUP
PEARS (CAN)	6.15	HALF
PEAS, BLACKEYED (CAN)	1.03	CUP
PEAS (CAN/DEL MONTE NO SODIUM)	13.5	OZ
PEAS, GREEN GIANT FROZEN, SWEET	1.77	CUP
PEAS, EDIBLE-PODDED	3.1	CUP
PINEAPPLE, FRESH/DICED	2.37	CUP
PINEAPPLE, DEL MONTE SNACK CAN (LITE)	2.65	3.5 OZ
PINEAPPLE (CAN/DOLE LITE SYRUP)	10.9	SLICE
PRUNES, DOLE, DRIED	2.65	OZ
PUMPKIN (CAN)	3.7	CUP
RAISINS	0.385	CUP
RED PEPPER	9.25	MEDIUM
STRAWBERRIES (FRESH)	1.9	PINT
STRAWBERRIES (FROZEN)	2.47	CUP
SQUASH, CAN, STOKLEY	1.85	CUP
SQUASH, FRESH BAKED	1.63	CUP
TANGERINE	5	2.5 INCH
TOMATO, CAN	17.2	OZ
TOMATO, FRESH	7.1	3 INCH
TOMATO, JUICE	29.5	OZ
VEGETABLES, MIXED (FROZEN)	2.5	CUP
WATERMELLON	1.22	1X10 INCH
ZUCCHINI, FRESH, SLICED	10.3	CUP

Yogurts and Desserts

DING DONG	1.16	DING
DREYERS FROZEN FAT FREE YOGURT	1.03	CUP
FRUIT ROLL-UP	2.65	ROLL-UP
POPCORN, WHITE	3.7	TBLSP
TCBY, SOFT SERVE/NONFAT/NO SUGAR	1.16	CUP
YOGURT, FAT FREE, MOUNTAIN HIGH	8	OZ
YOGURT, FAT FREE, DANNON	8	OZ
LUCERN, YOGURT, NONFAT, LITE	8	OZ

YOGURT, YOPLAIT, FAT FREE, LITE	6	OZ
YOGURT,YOPLAIT ORIGINAL/99% FAT FREE	6	OZ
YOGURT, HORIZON, FF / BLUEBERRY	6	OZ
PLANTER DRIED WALNUT PIECES	0.2	CUP
RAW ALMONDS, TOASTED	1	OZ
PECANS, DRIED	0.88	OZ
PEANUTS, DRY ROASTED	0.2	CUP
HOT CHOCOLATE	3	ENVEL.
ALMONDS, SHELLED	1	OZ

Cereals

CEREAL, CHEERIOS	1.69	CUP
CEREAL, COCOA KRISPIES	1.16	CUP
CEREAL, GRAPENUTS	0.462	CUP
CEREAL, HONEY NUT TOASTY O'S	1.68	CUP
CEREAL, WHEATIES	1.68	CUP
CEREAL, KELLOGG'S ALL BRAN	1.16	CUP
CEREAL, KELLOGG'S CORN FLAKES	1.68	CUP
CEREAL, KELLOGG'S RAISIN BRAN	1.09	CUP
CEREAL, KELLOGG'S CRACKLIN' OAT BRAN	0.7	CUP
CEREAL, NABISCO SHREDDED WHEAT	2.32	PIECE
CEREAL, NAB. SHREDDED WHEAT (SPOON)	1.09	CUP
CEREAL, RICE KRISPIES	2.1	CUP
CEREAL, BENEFIT NUTRITION, PROTEIN +	0.88	CUP
CREAM OF WHEAT	4.63	TBL/DRY
GRANOLA, CW POST HEARTY	0.44	CUP
GRANOLA, KELLOGG'S LOW FAT	3	CUP
OATMEAL (PRE-COOK MEASUREMENT)	0.66	CUP

Breads

BREAD, OROWHEAT LITE	4.63	SLICE
BREAD, SUSAN'S HOMEMADE/18 SLICES	2.05	SLICE
BREAD, SUSAN'S HOMEMADE	0.113	LOAF
BUN, WONDER REDUCED CALORIE LITE	2.31	BUN
CRACKER, ZESTA SALTINES	5.15	CRACKER
TORTILLA (CAROLYN)	1.09	TORT
TORTILLA, TORTILLA'S MEXICO, FLOUR	1.68	TORT

TORTILLA, TORTILLA'S MEXICO, CORN	2.06	TORT
TRISCUITS	1.32	OZ
WAFFLE, EGGO, HOMESTYLE	1.69	WAFFLE
WHOLE GRAIN/WHOLE WHEAT FLOUR	0.455	CUP

Rice/Potatoes/Beans

BLACK BEANS (BOILED)	0.82	CUP
BLACK BEANS (DRY)	0.66	CUP
CHICKPEAS/GARBANZO BEANS	0.22	CUP
KIDNEY BEANS (BOILED)	0.25	CUP
LIMA BEANS (BOILED)	0.89	CUP
NAVY BEANS (BOILED)	0.72	CUP
NAVY BEANS (CAN)	0.77	CUP
PINTO BEANS (BOILED)	0.79	CUP
PINTO BEANS (CAN)	0.975	CUP
PINTO BEANS (DRY)	0.309	CUP
PORK & BEANS/VAN CAMPS	0.84	CUP
POTATO, SWEET	1.57	5"X2"
POTATO	11	OZ
RICE CAKE	3.7	CAKE
RICE, WHITE, BASMATI	0.772	CUP (C)
RICE, BROWN LONG GRAIN	0.925	CUP (C)
RICE, INSTANT, MINUTE BRAND	0.58	CUP(UC)
RICE, WHITE, LONG GRAIN	0.29	CUP(UC)
SOYBEANS (BOILED)	0.75	CUP
YAM, BOILED OR BAKED	1.17	CUP

Pasta

MACARONI, DAVINI TWIST	0.7	CUP/DRY
MACARONI, HOSPITALITY ELBOW	0.385	CUP/DRY
MACARONI, AM. BEAUTY ELBOW	0.44	CUP/DRY
PASTA, CREAMETTE PLAIN	1.77	OZ
SPAGHETTI, EDEN WHOLE WHEAT	1.76	OZ/UC

Protein Sources 3200 Calories

White Meat

CHICKEN BREAST (HORMEL/CAN)	1.23	CAN
CHICKEN BREAST (SKINLESS)	6.18	OZ
CHICKEN (LEG W/SKIN & BONE)	0.7	
CHICKEN (THIGH W/SKIN & BONE)	1.21	
CHICKEN (LEG & THIGH W/SKIN & BONE)	0.443	
HAM, BAR S, XTRA LEAN, 96% FAT FREE	5.3	OZ
HAM, DAK CAN	6.15	OZ
PORK, SIRLOIN, LEAN W/FAT	1.85	OZ
TURKEY BREAST (SKINLESS)	3.47	OZ
TURKEY BREAST (HORMEL/CAN)	1.06	CAN
TURKEY BRST/OVEN ROAST/SFWY/89% FF	7.4	OZ
VENISON / ANTELOPE	4.15	OZ

Red Meat

HAMBURGER (10% FAT)	3.3	OZ
HAMBURGER (15% FAT)	2.73	OZ
HAMBURGER (20% FAT)	2.65	OZ
HAMBURGER (27% FAT)	2.24	OZ
LAMB, SHOULDER	2.1	OZ
STEAK, BOTTOM ROUND	3.13	OZ
STEAK, BRISKET (FLAT HALF)	2.95	OZ
STEAK, CHUCK, ARM	3.04	OZ
STEAK, CHUCK, BLADE	2.6	OZ
STEAK, EYE ROUND	3.9	OZ
STEAK, FLANK	3.16	OZ
STEAK, NEW YORK STRIP	3.7	OZ
STEAK, PORTERHOUSE	3	OZ
STEAK, RIBEYE	2.91	OZ
STEAK, ROUND TIP	3.55	OZ
STEAK, SHANK (CROSSCUTS)	3.25	OZ
STEAK, T-BONE	3.05	OZ
STEAK, TENDERLOIN	3.1	OZ
STEAK, TOP LOIN	3.15	OZ
STEAK, TOP ROUND	3.64	OZ

STEAK, TOP SIRLOIN	3.38	OZ
STEAK, TYSON SEASONED BEEF STRIPS	3.95	OZ
TACO/BURRITO MEAT/SMART GROUND	0.96	CUP
OSCAR MAYER BACON	6.15	SLICE
LITTLE SIZZLER BROWN/SERVE SAUSAGE	2.4	LINK

Sea Food

BASS, FRESHWATER, DRY HEAT	4.5	OZ
BASS, STRIPED, DRY HEAT	5.3	OZ
COD, ATLANTIC, DRY HEAT	6.25	OZ
CRAB, ALASKA KING, MOIST HEAT	6.8	OZ
CRAB, BLUE, MOIST HEAT	6.4	OZ
FLOUNDER, DRY HEAT	5.6	OZ
HADDOCK, DRY HEAT	5.85	OZ
HALIBUT, DRY HEAT	4.67	OZ
LOBSTER, NORTHERN, MOIST HEAT	6.7	OZ
MAHI MAHI	7.6	OZ
ORANGE ROUGHY, DRY HEAT	7.33	OZ
PERCH, DRY HEAT	5.6	OZ
PERCH, OCEAN/ATLANTIC, DRY HEAT	5.4	OZ
SALMON, ATLANTIC, DRY HEAT	3.57	OZ
SHRIMP, MOIST HEAT	6.6	OZ
TROUT, DRY HEAT	3.45	OZ
TUNA BURGER, AHI/OMEGA FOODS	6.6	OZ
TUNA, LOW SODIUM, CAN	1.06	CAN
TUNA, WATER, CAN	1.23	CAN
TUNA, WHITE/LOW SALT, CAN (5 OZ)	1.06	CAN
TUNA, WHITE, CAN (5 OZ)	1.06	CAN
TUNA, FILLET/STEAK	4.2	OZ
WALLEYE, BAKED/BROILED/MICRO	5.5	OZ

Vegetarian

IVES VEG. COUSINE VEGGY DOG	3.08	DOG
SOY MILK (TRIS)	2	CUP
SOY MILK (SYLVIA)	1.75	CUP

Eggs/Dairy

1% COTTAGE CHEESE, NORDICA	1.16	CUP
2% COTTAGE CHEESE (LOW FAT)	0.925	CUP
COTTAGE CHEESE (LUCERNE FAT FREE)	1.16	CUP
COTT CHEESE MARIGOLD/DRY CURD	1.77	CUP
COTT CHEESE MARIGOLD/DRY CURD	28.3	TBLSP
COTT CHEESE BREAKSTONES FAT FREE	1.16	CUP
CHEDDER, SHREDDED, FAT FREE, KHF	1.03	CUP
CHEDDER, SHREDDED, 94% FAT FREE, HC	0.925	CUP
CHEESE, COLBY/MOZZARELLA	1.69	OZ
EGG WHITE	10.9	
EGG, WHOLE	2.46	
EGG BEATERS	1.54	CUP
MOZZARELLA SHREDDED, FAT FREE, KHF	0.92	CUP
SKIM MOZZARELLA STRING CHEESE	2.32	OZ

Free Carbs, Supplements, Fast Foods
3200 calories

Free Carbs

ASPARAGUS
BROCCOLI
CABBAGE
CAULIFLOWER
CELERY
CUCUMBER
GREEN BEANS
GREEN PEPPERS
GREEN SQUASH
LETTUCE, ICEBERG
LETTUCE, LEAF/SHREDDED
MUSHROOMS
ONION
PICKLES (DILL)

RADISH
RED PEPPERS
SPINACH (CAN/NO SALT)
SPINACH (FRESH)
TOMATO (EXCLUDING JUICE)
ZUCCHINI

Supplements/Fast Foods

ATKINS BAR	0.75	BAR
EAS ADVANTEDGE, C&C/LEM/BLUE	0.75	BAR
BAR, ZONE	0.75	BAR
BAR, PURE PROTEIN, 50 G.	1	BAR
BAR, W.W. PURE PROTEIN, 78 G.	0.5	BAR
BAR, PROTEIN REVOLUTION, PBJ	0.75	BAR
BAR, FIBAR, PEANUT BUTTER, 1.2 OZ	1.25	BAR
BAR, PREMIER 1, PROTEIN 8, CHOC/COCO	0.5	BAR
BAR, PREFERRED BAR, CHOC./FUDG/RAS	0.75	BAR
BAR, PREFERRED BAR, CHOC./FUDG/BROW	0.75	BAR
ALIVE, HI CARB POWDER	1	TBLSP
POWERADE	2	SERVING
PROTEIN,GNC P.P. EGG/WHEY	1.5	SERVING
PROTEIN. GNC P.PERF. WHEY	4	SCOOP
OPTIMUM NUTRITION WHEY	1.5	SCOOP
SYNTRAX WHEY PROTEIN	2	SCOOP
TRI PROTEIN PLUS POWDER	1.25	SERVING
HW STRAWBERRY PROT. POWD.	1.75	SCOOP
BIOCHEM WHEY PRO 290	2.25	SCOOP
HUMAN DEV. TECH. WHEY	1.25	SCOOP
NATURADE 100% SOY PROTEIN	0.5	CUP
SUPER GREEN PRO 96 - SOY	0.5	CUP
100% PURE WHEY, PROLAB	1.25	SCOOP
ECLIPSE BULK UP WHEY	1.75	SCOOP
VITAMIN WORLD WHEY 100%	1.5	SCOOP
ULT. NUT. PROSTAR WHEY	1.5	SCOOP
RED WINE	7	OZ
MET RX CH.RST.PNT.PRO + BAR	0.5	BAR
MET RX BAV. MINT. PRO + BAR	0.75	BAR
MET AFTER FX BAR	0.75	BAR

MET RX CH. CH. CHIP PRO + BAR	0.5	BAR
MET RX SOURCE ONE BAR	0.75	BAR
MET RX CHOC. GRAHCRK CHIP BAR	0.5	BAR
MET RX PEANUT BUTTER BAR	0.5	BAR
MET RX DRINK MIX, MRP	0.75	SERVING
MET RX PRO 50, ANABOLIC DRIVE	0.5	SERVING
MET RX PRO 60, ANABOLIC DRIVE	0.5	SERVING
MET RX PROTEIN PLUS	2.25	SCOOP
MET RX KETO PRO	2.25	SCOOP
NUTRI FORCE DRINK MIX, MRP	0.5	SERVING
EAS MYO. DEL. CH/PB BAR	0.5	BAR
EAS MYOPLEX + DELUXE	0.5	SERVING
EAS MYOPLEX LITE	0.75	SERVING
ADVANT EDGE QUICK STIR PROTEIN DRINK	0.75	SERVING
EAS NEUROGAIN	1	SCOOP
EAS PHOSPHAGEN HP	1.25	SCOOP
EAS PRECISION PROTEIN	1.75	SCOOP
EAS SIMPLY PROTEIN	3	SCOOP
EAS WHEY PROTEIN	1.5	SCOOP
EAS SUPPER SHAKE	0.33	SHAKE
VITAMIN WORLD DAILY RX, MRP	0.5	SHAKE
VITAMIN WORLD PROTOPLEX DELUXE, MRP	0.5	SHAKE
VITAMIN WORLD PRE. ENG. WHEY PROT.	1.75	SCOOP
PERFECT RX, MRP, CHOCOLATE	0.75	SHAKE
OPTI PRO	0.5	SHAKE
ARBY'S CHICK. SAND. R.DELX.LITE	0.5	BURGER
ARBY'S SIDE SALAD	1	SALAD
ARBY'S GARDEN SALAD	1	SALAD
ARBY'S RST. CHCK. SALAD	1	SALAD
ARBY'S RED. CAL. ITAL. DRESSING	1	PACKET
ARBY'S RED RANCH DRESSING	1	PACKET
MCD'S VINEG. LITE SALAD DR.	1	PACKET
MCD'S GARDEN SALAD	1	SALAD
MCD'S VINEG. LITE SALAD DR.	1	PACKET
P.HUT. HAND-TOSS CHEESE	0.5	SLICE
P.HUT. HAND-TOSS HAM	0.75	SLICE
P.HUT. HAND-TOSS VEG. LUV.	0.75	SLICE
P.HUT. HAND-TOSS PEPPERON	0.75	SLICE

P.HUT. THIN/CRISP CHEESE	0.75	SLICE
P.HUT. THIN/CRISP HAM	1	SLICE
P.HUT. THIN/CRISP VEG. LUV.	1	SLICE
P.HUT. THIN/CRISP PEPPERON	0.75	SLICE
SW 6" COLD SUB/VEGG. DELIT	1	SUB
SW 6" COLD SUB/TURK. BRST.	1	SUB
SW 6" COLD SUB/TURK.B/HAM	1	SUB
SW 6" COLD SUB/HAM	1	SUB
SW 6" COLD SUB/ROAST BEEF	1	SUB
SW 6" COLD SUB/SFOOD,CRAB	1	SUB
SW 6" COLD SUB/COLD CUT 3	1	SUB
SW 6" COLD SUB/TUNA	1	SUB
SW 6" HOT SUB/RST.CHICK.BR.	1	SUB
SW 6" HOT SUB/STAK/CHEESE	1	SUB
SW 6" HOT SUB/SUB MELT	1	SUB
SW VEGGIE DELITE SALAD	1	SALAD
SW TURKEY BREAST SALAD	1	SALAD
SW ROAST BEEF SALAD	1	SALAD
SW TURK. BRST/HAM SALAD	1	SALAD
SW RST. CHICK. BR. SALAD	0.75	SALAD
SW SEAFOOD/CRAB SALAD	0.75	SALAD
SW STEAK/CHEESE SALAD	0.75	SALAD
SW SUBWAY MELT SALAD	0.75	SALAD
SW COLD CUT 3 SALAD	0.75	SALAD
SW FAT FREE ITALIAN DRESS	1	OZ
SW FAT FREE FRENCH DRESS	1	OZ
SW FAT FREE RANCH DRESS	1	OZ
SW DELI STYLE TURKEY BR.	0.75	SNDWCH
SW DELI STYLE HAM	0.75	SNDWCH
SW DELI STYLE ROAST BEEF	0.75	SNDWCH
TB GRILLED STEAK SOFT TACO	0.75	TACO
WAHOO'S CHBROIL FISH TACO	0.5	TACO
WENDI'S SIDE SALAD	1	SALAD
WENDI'S FF FRENCH DRESSING	1	OZ
WENDI'S ITALIAN RED. F/C DRESS	1	OZ
WENDI'S SMALL CHILI	0.75	BOWL
WENDI'S GRILLED CHICK. FILLET	1	MEAT

	3300 Calories/Day Eating Plan	
	What Does Your Doctor Look Like Naked?	
Name: _____		
Date: _____		
Exercise: 30-40 min in a.m. before food		Write what you eat here:
Meal 1 Time: _____	2 Protein Sources 4 Active Carbohydrates	
Meal 2 Time:	3 oz Raw Almonds	
Meal 3 Time: _____	2 Protein Source 2 Active Carbohydrates Free Carbohydrates (as much as you want)	
Meal 4 Time: _____	1 LOW CARB protein bar (OR) 2 scoops Whey Protein Powder in water AND 1 oz String Cheese 1 oz Raw Almonds	
Meal 5 Time: _____	2 Protein Source 0 Active Carbohydrates Free Carbohydrates (as much as you want)	
Bedtime Meal (Optional)	Sugar Free Jell-O 1 cup	

Add fiber supplement in evening, such as Metamucil or other (sugar FREE).
Add spices, pepper, etc. as needed.
Try to eat every two to three hours
Drink 1 ½ gallons of water EVERY DAY!
May have up to 2 diet pops (or) 2 cups a coffee a day

Active Carbohydrates 3300 Calories

Fruit and Vegetables

APPLE	2.35	3 INCH
APPLESAUCE, MOTT'S	0.865	CUP
APRICOTS (CAN/DEL MONTE LITE)	1.59	CUP
APRICOTS (DRIED)	2.72	OZ
APRICOTS (FRESH 12/LB)	11.2	MEDIUM
ASPARAGUS	51.5	OZ
BANANA	1.81	MEDIUM
BLUEBERRIES (FRESH)	2.32	CUP
BRUSSELS SPROUTS, BOILED	3.18	CUP
CABBAGE, SHREDDED	10.6	CUP
CANTALOUPE	1.01	5 INCH
CARROT (FRESH)	17.2	OZ
CAULIFLOWER	7.34	CUP
CELERY	47.5	OZ
CHERRIES, FRESH, SWEET W/PIT	1.83	CUP
CHERRIES, DARK (CAN/DEL MONTE)	0.95	CUP
COLLARD GREENS (CAN)	3.18	CUP
COLLARD GREENS (FRESH)	15.9	CUP
CORN CAKE	5.45	CAKE
CORN (CAN/DEL MONTE NO SODIUM)	13.9	OZ
CUCUMBER, SLICED	13.6	CUP
EGGPLANT	8.65	CUP
FRUIT, MIXED FROZEN	2.12	CUP
GARLIC, 1 CLOVE	47.5	CLOVE
GARLIC, TRIMMED	4.53	OZ
GRAPES	1.67	CUP
GRAPE JUICE/VERYFINE	10.18	OZ
GRAPEFRUIT	2.07	4 INCH
GREEN BEANS (CAN/DEL MONTE NO SALT)	4.75	CUP
GREEN PEPPER	9.5	MEDIUM
KIWI	12.8	OZ
MUSHROOMS, FRESH	10.6	CUP
ONION, FRESH/CHOPPED	3.17	CUP
ORANGE, NAVAL	2.93	3 INCH

ORANGE, JUICE	13.85	OZ
PAPAYA	1.63	LB.
PAPAYA, PEELED/CUBED	3.52	CUP
PEACH, FRESH, SLICED	2.58	CUP
PEACH (CAN/DEL MONTE EXTRA LITE)	1.59	CUP
PEARS (CAN)	6.35	HALF
PEAS, BLACKEYED (CAN)	1.06	CUP
PEAS (CAN/DEL MONTE NO SODIUM)	13.9	OZ
PEAS, GREEN GIANT FROZEN, SWEET	1.84	CUP
PEAS, EDIBLE-PODDED	3.18	CUP
PINEAPPLE, FRESH/DICED	2.44	CUP
PINEAPPLE, DEL MONTE SNACK CAN (LITE)	2.72	3.5 OZ
PINEAPPLE (CAN/DOLE LITE SYRUP)	11.2	SLICE
PRUNES, DOLE, DRIED	2.72	OZ
PUMPKIN (CAN)	3.8	CUP
RAISINS	0.397	CUP
RED PEPPER	9.5	MEDIUM
STRAWBERRIES (FRESH)	1.96	PINT
STRAWBERRIES (FROZEN)	2.54	CUP
SQUASH, CAN, STOKLEY	1.9	CUP
SQUASH, FRESH BAKED	1.67	CUP
TANGERINE	5.15	2.5 INCH
TOMATO, CAN	17.8	OZ
TOMATO, FRESH	7.33	3 INCH
TOMATO, JUICE	30.4	OZ
VEGETABLES, MIXED (FROZEN)	2.12	CUP
WATERMELLON	1.25	1X10 INCH
ZUCCHINI, FRESH, SLICED	10.6	CUP

Yogurts and Desserts

DING DONG	1.19	DING
DREYERS FROZEN FAT FREE YOGURT	1.06	CUP
FRUIT ROLL-UP	2.72	ROLL-UP
POPCORN, WHITE	3.8	TBLSP
TCBY, SOFT SERVE/NONFAT/NO SUGAR	1.19	CUP
YOGURT, FAT FREE, MOUNTAIN HIGH	8	OZ
YOGURT, FAT FREE, DANNON	8	OZ
LUCERN, YOGURT, NONFAT, LITE	8	OZ

YOGURT, YOPLAIT, FAT FREE, LITE	6	OZ
YOGURT, YOPLAIT ORIGINAL/99% FAT FREE	6	OZ
YOGURT, HORIZON, FF / BLUEBERRY	6	OZ
PLANTER DRIED WALNUT PIECES	0.2	CUP
RAW ALMONDS, TOASTED	1	OZ
PECANS, DRIED	0.88	OZ
PEANUTS, DRY ROASTED	0.2	CUP
HOT CHOCOLATE	3	ENVEL.
ALMONDS, SHELLED	1	OZ

Cereals

CEREAL, CHEERIOS	1.73	CUP
CEREAL, COCOA KRISPIES	1.19	CUP
CEREAL, GRAPENUTS	0.475	CUP
CEREAL, HONEY NUT TOASTY O'S	1.73	CUP
CEREAL, WHEATIES	1.73	CUP
CEREAL, KELLOGG'S ALL BRAN	1.19	CUP
CEREAL, KELLOGG'S CORN FLAKES	1.73	CUP
CEREAL, KELLOGG'S RAISIN BRAN	1.12	CUP
CEREAL, KELLOGG'S CRACKLIN' OAT BRAN	0.72	CUP
CEREAL, NABISCO SHREDDED WHEAT	2.38	PIECE
CEREAL, NAB. SHREDDED WHEAT (SPOON)	1.12	CUP
CEREAL, RICE KRISPIES	2.17	CUP
CEREAL, BENEFIT NUTRITION, PROTEIN +	0.91	CUP
CREAM OF WHEAT	4.75	TBL/DRY
GRANOLA, CW POST HEARTY	0.453	CUP
GRANOLA, KELLOGG'S LOW FAT	4	CUP
OATMEAL (PRE-COOK MEASUREMENT)	0.68	CUP

Breads

BREAD, OROWHEAT LITE	4.75	SLICE
BREAD, SUSAN'S HOMEMADE/18 SLICES	2.1	SLICE
BREAD, SUSAN'S HOMEMADE	0.117	LOAF
BUN, WONDER REDUCED CALORIE LITE	2.38	BUN
CRACKER, ZESTA SALTINES	15.9	CRACKER
TORTILLA (CAROLYN)	1.12	TORT
TORTILLA, TORTILLA'S MEXICO, FLOUR	1.73	TORT

TORTILLA, TORTILLA'S MEXICO, CORN	2.12	TORT
TRISCUITS	1.36	OZ
WAFFLE, EGGO, HOMESTYLE	1.73	WAFFLE
WHOLE GRAIN/WHOLE WHEAT FLOUR	0.467	CUP

Rice/Potatoes/Beans

BLACK BEANS (BOILED)	0.845	CUP
BLACK BEANS (DRY)	0.68	CUP
CHICKPEAS/GARBANZO BEANS	0.22	CUP
KIDNEY BEANS (BOILED)	0.25	CUP
LIMA BEANS (BOILED)	0.915	CUP
NAVY BEANS (BOILED)	0.74	CUP
NAVY BEANS (CAN)	0.795	CUP
PINTO BEANS (BOILED)	0.815	CUP
PINTO BEANS (CAN)	1	CUP
PINTO BEANS (DRY)	0.318	CUP
PORK & BEANS/VAN CAMPS	0.865	CUP
POTATO, SWEET	1.615	5"X2"
POTATO	11.3	OZ
RICE CAKE	3.8	CAKE
RICE, WHITE, BASMATI	0.795	CUP (C)
RICE, BROWN LONG GRAIN	0.95	CUP (C)
RICE, INSTANT, MINUTE BRAND	0.595	CUP(UC)
RICE, WHITE, LONG GRAIN	0.297	CUP(UC)
SOYBEANS (BOILED)	0.75	CUP
YAM, BOILED OR BAKED	1.2	CUP

Pasta

MACARONI, DAVINI TWIST	0.725	CUP/DRY
MACARONI, HOSPITALITY ELBOW	0.396	CUP/DRY
MACARONI, AM. BEAUTY ELBOW	0.454	CUP/DRY
PASTA, CREAMETTE PLAIN	1.81	OZ
SPAGHETTI, EDEN WHOLE WHEAT	1.81	OZ/UC

Protein Sources 3300 Calories

White Meat

CHICKEN BREAST (HORMEL/CAN)	1.27	CAN
CHICKEN BREAST (SKINLESS)	6.35	OZ
CHICKEN (LEG W/SKIN & BONE)	0.72	
CHICKEN (THIGH W/SKIN & BONE)	1.245	
CHICKEN (LEG & THIGH W/SKIN & BONE)	0.455	
HAM, BAR S, XTRA LEAN, 96% FAT FREE	5.45	OZ
HAM, DAK CAN	6.34	OZ
PORK, SIRLOIN, LEAN W/FAT	1.9	OZ
TURKEY BREAST (SKINLESS)	3.56	OZ
TURKEY BREAST (HORMEL/CAN)	1.09	CAN
TURKEY BRST/OVEN ROAST/SFWY/89% FF	7.6	OZ
VENISON/ANTELOPE	4.25	OZ

Red Meat

HAMBURGER (10% FAT)	3.39	OZ
HAMBURGER (15% FAT)	2.8	OZ
HAMBURGER (20% FAT)	2.72	OZ
HAMBURGER (27% FAT)	2.3	OZ
LAMB, SHOULDER	2.17	OZ
STEAK, BOTTOM ROUND	3.21	OZ
STEAK, BRISKET (FLAT HALF)	3.02	OZ
STEAK, CHUCK, ARM	3.12	OZ
STEAK, CHUCK, BLADE	2.69	OZ
STEAK, EYE ROUND	4	OZ
STEAK, FLANK	3.25	OZ
STEAK, NEW YORK STRIP	3.8	OZ
STEAK, PORTERHOUSE	3.09	OZ
STEAK, RIBEYE	2.99	OZ
STEAK, ROUND TIP	3.64	OZ
STEAK, SHANK (CROSSCUTS)	3.35	OZ
STEAK, T-BONE	3.14	OZ
STEAK, TENDERLOIN	3.2	OZ
STEAK, TOP LOIN	3.25	OZ
STEAK, TOP ROUND	3.74	OZ

STEAK, TOP SIRLOIN	3.47	OZ
STEAK, TYSON SEASONED BEEF STRIPS	4.08	OZ
TACO/BURRITO MEAT/SMART GROUND	0.99	CUP
OSCAR MAYER BACON	6.34	SLICE
LITTLE SIZZLER BROWN/SERVE SAUSAGE	2.47	LINK

Sea Food

BASS, FRESHWATER, DRY HEAT	4.6	OZ
BASS, STRIPED, DRY HEAT	5.45	OZ
COD, ATLANTIC, DRY HEAT	6.43	OZ
CRAB, ALASKA KING, MOIST HEAT	7	OZ
CRAB, BLUE, MOIST HEAT	6.58	OZ
FLOUNDER, DRY HEAT	5.78	OZ
HADDOCK, DRY HEAT	6	OZ
HALIBUT, DRY HEAT	4.8	OZ
LOBSTER, NORTHERN, MOIST HEAT	6.9	OZ
MAHI MAHI	7.84	OZ
ORANGE ROUGHY, DRY HEAT	7.52	OZ
PERCH, DRY HEAT	5.78	OZ
PERCH, OCEAN/ATLANTIC, DRY HEAT	5.55	OZ
SALMON, ATLANTIC, DRY HEAT	3.66	OZ
SHRIMP, MOIST HEAT	6.8	OZ
TROUT, DRY HEAT	3.55	OZ
TUNA BURGER, AHI/OMEGA FOODS	6.8	OZ
TUNA, LOW SODIUM, CAN	1.09	CAN
TUNA, WATER, CAN	1.27	CAN
TUNA, WHITE/LOW SALT, CAN (5 OZ)	1.09	CAN
TUNA, WHITE, CAN (5 OZ)	1.09	CAN
TUNA, FILLET/STEAK	4.32	OZ
WALLEYE, BAKED/BROILED/MICRO	5.63	OZ

Vegetarian

IVES VEG. COUSINE VEGGY DOG	3.17	DOG
SOY MILK (TRIS)	2	CUP
SOY MILK (SYLVIA)	1.75	CUP

Eggs/Dairy

1% COTTAGE CHEESE, NORDICA	1.19	CUP
2% COTTAGE CHEESE (LOW FAT)	0.95	CUP
COTTAGE CHEESE (LUCERNE FAT FREE)	1.19	CUP
COTT CHEESE MARIGOLD/DRY CURD	1.81	CUP
COTT CHEESE MARIGOLD/DRY CURD	29	TBLSP
COTT CHEESE BREAKSTONES FAT FREE	1.19	CUP
CHEDDER, SHREDDED, FAT FREE, KHF	1.06	CUP
CHEDDER, SHREDDED, 94% FAT FREE, HC	0.95	CUP
CHEESE, COLBY/MOZZARELLA	1.73	OZ
EGG WHITE	11.2	
EGG, WHOLE	2.54	
EGG BEATERS	1.59	CUP
MOZZARELLA SHREDDED, FAT FREE, KHF	0.95	CUP
SKIM MOZZARELLA STRING CHEESE	2.38	OZ

Free Carbs, Supplements, Fast Foods
3300 calories

Free Carbs

ASPARAGUS
BROCCOLI
CABBAGE
CAULIFLOWER
CELERY
CUCUMBER
GREEN BEANS
GREEN PEPPERS
GREEN SQUASH
LETTUCE, ICEBERG
LETTUCE, LEAF/SHREDDED
MUSHROOMS
ONION
PICKLES (DILL)
RADISH

RED PEPPERS
SPINACH (CAN/NO SALT)
SPINACH (FRESH)
TOMATO (EXCLUDING JUICE)
ZUCCHINI

Supplements/Fast Foods

ATKINS BAR	0.75	BAR
EAS ADVANTEDGE, C&C/LEM/BLUE	0.75	BAR
BAR, ZONE	0.75	BAR
BAR, PURE PROTEIN, 50 G.	1	BAR
BAR, W.W. PURE PROTEIN, 78 G.	0.5	BAR
BAR, PROTEIN REVOLUTION, PBJ	0.75	BAR
BAR, FIBAR, PEANUT BUTTER, 1.2 OZ	1.25	BAR
BAR, PREMIER 1, PROTEIN 8, CHOC/COCO	0.5	BAR
BAR, PREFERRED BAR, CHOC./FUDG/RAS	0.75	BAR
BAR, PREFERRED BAR, CHOC./FUDG/BROW	0.75	BAR
ALIVE, HI CARB POWDER	3	TBLSP
POWERADE	2	SERVING
PROTEIN,GNC P.P. EGG/WHEY	1.5	SERVING
PROTEIN. GNC P.PERF. WHEY	4	SCOOP
OPTIMUM NUTRITION WHEY	1.5	SCOOP
SYNTRAX WHEY PROTEIN	2	SCOOP
TRI PROTEIN PLUS POWDER	1.25	SERVING
HW STRAWBERRY PROT. POWD.	1.75	SCOOP
BIOCHEM WHEY PRO 290	2.25	SCOOP
HUMAN DEV. TECH. WHEY	1.25	SCOOP
NATURADE 100% SOY PROTEIN	0.5	CUP
SUPER GREEN PRO 96 - SOY	0.5	CUP
100% PURE WHEY, PROLAB	1.25	SCOOP
ECLIPSE BULK UP WHEY	1.75	SCOOP
VITAMIN WORLD WHEY 100%	1.5	SCOOP
ULT. NUT. PROSTAR WHEY	1.5	SCOOP
RED WINE	7	OZ
MET RX CH.RST.PNT.PRO + BAR	0.5	BAR
MET RX BAV. MINT. PRO + BAR	0.75	BAR
MET AFTER FX BAR	0.75	BAR
MET RX CH. CH. CHIP PRO + BAR	0.5	BAR

MET RX SOURCE ONE BAR	0.75	BAR
MET RX CHOC. GRAHCRK CHIP BAR	0.5	BAR
MET RX PEANUT BUTTER BAR	0.5	BAR
MET RX DRINK MIX, MRP	0.75	SERVING
MET RX PRO 50, ANABOLIC DRIVE	0.5	SERVING
MET RX PRO 60, ANABOLIC DRIVE	0.5	SERVING
MET RX PROTEIN PLUS	2.25	SCOOP
MET RX KETO PRO	2.25	SCOOP
NUTRI FORCE DRINK MIX, MRP	0.5	SERVING
EAS MYO. DEL. CH/PB BAR	0.5	BAR
EAS MYOPLEX + DELUXE	0.5	SERVING
EAS MYOPLEX LITE	0.75	SERVING
ADVANT EDGE QUICK STIR PROTEIN DRINK	0.75	SERVING
EAS NEUROGAIN	3.5	SCOOP
EAS PHOSPHAGEN HP	1	SCOOP
EAS PRECISION PROTEIN	1.75	SCOOP
EAS SIMPLY PROTEIN	3	SCOOP
EAS WHEY PROTEIN	1.5	SCOOP
EAS SUPPER SHAKE	0.33	SHAKE
VITAMIN WORLD DAILY RX, MRP	0.5	SHAKE
VITAMIN WORLD PROTOPLEX DELUXE, MRP	0.5	SHAKE
VITAMIN WORLD PRE. ENG. WHEY PROT.	1.75	SCOOP
PERFECT RX, MRP, CHOCOLATE	0.75	SHAKE
OPTI PRO	0.5	SHAKE
ARBY'S CHICK. SAND. R.DELX.LITE	0.5	BURGER
ARBY'S SIDE SALAD	1	SALAD
ARBY'S GARDEN SALAD	1	SALAD
ARBY'S RST. CHCK. SALAD	1	SALAD
ARBY'S RED. CAL. ITAL. DRESSING	1	PACKET
ARBY'S RED RANCH DRESSING	1	PACKET
MCD'S VINEG. LITE SALAD DR.	1	PACKET
MCD'S GARDEN SALAD	1	SALAD
MCD'S VINEG. LITE SALAD DR.	1	PACKET
P.HUT. HAND-TOSS CHEESE	0.75	SLICE
P.HUT. HAND-TOSS HAM	0.75	SLICE
P.HUT. HAND-TOSS VEG. LUV.	0.75	SLICE
P.HUT. HAND-TOSS PEPPERON	0.75	SLICE
P.HUT. THIN/CRISP CHEESE	0.75	SLICE

P.HUT. THIN/CRISP HAM	1	SLICE
P.HUT. THIN/CRISP VEG. LUV.	1	SLICE
P.HUT. THIN/CRISP PEPPERON	0.75	SLICE
SW 6" COLD SUB/VEGG. DELIT	1	SUB
SW 6" COLD SUB/TURK. BRST.	1	SUB
SW 6" COLD SUB/TURK.B/HAM	1	SUB
SW 6" COLD SUB/HAM	1	SUB
SW 6" COLD SUB/ROAST BEEF	1	SUB
SW 6" COLD SUB/SFOOD,CRAB	1	SUB
SW 6" COLD SUB/COLD CUT 3	1	SUB
SW 6" COLD SUB/TUNA	1	SUB
SW 6" HOT SUB/RST.CHICK.BR.	1	SUB
SW 6" HOT SUB/STAK/CHEESE	1	SUB
SW 6" HOT SUB/SUB MELT	1	SUB
SW VEGGIE DELITE SALAD	1	SALAD
SW TURKEY BREAST SALAD	1	SALAD
SW ROAST BEEF SALAD	1	SALAD
SW TURK. BRST/HAM SALAD	1	SALAD
SW RST. CHICK. BR. SALAD	1	SALAD
SW SEAFOOD/CRAB SALAD	1	SALAD
SW STEAK/CHEESE SALAD	0.75	SALAD
SW SUBWAY MELT SALAD	1	SALAD
SW COLD CUT 3 SALAD	1	SALAD
SW FAT FREE ITALIAN DRESS	1	OZ
SW FAT FREE FRENCH DRESS	1	OZ
SW FAT FREE RANCH DRESS	1	OZ
SW DELI STYLE TURKEY BR.	0.75	SNDWCH
SW DELI STYLE HAM	0.75	SNDWCH
SW DELI STYLE ROAST BEEF	0.75	SNDWCH
TB GRILLED STEAK SOFT TACO	0.75	TACO
WAHOO'S CHBROIL FISH TACO	0.5	TACO
WENDI'S SIDE SALAD	1	SALAD
WENDI'S FF FRENCH DRESSING	1	OZ
WENDI'S ITALIAN RED. F/C DRESS	1	OZ
WENDI'S SMALL CHILI	0.75	BOWL
WENDI'S GRILLED CHICK. FILLET	1	MEAT

3400 Calories/Day Eating Plan		
What Does Your Doctor Look Like Naked?		
Name: _____		
Date: _____		
Exercise: 30-40 min in a.m. before food		
		Write what you eat here:
Meal 1 Time: _____	2 Protein Sources 4 Active Carbohydrates	
Meal 2 Time: _____	3 oz Raw Almonds	
Meal 3 Time: _____	2 Protein Source 2 Active Carbohydrates Free Carbohydrates (as much as you want)	
Meal 4 Time: _____	1 LOW CARB protein bar (OR) 2 scoops Whey Protein Powder in water AND 1 oz String Cheese 1 oz Raw Almonds	
Meal 5 Time: _____	2 Protein Source 0 Active Carbohydrates Free Carbohydrates (as much as you want)	
Bedtime Meal (Optional)	Sugar Free Jell-O 1 cup	

Add fiber supplement in evening, such as Metamucil or other (sugar FREE).
Add spices, pepper, etc. as needed.
Try to eat every two to three hours.
Drink 1½ gallons of water EVERY DAY!
May have up to 2 diet pops (or) 2 cups a coffee a day.

Active Carbohydrates 3400 Calories

Fruit and Vegetables

APPLE	2.49	3 INCH
APPLESAUCE, MOTT'S	0.91	CUP
APRICOTS (CAN/DEL MONTE LITE)	1.68	CUP
APRICOTS (DRIED)	2.88	OZ
APRICOTS (FRESH 12/LB)	11.8	MEDIUM
ASPARAGUS	54.4	OZ
BANANA	1.92	MEDIUM
BLUEBERRIES (FRESH)	2.46	CUP
BRUSSELS SPROUTS, BOILED	3.35	CUP
CABBAGE, SHREDDED	11.2	CUP
CANTALOUPE	1.07	5 INCH
CARROT (FRESH)	18.1	OZ
CAULIFLOWER	7.75	CUP
CELERY	50	OZ
CHERRIES, FRESH, SWEET W/PIT	1.94	CUP
CHERRIES, DARK (CAN/DEL MONTE)	1	CUP
COLLARD GREENS (CAN)	3.36	CUP
COLLARD GREENS (FRESH)	16.8	CUP
CORN CAKE	5.75	CAKE
CORN (CAN/DEL MONTE NO SODIUM)	14.7	OZ
CUCUMBER, SLICED	14.4	CUP
EGGPLANT	9.1	CUP
FRUIT, MIXED FROZEN	2.24	CUP
GARLIC, 1 CLOVE	50	CLOVE
GARLIC, TRIMMED	4.8	OZ
GRAPES	1.77	CUP
GRAPE JUICE/VERYFINE	10.7	OZ
GRAPEFRUIT	2.19	4 INCH
GREEN BEANS (CAN/DEL MONTE NO SALT)	5	CUP
GREEN PEPPER	10	MEDIUM
KIWI	13.5	OZ
MUSHROOMS, FRESH	11.2	CUP
ONION, FRESH/CHOPPED	3.36	CUP
ORANGE, NAVAL	3.1	3 INCH

ORANGE, JUICE	14.6	OZ
PAPAYA	1.72	LB.
PAPAYA, PEELED/CUBED	3.74	CUP
PEACH, FRESH, SLICED	2.72	CUP
PEACH (CAN/DEL MONTE EXTRA LITE)	1.68	CUP
PEARS (CAN)	6.7	HALF
PEAS, BLACKEYED (CAN)	1.12	CUP
PEAS (CAN/DEL MONTE NO SODIUM)	14.7	OZ
PEAS, GREEN GIANT FROZEN, SWEET	1.92	CUP
PEAS, EDIBLE-PODDED	3.35	CUP
PINEAPPLE, FRESH/DICED	2.58	CUP
PINEAPPLE, DEL MONTE SNACK CAN (LITE)	2.88	3.5 OZ
PINEAPPLE (CAN/DOLE LITE SYRUP)	11.88	SLICE
PRUNES, DOLE, DRIED	2.88	OZ
PUMPKIN (CAN)	4	CUP
RAISINS	0.42	CUP
RED PEPPER	10	MEDIUM
STRAWBERRIES (FRESH)	2.08	PINT
STRAWBERRIES (FROZEN)	2.69	CUP
SQUASH, CAN, STOKLEY	2	CUP
SQUASH, FRESH BAKED	1.77	CUP
TANGERINE	5.45	2.5 INCH
TOMATO, CAN	18.8	OZ
TOMATO, FRESH	7.7	3 INCH
TOMATO, JUICE	32	OZ
VEGETABLES, MIXED (FROZEN)	2.24	CUP
WATERMELLON	1.32	1X10 INCH
ZUCCHINI, FRESH, SLICED	11.2	CUP

Yogurts and Desserts

DING DONG	1.26	DING
DREYERS FROZEN FAT FREE YOGURT	1.12	CUP
FRUIT ROLL-UP	2.88	ROLL-UP
POPCORN, WHITE	4	TBLSP
TCBY, SOFT SERVE/NONFAT/NO SUGAR	1.26	CUP
YOGURT, FAT FREE, MOUNTAIN HIGH	8	OZ
YOGURT, FAT FREE, DANNON	8	OZ
LUCERN, YOGURT, NONFAT, LITE	8	OZ

YOGURT, YOPLAIT, FAT FREE, LITE	6	OZ
YOGURT,YOPLAIT ORIGINAL/99% FAT FREE	6	OZ
YOGURT, HORIZON, FF / BLUEBERRY	6	OZ
PLANTER DRIED WALNUT PIECES	0.25	CUP
RAW ALMONDS, TOASTED	1.19	OZ
PECANS, DRIED	1	OZ
PEANUTS, DRY ROASTED	0.2	CUP
HOT CHOCOLATE	4	ENVEL.
ALMONDS, SHELLED	1	OZ

Cereals

CEREAL, CHEERIOS	1.83	CUP
CEREAL, COCOA KRISPIES	1.26	CUP
CEREAL, GRAPENUTS	0.5	CUP
CEREAL, HONEY NUT TOASTY O'S	1.83	CUP
CEREAL, WHEATIES	1.83	CUP
CEREAL, KELLOGG'S ALL BRAN	1.26	CUP
CEREAL, KELLOGG'S CORN FLAKES	1.83	CUP
CEREAL, KELLOGG'S RAISIN BRAN	1.18	CUP
CEREAL, KELLOGG'S CRACKLIN' OAT BRAN	0.76	CUP
CEREAL, NABISCO SHREDDED WHEAT	2.5	PIECE
CEREAL, NAB. SHREDDED WHEAT (SPOON)	1.18	CUP
CEREAL, RICE KRISPIES	2.29	CUP
CEREAL, BENEFIT NUTRITION, PROTEIN +	0.96	CUP
CREAM OF WHEAT	5	TBL/DRY
GRANOLA, CW POST HEARTY	0.48	CUP
GRANOLA, KELLOGG'S LOW FAT	4	CUP
OATMEAL (PRE-COOK MEASUREMENT)	0.72	CUP

Breads

BREAD, OROWHEAT LITE	5	SLICE
BREAD, SUSAN'S HOMEMADE/18 SLICES	2.22	SLICE
BREAD, SUSAN'S HOMEMADE	0.123	LOAF
BUN, WONDER REDUCED CALORIE LITE	2.5	BUN
CRACKER, ZESTA SALTINES	16.8	CRACKER
TORTILLA (CAROLYN)	1.18	TORT
TORTILLA, TORTILLA'S MEXICO, FLOUR	1.83	TORT

TORTILLA, TORTILLA'S MEXICO, CORN	2.24	TORT
TRISCUITS	1.44	OZ
WAFFLE, EGGO, HOMESTYLE	1.83	WAFFLE
WHOLE GRAIN/WHOLE WHEAT FLOUR	0.495	CUP

Rice/Potatoes/Beans

BLACK BEANS (BOILED)	0.89	CUP
BLACK BEANS (DRY)	0.72	CUP
CHICKPEAS/GARBANZO BEANS	0.25	CUP
KIDNEY BEANS (BOILED)	0.25	CUP
LIMA BEANS (BOILED)	0.568	CUP
NAVY BEANS (BOILED)	0.78	CUP
NAVY BEANS (CAN)	0.838	CUP
PINTO BEANS (BOILED)	0.86	CUP
PINTO BEANS (CAN)	1.06	CUP
PINTO BEANS (DRY)	0.335	CUP
PORK & BEANS/VAN CAMPS	0.91	CUP
POTATO, SWEET	1.71	5"X2"
POTATO	12	OZ
RICE CAKE	4	CAKE
RICE, WHITE, BASMATI	0.84	CUP (C)
RICE, BROWN LONG GRAIN	1	CUP (C)
RICE, INSTANT, MINUTE BRAND	0.63	CUP(UC)
RICE, WHITE, LONG GRAIN	0.315	CUP(UC)
SOYBEANS (BOILED)	0.75	CUP
YAM, BOILED OR BAKED	1.27	CUP

Pasta

MACARONI, DAVINI TWIST	0.765	CUP/DRY
MACARONI, HOSPITALITY ELBOW	0.42	CUP/DRY
MACARONI, AM. BEAUTY ELBOW	0.48	CUP/DRY
PASTA, CREAMETTE PLAIN	1.92	OZ
SPAGHETTI, EDEN WHOLE WHEAT	1.92	OZ/UC

Protein Sources 3400 Calories

White Meat

CHICKEN BREAST (HORMEL/CAN)	1.34	CAN
CHICKEN BREAST (SKINLESS)	6.7	OZ
CHICKEN (LEG W/ SKIN & BONE)	0.76	
CHICKEN (THIGH W/SKIN & BONE)	1.32	
CHICKEN (LEG & THIGH W/SKIN & BONE)	0.48	
HAM, BAR S, XTRA LEAN, 96% FAT FREE	5.75	OZ
HAM, DAK CAN	6.7	OZ
PORK, SIRLOIN, LEAN W/FAT	2	OZ
TURKEY BREAST (SKINLESS)	3.76	OZ
TURKEY BREAST (HORMEL/CAN)	1.15	CAN
TURKEY BRST/OVEN ROAST/SFWY/89% FF	8	OZ
VENISON/ANTELOPE	4.5	OZ

Red Meat

HAMBURGER (10% FAT)	3.58	OZ
HAMBURGER (15% FAT)	2.96	OZ
HAMBURGER (20% FAT)	2.88	OZ
HAMBURGER (27% FAT)	2.44	OZ
LAMB, SHOULDER	2.29	OZ
STEAK, BOTTOM ROUND	3.4	OZ
STEAK, BRISKET (FLAT HALF)	3.2	OZ
STEAK, CHUCK, ARM	3.3	OZ
STEAK, CHUCK, BLADE	2.84	OZ
STEAK, EYE ROUND	4.22	OZ
STEAK, FLANK	3.44	OZ
STEAK, NEW YORK STRIP	4	OZ
STEAK, PORTERHOUSE	3.27	OZ
STEAK, RIBEYE	3.16	OZ
STEAK, ROUND TIP	3.85	OZ
STEAK, SHANK (CROSSCUTS)	3.53	OZ
STEAK, T-BONE	3.32	OZ
STEAK, TENDERLOIN	3.38	OZ
STEAK, TOP LOIN	3.44	OZ
STEAK, TOP ROUND	3.95	OZ

STEAK, TOP SIRLOIN	3.67	OZ
STEAK, TYSON SEASONED BEEF STRIPS	4.3	OZ
TACO/BURRITO MEAT/SMART GROUND	1.05	CUP
OSCAR MAYER BACON	6.7	SLICE
LITTLE SIZZLER BROWN/SERVE SAUSAGE	2.62	LINK

Sea Food

BASS, FRESHWATER, DRY HEAT	4.9	OZ
BASS, STRIPED, DRY HEAT	5.75	OZ
COD, ATLANTIC, DRY HEAT	6.8	OZ
CRAB, ALASKA KING, MOIST HEAT	7.38	OZ
CRAB, BLUE, MOIST HEAT	6.95	OZ
FLOUNDER, DRY HEAT	6.1	OZ
HADDOCK, DRY HEAT	6.35	OZ
HALIBUT, DRY HEAT	5.08	OZ
LOBSTER, NORTHERN, MOIST HEAT	7.3	OZ
MAHI MAHI	8.3	OZ
ORANGE ROUGHY, DRY HEAT	7.9	OZ
PERCH, DRY HEAT	6.1	OZ
PERCH, OCEAN/ATLANTIC, DRY HEAT	5.86	OZ
SALMON, ATLANTIC, DRY HEAT	3.87	OZ
SHRIMP, MOIST HEAT	7.2	OZ
TROUT, DRY HEAT	3.75	OZ
TUNA BURGER, AHI/OMEGA FOODS	7.2	OZ
TUNA, LOW SODIUM, CAN	1.15	CAN
TUNA, WATER, CAN	1.34	CAN
TUNA, WHITE/LOW SALT, CAN (5 OZ)	1.15	CAN
TUNA, WHITE, CAN (5 OZ)	1.15	CAN
TUNA, FILLET/STEAK	4.57	OZ
WALLEYE, BAKED/BROILED/MICRO	5.97	OZ

Vegetarian

IVES VEG. COUSINE VEGGY DOG	3.35	DOG
SOY MILK (TRIS)	2.25	CUP
SOY MILK (SYLVIA)	2	CUP

Eggs/Dairy

1% COTTAGE CHEESE, NORDICA	1.26	CUP
2% COTTAGE CHEESE (LOW FAT)	1	CUP
COTTAGE CHEESE (LUCERNE FAT FREE)	1.26	CUP
COTT CHEESE MARIGOLD/DRY CURD	1.92	CUP
COTT CHEESE MARIGOLD/DRY CURD	30.5	TBLSP
COTT CHEESE BREAKSTONES FAT FREE	1.26	CUP
CHEDDER, SHREDDED, FAT FREE, KHF	1.12	CUP
CHEDDER, SHREDDED, 94% FAT FREE, HC	1	CUP
CHEESE, COLBY/MOZZARELLA	1.83	OZ
EGG WHITE	11.8	
EGG, WHOLE	2.69	
EGG BEATERS	1.68	CUP
MOZZARELLA SHREDDED, FAT FREE, KHF	1	CUP
SKIM MOZZARELLA STRING CHEESE	2.5	OZ

Free Carbs, Supplements, Fast Foods
3400 calories

Free Carbs

ASPARAGUS
BROCCOLI
CABBAGE
CAULIFLOWER
CELERY
CUCUMBER
GREEN BEANS
GREEN PEPPERS
GREEN SQUASH
LETTUCE, ICEBERG
LETTUCE, LEAF/SHREDDED
MUSHROOMS
ONION
PICKLES (DILL)

RADISH
RED PEPPERS
SPINACH (CAN/NO SALT)
SPINACH (FRESH)
TOMATO (EXCLUDING JUICE)
ZUCCHINI

Supplements/Fast Foods

ATKINS BAR	0.75	BAR
EAS ADVANTEDGE, C&C/LEM/BLUE	0.75	BAR
BAR, ZONE	0.88	BAR
BAR, PURE PROTEIN, 50 G.	1	BAR
BAR, W.W. PURE PROTEIN, 78 G.	0.5	BAR
BAR, PROTEIN REVOLUTION, PBJ	0.88	BAR
BAR, FIBAR, PEANUT BUTTER, 1.2 OZ	1.33	BAR
BAR, PREMIER 1, PROTEIN 8, CHOC/COCO	0.75	BAR
BAR, PREFERRED BAR, CHOC./FUDG/RAS	0.88	BAR
BAR, PREFERRED BAR, CHOC./FUDG/BROW	0.88	BAR
ALIVE, HI CARB POWDER	5	TBLSP
POWERADE	2	SERVING
PROTEIN,GNC P.P. EGG/WHEY	1.5	SERVING
PROTEIN. GNC P.PERF. WHEY	4	SCOOP
OPTIMUM NUTRITION WHEY	1.75	SCOOP
SYNTRAX WHEY PROTEIN	2.25	SCOOP
TRI PROTEIN PLUS POWDER	1.5	SERVING
HW STRAWBERRY PROT. POWD.	2	SCOOP
BIOCHEM WHEY PRO 290	2.5	SCOOP
HUMAN DEV. TECH. WHEY	1.5	SCOOP
NATURADE 100% SOY PROTEIN	0.5	CUP
SUPER GREEN PRO 96 - SOY	0.5	CUP
100% PURE WHEY, PROLAB	0.75	SCOOP
ECLIPSE BULK UP WHEY	2	SCOOP
VITAMIN WORLD WHEY 100%	1.75	SCOOP
ULT. NUT. PROSTAR WHEY	1.75	SCOOP
RED WINE	8	OZ
MET RX CH.RST.PNT.PRO + BAR	0.5	BAR
MET RX BAV. MINT. PRO + BAR	0.75	BAR
MET AFTER FX BAR	0.75	BAR

MET RX CH. CH. CHIP PRO + BAR	0.75	BAR
MET RX SOURCE ONE BAR	0.75	BAR
MET RX CHOC. GRAHCRK CHIP BAR	0.5	BAR
MET RX PEANUT BUTTER BAR	0.5	BAR
MET RX DRINK MIX, MRP	0.75	SERVING
MET RX PRO 50, ANABOLIC DRIVE	0.75	SERVING
MET RX PRO 60, ANABOLIC DRIVE	0.5	SERVING
MET RX PROTEIN PLUS	2.5	SCOOP
MET RX KETO PRO	2.5	SCOOP
NUTRI FORCE DRINK MIX, MRP	0.75	SERVING
EAS MYO. DEL. CH/PB BAR	0.5	BAR
EAS MYOPLEX + DELUXE	0.5	SERVING
EAS MYOPLEX LITE	0.75	SERVING
ADVANT EDGE QUICK STIR PROTEIN DRINK	0.75	SERVING
EAS NEUROGAIN	4	SCOOP
EAS PHOSPHAGEN HP	1	SCOOP
EAS PRECISION PROTEIN	1.75	SCOOP
EAS SIMPLY PROTEIN	3	SCOOP
EAS WHEY PROTEIN	1.75	SCOOP
EAS SUPPER SHAKE	0.33	SHAKE
VITAMIN WORLD DAILY RX, MRP	0.75	SHAKE
VITAMIN WORLD PROTOPLEX DELUXE, MRP	0.5	SHAKE
VITAMIN WORLD PRE. ENG. WHEY PROT.	2	SCOOP
PERFECT RX, MRP, CHOCOLATE	0.75	SHAKE
OPTI PRO	0.75	SHAKE
ARBY'S CHICK. SAND. R.DELX.LITE	0.5	BURGER
ARBY'S SIDE SALAD	1	SALAD
ARBY'S GARDEN SALAD	1	SALAD
ARBY'S RST. CHCK. SALAD	1	SALAD
ARBY'S RED. CAL. ITAL. DRESSING	1	PACKET
ARBY'S RED RANCH DRESSING	1	PACKET
MCD'S VINEG. LITE SALAD DR.	1	PACKET
MCD'S GARDEN SALAD	1	SALAD
MCD'S VINEG. LITE SALAD DR.	1	PACKET
P.HUT. HAND-TOSS CHEESE	0.75	SLICE
P.HUT. HAND-TOSS HAM	0.75	SLICE
P.HUT. HAND-TOSS VEG. LUV.	0.75	SLICE
P.HUT. HAND-TOSS PEPPERON	0.75	SLICE

P.HUT. THIN/CRISP CHEESE	1	SLICE
P.HUT. THIN/CRISP HAM	1	SLICE
P.HUT. THIN/CRISP VEG. LUV.	1	SLICE
P.HUT. THIN/CRISP PEPPERON	0.75	SLICE
SW 6" COLD SUB/VEGG. DELIT	1	SUB
SW 6" COLD SUB/TURK. BRST.	1	SUB
SW 6" COLD SUB/TURK.B/HAM	1	SUB
SW 6" COLD SUB/HAM	1	SUB
SW 6" COLD SUB/ROAST BEEF	1	SUB
SW 6" COLD SUB/SFOOD,CRAB	1	SUB
SW 6" COLD SUB/COLD CUT 3	1	SUB
SW 6" COLD SUB/TUNA	1	SUB
SW 6" HOT SUB/RST.CHICK.BR.	1	SUB
SW 6" HOT SUB/STAK/CHEESE	1	SUB
SW 6" HOT SUB/SUB MELT	1	SUB
SW VEGGIE DELITE SALAD	1	SALAD
SW TURKEY BREAST SALAD	1	SALAD
SW ROAST BEEF SALAD	1	SALAD
SW TURK. BRST/HAM SALAD	1	SALAD
SW RST. CHICK. BR. SALAD	1	SALAD
SW SEAFOOD/CRAB SALAD	1	SALAD
SW STEAK/CHEESE SALAD	0.75	SALAD
SW SUBWAY MELT SALAD	1	SALAD
SW COLD CUT 3 SALAD	1	SALAD
SW FAT FREE ITALIAN DRESS	1	OZ
SW FAT FREE FRENCH DRESS	1	OZ
SW FAT FREE RANCH DRESS	1	OZ
SW DELI STYLE TURKEY BR.	0.75	SNDWCH
SW DELI STYLE HAM	0.75	SNDWCH
SW DELI STYLE ROAST BEEF	0.75	SNDWCH
TB GRILLED STEAK SOFT TACO	0.75	TACO
WAHOO'S CHBROIL FISH TACO	1	TACO
WENDI'S SIDE SALAD	1	SALAD
WENDI'S FF FRENCH DRESSING	1	OZ
WENDI'S ITALIAN RED. F/C DRESS	1	OZ
WENDI'S SMALL CHILI	1	BOWL
WENDI'S GRILLED CHICK. FILLET	1.5	MEAT

3500 Calories/Day Eating Plan		
What Does Your Doctor Look Like Naked?		

Name: _____		
Date: _____		

Exercise: 30-40 min in a.m. before food		Write what you eat here:
Meal 1 Time: _____	2 Protein Sources 4 Active Carbohydrates	
Meal 2 Time:	3 oz Raw Almonds	
Meal 3 Time: _____	2 Protein Source 2 Active Carbohydrates Free Carbohydrates (as much as you want)	
Meal 4 Time: _____	1 LOW CARB protein bar (OR) 2 scoops Whey Protein Powder in water AND 1 oz String Cheese 1 oz Raw Almonds	
Meal 5 Time: _____	2 Protein Source 0 Active Carbohydrates Free Carbohydrates (as much as you want)	
Bedtime Meal (Optional)	Sugar Free Jell-O 1 cup	

Add fiber supplement in evening, such as Metamucil or other (sugar FREE).
Add spices, pepper, etc. as needed.
Try to eat every two to three hours.
Drink 1½ gallons of water EVERY DAY!
May have up to 2 diet pops (or) 2 cups a coffee a day.

Active Carbohydrates 3500 Calories

Fruit and Vegetables

APPLE	2.56	3 INCH
APPLESAUCE, MOTT'S	0.945	CUP
APRICOTS (CAN/DEL MONTE LITE)	1.73	CUP
APRICOTS (DRIED)	2.96	OZ
APRICOTS (FRESH 12/LB)	12.2	MEDIUM
ASPARAGUS	56	OZ
BANANA	1.98	MEDIUM
BLUEBERRIES (FRESH)	2.53	CUP
BRUSSELS SPROUTS, BOILED	3.45	CUP
CABBAGE, SHREDDED	11.5	CUP
CANTALOUPE	1.1	5 INCH
CARROT (FRESH)	18.7	OZ
CAULIFLOWER	7.97	CUP
CELERY	51.8	OZ
CHERRIES, FRESH, SWEET W/PIT	1.99	CUP
CHERRIES, DARK (CAN/DEL MONTE)	1.035	CUP
COLLARD GREENS (CAN)	3.45	CUP
COLLARD GREENS (FRESH)	17.3	CUP
CORN CAKE	5.94	CAKE
CORN (CAN/DEL MONTE NO SODIUM)	15.15	OZ
CUCUMBER, SLICED	14.8	CUP
EGGPLANT	14.8	CUP
FRUIT, MIXED FROZEN	2.3	CUP
GARLIC, 1 CLOVE	51.8	CLOVE
GARLIC, TRIMMED	4.95	OZ
GRAPES	1.82	CUP
GRAPE JUICE/VERYFINE	11.05	OZ
GRAPEFRUIT	2.25	4 INCH
GREEN BEANS (CAN/DEL MONTE NO SALT)	5.18	CUP
GREEN PEPPER	10.35	MEDIUM
KIWI	13.95	OZ
MUSHROOMS, FRESH	11.5	CUP
ONION, FRESH/CHOPPED	3.45	CUP

ORANGE, NAVAL	3.19	3 INCH
ORANGE, JUICE	15.1	OZ
PAPAYA	3.85	LB.
PAPAYA, PEELED/CUBED	1.98	CUP
PEACH, FRESH, SLICED	2.8	CUP
PEACH (CAN/DEL MONTE EXTRA LITE)	1.73	CUP
PEARS (CAN)	6.9	HALF
PEAS, BLACKEYED (CAN)	1.15	CUP
PEAS (CAN/DEL MONTE NO SODIUM)	15.15	OZ
PEAS, GREEN GIANT FROZEN, SWEET	1.98	CUP
PEAS, EDIBLE-PODDED	3.45	CUP
PINEAPPLE, FRESH/DICED	2.66	CUP
PINEAPPLE, DEL MONTE SNACK CAN (LITE)	2.96	3.5 OZ
PINEAPPLE (CAN/DOLE LITE SYRUP)	12.2	SLICE
PRUNES, DOLE, DRIED	2.96	OZ
PUMPKIN (CAN)	4.14	CUP
RAISINS	0.433	CUP
RED PEPPER	10.35	MEDIUM
STRAWBERRIES (FRESH)	2.14	PINT
STRAWBERRIES (FROZEN)	2.76	CUP
SQUASH, CAN, STOKLEY	2.07	CUP
SQUASH, FRESH BAKED	1.82	CUP
TANGERINE	5.6	2.5 INCH
TOMATO, CAN	19.4	OZ
TOMATO, FRESH	8	3 INCH
TOMATO, JUICE	33	OZ
VEGETABLES, MIXED (FROZEN)	2.3	CUP
WATERMELLON	1.36	1X10 INCH
ZUCCHINI, FRESH, SLICED	11.5	CUP

Yogurts and Desserts

DING DONG	1.29	DING
DREYERS FROZEN FAT FREE YOGURT	1.15	CUP
FRUIT ROLL-UP	2.96	ROLL-UP
POPCORN, WHITE	4.15	TBLSP
TCBY, SOFT SERVE/NONFAT/NO SUGAR	1.29	CUP
YOGURT, FAT FREE, MOUNTAIN HIGH	8	OZ

YOGURT, FAT FREE, DANNON	8	OZ
LUCERN, YOGURT, NONFAT, LITE	8	OZ
YOGURT, YOPLAIT, FAT FREE, LITE	6	OZ
YOGURT,YOPLAIT ORIGINAL/99% FAT FREE	6	OZ
YOGURT, HORIZON, FF/BLUEBERRY	6	OZ
PLANTER DRIED WALNUT PIECES	0.25	CUP
RAW ALMONDS, TOASTED	1.25	OZ
PECANS, DRIED	1	OZ
PEANUTS, DRY ROASTED	0.25	CUP
HOT CHOCOLATE	4	ENVEL.
ALMONDS, SHELLED	1.25	OZ

Cereals

CEREAL, CHEERIOS	1.89	CUP
CEREAL, COCOA KRISPIES	1.295	CUP
CEREAL, GRAPENUTS	0.518	CUP
CEREAL, HONEY NUT TOASTY O'S	1.89	CUP
CEREAL, WHEATIES	1.89	CUP
CEREAL, KELLOGG'S ALL BRAN	1.295	CUP
CEREAL, KELLOGG'S CORN FLAKES	1.89	CUP
CEREAL, KELLOGG'S RAISIN BRAN	1.22	CUP
CEREAL, KELLOGG'S CRACKLIN' OAT BRAN	0.785	CUP
CEREAL, NABISCO SHREDDED WHEAT	2.59	PIECE
CEREAL, NAB. SHREDDED WHEAT (SPOON)	1.22	CUP
CEREAL, RICE KRISPIES	2.36	CUP
CEREAL, BENEFIT NUTRITION, PROTEIN +	0.99	CUP
CREAM OF WHEAT	5.18	TBL/DRY
GRANOLA, CW POST HEARTY	0.495	CUP
GRANOLA, KELLOGG'S LOW FAT	4	CUP
OATMEAL (PRE-COOK MEASUREMENT)	0.74	CUP

Breads

BREAD, OROWHEAT LITE	5.18	SLICE
BREAD, SUSAN'S HOMEMADE/18 SLICES	2.29	SLICE
BREAD, SUSAN'S HOMEMADE	0.127	LOAF
BUN, WONDER REDUCED CALORIE LITE	2.59	BUN
CRACKER, ZESTA SALTINES	17.3	CRACKER

TORTILLA (CAROLYN)	1.22	TORT
TORTILLA, TORTILLA'S MEXICO, FLOUR	1.89	TORT
TORTILLA, TORTILLA'S MEXICO, CORN	2.3	TORT
TRISCUITS	1.48	OZ
WAFFLE, EGGO, HOMESTYLE	1.89	WAFFLE
WHOLE GRAIN/WHOLE WHEAT FLOUR	0.51	CUP

Rice/Potatoes/Beans

BLACK BEANS (BOILED)	0.92	CUP
BLACK BEANS (DRY)	0.74	CUP
CHICKPEAS/GARBANZO BEANS	0.25	CUP
KIDNEY BEANS (BOILED)	0.33	CUP
LIMA BEANS (BOILED)	1	CUP
NAVY BEANS (BOILED)	0.8	CUP
NAVY BEANS (CAN)	0.865	CUP
PINTO BEANS (BOILED)	0.886	CUP
PINTO BEANS (CAN)	1.09	CUP
PINTO BEANS (DRY)	0.345	CUP
PORK & BEANS/VAN CAMPS	0.945	CUP
POTATO, SWEET	1.76	5"X2"
POTATO	12.3	OZ
RICE CAKE	4.14	CAKE
RICE, WHITE, BASMATI	0.865	CUP (C)
RICE, BROWN LONG GRAIN	1.035	CUP (C)
RICE, INSTANT, MINUTE BRAND	0.645	CUP(UC)
RICE, WHITE, LONG GRAIN	0.324	CUP(UC)
SOYBEANS (BOILED)	0.75	CUP
YAM, BOILED OR BAKED	1.31	CUP

Pasta

MACARONI, DAVINI TWIST	0.79	CUP/DRY
MACARONI, HOSPITALITY ELBOW	0.433	CUP/DRY
MACARONI, AM. BEAUTY ELBOW	0.495	CUP/DRY
PASTA, CREAMETTE PLAIN	1.98	OZ
SPAGHETTI, EDEN WHOLE WHEAT	1.98	OZ/UC

Protein Sources 3500 Calories

White Meat

CHICKEN BREAST (HORMEL/CAN)	1.38	CAN
CHICKEN BREAST (SKINLESS)	6.9	OZ
CHICKEN (LEG W/SKIN & BONE)	0.78	
CHICKEN (THIGH W/SKIN & BONE)	1.355	
CHICKEN (LEG & THIGH W/SKIN & BONE)	0.496	
HAM, BAR S, XTRA LEAN, 96% FAT FREE	5.93	OZ
HAM, DAK CAN	6.9	OZ
PORK, SIRLOIN, LEAN W/FAT	2.07	OZ
TURKEY BREAST (SKINLESS)	3.87	OZ
TURKEY BREAST (HORMEL/CAN)	1.185	CAN
TURKEY BRST/OVEN ROAST/SFWY/89% FF	8.3	OZ
VENISON / ANTELOPE	4.64	OZ

Red Meat

HAMBURGER (10% FAT)	3.68	OZ
HAMBURGER (15% FAT)	3.05	OZ
HAMBURGER (20% FAT)	2.96	OZ
HAMBURGER (27% FAT)	2.51	OZ
LAMB, SHOULDER	2.36	OZ
STEAK, BOTTOM ROUND	3.5	OZ
STEAK, BRISKET (FLAT HALF)	3.3	OZ
STEAK, CHUCK, ARM	3.4	OZ
STEAK, CHUCK, BLADE	2.92	OZ
STEAK, EYE ROUND	4.35	OZ
STEAK, FLANK	3.54	OZ
STEAK, NEW YORK STRIP	4.14	OZ
STEAK, PORTERHOUSE	3.36	OZ
STEAK, RIBEYE	3.26	OZ
STEAK, ROUND TIP	3.97	OZ
STEAK, SHANK (CROSSCUTS)	3.64	OZ
STEAK, T-BONE	3.42	OZ
STEAK, TENDERLOIN	3.48	OZ
STEAK, TOP LOIN	3.54	OZ
STEAK, TOP ROUND	4.07	OZ

STEAK, TOP SIRLOIN	3.78	OZ
STEAK, TYSON SEASONED BEEF STRIPS	4.45	OZ
TACO/BURRITO MEAT/SMART GROUND	1.08	CUP
OSCAR MAYER BACON	6.9	SLICE
LITTLE SIZZLER BROWN/SERVE SAUSAGE	2.7	LINK

Sea Food

BASS, FRESHWATER, DRY HEAT	5	OZ
BASS, STRIPED, DRY HEAT	5.93	OZ
COD, ATLANTIC, DRY HEAT	7	OZ
CRAB, ALASKA KING, MOIST HEAT	7.6	OZ
CRAB, BLUE, MOIST HEAT	7.15	OZ
FLOUNDER, DRY HEAT	6.3	OZ
HADDOCK, DRY HEAT	6.56	OZ
HALIBUT, DRY HEAT	5.23	OZ
LOBSTER, NORTHERN, MOIST HEAT	7.5	OZ
MAHI MAHI	8.55	OZ
ORANGE ROUGHY, DRY HEAT	8.2	OZ
PERCH, DRY HEAT	6.3	OZ
PERCH, OCEAN/ATLANTIC, DRY HEAT	6.04	OZ
SALMON, ATLANTIC, DRY HEAT	3.99	OZ
SHRIMP, MOIST HEAT	7.4	OZ
TROUT, DRY HEAT	3.86	OZ
TUNA BURGER, AHI/OMEGA FOODS	7.4	OZ
TUNA, LOW SODIUM, CAN	1.185	CAN
TUNA, WATER, CAN	1.38	CAN
TUNA, WHITE/LOW SALT, CAN (5 OZ)	1.18	CAN
TUNA, WHITE, CAN (5 OZ)	1.18	CAN
TUNA, FILLET/STEAK	4.72	OZ
WALLEYE, BAKED/BROILED/MICRO	6.15	OZ

Vegetarian

IVES VEG. COUSINE VEGGY DOG	3.45	DOG
SOY MILK (TRIS)	2.25	CUP
SOY MILK (SYLVIA)	2	CUP

Eggs/Dairy

1% COTTAGE CHEESE, NORDICA	1.295	CUP
2% COTTAGE CHEESE (LOW FAT)	1.035	CUP
COTTAGE CHEESE (LUCERNE FAT FREE)	1.29	CUP
COTT CHEESE MARIGOLD/DRY CURD	1.98	CUP
COTT CHEESE MARIGOLD/DRY CURD	31.6	TBLSP
COTT CHEESE BREAKSTONES FAT FREE	1.295	CUP
CHEDDER, SHREDDED, FAT FREE, KHF	1.15	CUP
CHEDDER, SHREDDED, 94% FAT FREE, HC	1.035	CUP
CHEESE, COLBY/MOZZARELLA	1.89	OZ
EGG WHITE	12.2	
EGG, WHOLE	2.76	
EGG BEATERS	1.73	CUP
MOZZARELLA SHREDDED, FAT FREE, KHF	1.03	CUP
SKIM MOZZARELLA STRING CHEESE	2.59	OZ

Free Carbs, Supplements, Fast Foods
3500 calories

Free Carbs
ASPARAGUS
BROCCOLI
CABBAGE
CAULIFLOWER
CELERY
CUCUMBER
GREEN BEANS
GREEN PEPPERS
GREEN SQUASH
LETTUCE, ICEBERG
LETTUCE, LEAF/SHREDDED
MUSHROOMS
ONION
PICKLES (DILL)
RADISH

RED PEPPERS
SPINACH (CAN/NO SALT)
SPINACH (FRESH)
TOMATO (EXCLUDING JUICE)
ZUCCHINI

Supplements/Fast Foods

ATKINS BAR	1	BAR
EAS ADVANTEDGE, C&C/LEM/BLUE	1	BAR
BAR, ZONE	1	BAR
BAR, PURE PROTEIN, 50 G.	1	BAR
BAR, W.W. PURE PROTEIN, 78 G.	0.5	BAR
BAR, PROTEIN REVOLUTION, PBJ	0.88	BAR
BAR, FIBAR, PEANUT BUTTER, 1.2 OZ	1.5	BAR
BAR, PREMIER 1, PROTEIN 8, CHOC/COCO	0.75	BAR
BAR, PREFERRED BAR, CHOC./FUDG/RAS	1	BAR
BAR, PREFERRED BAR, CHOC./FUDG/BROW	1	BAR
ALIVE, HI CARB POWDER	5	TBLSP
POWERADE	2.5	SERVING
PROTEIN,GNC P.P. EGG/WHEY	1.75	SERVING
PROTEIN. GNC P.PERF. WHEY	5	SCOOP
OPTIMUM NUTRITION WHEY	1.75	SCOOP
SYNTRAX WHEY PROTEIN	2.33	SCOOP
TRI PROTEIN PLUS POWDER	1.5	SERVING
HW STRAWBERRY PROT. POWD.	2.25	SCOOP
BIOCHEM WHEY PRO 290	2.5	SCOOP
HUMAN DEV. TECH. WHEY	1.5	SCOOP
NATURADE 100% SOY PROTEIN	0.5	CUP
SUPER GREEN PRO 96 - SOY	0.5	CUP
100% PURE WHEY, PROLAB	1.5	SCOOP
ECLIPSE BULK UP WHEY	2	SCOOP
VITAMIN WORLD WHEY 100%	1.88	SCOOP
ULT. NUT. PROSTAR WHEY	1.88	SCOOP
RED WINE	8	OZ
MET RX CH.RST.PNT.PRO + BAR	0.5	BAR
MET RX BAV. MINT. PRO + BAR	0.75	BAR
MET AFTER FX BAR	0.75	BAR
MET RX CH. CH. CHIP PRO + BAR	0.75	BAR

MET RX SOURCE ONE BAR	1	BAR
MET RX CHOC. GRAHCRK CHIP BAR	0.5	BAR
MET RX PEANUT BUTTER BAR	0.5	BAR
MET RX DRINK MIX, MRP	0.75	SERVING
MET RX PRO 50, ANABOLIC DRIVE	0.75	SERVING
MET RX PRO 60, ANABOLIC DRIVE	0.5	SERVING
MET RX PROTEIN PLUS	3	SCOOP
MET RX KETO PRO	2.75	SCOOP
NUTRI FORCE DRINK MIX, MRP	0.75	SERVING
EAS MYO. DEL. CH/PB BAR	0.5	BAR
EAS MYOPLEX + DELUXE	0.5	SERVING
EAS MYOPLEX LITE	0.5	SERVING
ADVANT EDGE QUICK STIR PROTEIN DRINK	0.88	SERVING
EAS NEUROGAIN	4.5	SCOOP
EAS PHOSPHAGEN HP	1.5	SCOOP
EAS PRECISION PROTEIN	2	SCOOP
EAS SIMPLY PROTEIN	3.5	SCOOP
EAS WHEY PROTEIN	1.75	SCOOP
EAS SUPPER SHAKE	0.33	SHAKE
VITAMIN WORLD DAILY RX, MRP	0.75	SHAKE
VITAMIN WORLD PROTOPLEX DELUXE, MRP	0.5	SHAKE
VITAMIN WORLD PRE. ENG. WHEY PROT.	2.5	SCOOP
PERFECT RX, MRP, CHOCOLATE	0.75	SHAKE
OPTI PRO	0.75	SHAKE
ARBY'S CHICK. SAND. R.DELX.LITE	0.75	BURGER
ARBY'S SIDE SALAD	1	SALAD
ARBY'S GARDEN SALAD	1	SALAD
ARBY'S RST. CHCK. SALAD	1	SALAD
ARBY'S RED. CAL. ITAL. DRESSING	1	PACKET
ARBY'S RED RANCH DRESSING	1	PACKET
MCD'S VINEG. LITE SALAD DR.	1	PACKET
MCD'S GARDEN SALAD	1	SALAD
MCD'S VINEG. LITE SALAD DR.	1	PACKET
P.HUT. HAND-TOSS CHEESE	0.88	SLICE
P.HUT. HAND-TOSS HAM	1	SLICE
P.HUT. HAND-TOSS VEG. LUV.	0.88	SLICE
P.HUT. HAND-TOSS PEPPERON	0.75	SLICE
P.HUT. THIN/CRISP CHEESE	1	SLICE

P.HUT. THIN/CRISP HAM	1	SLICE
P.HUT. THIN/CRISP VEG. LUV.	1	SLICE
P.HUT. THIN/CRISP PEPPERON	1	SLICE
SW 6" COLD SUB/VEGG. DELIT	1	SUB
SW 6" COLD SUB/TURK. BRST.	1	SUB
SW 6" COLD SUB/TURK.B/HAM	1	SUB
SW 6" COLD SUB/HAM	1	SUB
SW 6" COLD SUB/ROAST BEEF	1	SUB
SW 6" COLD SUB/SFOOD,CRAB	1	SUB
SW 6" COLD SUB/COLD CUT 3	1	SUB
SW 6" COLD SUB/TUNA	1	SUB
SW 6" HOT SUB/RST.CHICK.BR.	1	SUB
SW 6" HOT SUB/STAK/CHEESE	1	SUB
SW 6" HOT SUB/SUB MELT	1	SUB
SW VEGGIE DELITE SALAD	1	SALAD
SW TURKEY BREAST SALAD	1	SALAD
SW ROAST BEEF SALAD	1	SALAD
SW TURK. BRST/HAM SALAD	1	SALAD
SW RST. CHICK. BR. SALAD	1	SALAD
SW SEAFOOD/CRAB SALAD	1	SALAD
SW STEAK/CHEESE SALAD	1	SALAD
SW SUBWAY MELT SALAD	1	SALAD
SW COLD CUT 3 SALAD	1	SALAD
SW FAT FREE ITALIAN DRESS	1	OZ
SW FAT FREE FRENCH DRESS	1	OZ
SW FAT FREE RANCH DRESS	1	OZ
SW DELI STYLE TURKEY BR.	0.88	SNDWCH
SW DELI STYLE HAM	0.88	SNDWCH
SW DELI STYLE ROAST BEEF	0.75	SNDWCH
TB GRILLED STEAK SOFT TACO	0.88	TACO
WAHOO'S CHBROIL FISH TACO	1	TACO
WENDI'S SIDE SALAD	1	SALAD
WENDI'S FF FRENCH DRESSING	1	OZ
WENDI'S ITALIAN RED. F/C DRESS	1	OZ
WENDI'S SMALL CHILI	1	BOWL
WENDI'S GRILLED CHICK. FILLET	1	MEAT

Condiments

Feel free to use two active condiments each day before 3:00 pm.
Use the free condiments as needed.

Active Condiments

Food Type	Serving Size
Butter, unsalted	1 Tspn
Dressing, kraft fat free ranch	1 Tblsp
Hidden val. Orig. F.F. Ranch w/ bacon	1 Tblsp
Dressing, kraft free,blue cheese	1 Tblsp
Kraft lite done r. Roka blue cheese	1 Tblsp
Wishbone just 2 good blue cheese	1 Tblsp
Knorr spring veggy soup/dip mix	1 Tblsp
Jam, smuckers reduced sugar	1 Tblsp
Ketchup, heinz	1 Tblsp
Ketchup, hunts	1 Tblsp
Ketchup, del monte	1 Tblsp
Mayonnaise, best foods, low fat	1 Tblsp
Pasta sauce, hunt's homestyle	0.5 Cup
Psta sauce, sw verdi sel., mush/onion	0.5 Cup
Peanut butter, peter pan creamy	1 Tspn
Soy nut butter	1 Tspn
Tartar sauce, best foods, low fat	1 Tblsp
Cocktail sauce, kraft	0.25 Cup
Cocktail sauce, heinz	0.25 Cup
Kraft fat free parmesan	1 Tsp

Free Condiments

Food Type	Serving Size
Apple cider vinegar	1 Tblsp
Chicken broth, sfwy, ff, lo sodium	1 Cup
Dressing, kraft free, italian	1 Tblsp
Dress, kraft free,red wine vinegar	1 Tblsp
Bernstein's ff parmes cheese dress	1 Tblsp
Kraft fat free mayo	1 Tblsp
Mustard	1 Tblsp
Cinnamon, ground	1 Tspn
Picante sauce, pace	1 Tblsp
Lavictoria salsa supreme	1 Tblsp
Tostitos salsa	1 Tblsp
Rotel xtra hot tomatoes	1 Oz
Rotel mild tomatoes	1 Oz

Appendix II

Preventative Medicine Screening

Adapted from the Agency for Healthcare Research and Quality (AHRQ) (www.ahrq.gov) Internet Citation: *Clinical Preventive Services for Normal–Risk Adults Recommended by the U.S. Preventive Services Task Force*. Put Prevention into Practice, January 2003. Agency for Healthcare Research and Quality, Rockville, MD. http://www.ahrq.gov/ppip/adulttm.htm

Men

Screening tests, what you need and when:

Screening tests, such as colorectal cancer tests, can find diseases early when they are easier to treat. Some men need certain screening tests earlier, or more often, than others. Talk to your doctor about which of the tests listed below are right for you, when you should have them, and how often. The Task Force has made the following recommendations, based on scientific evidence, about which screening tests you should have.

- Cholesterol Checks: Have your cholesterol checked at least every 5 years, starting at age 35. If you smoke, have diabetes, or if heart disease runs in your family, start having your cholesterol checked at age 20.

- Blood Pressure: Have your blood pressure checked at least every 2 years.
- Colorectal Cancer Tests: Begin regular screening for colorectal cancer starting at age 50. Your doctor can help you decide which test is right for you. How often you need to be tested will depend on which test you have.
- Diabetes Tests: Have a test to screen for diabetes if you have high blood pressure or high cholesterol.
- Depression: If you've felt "down," sad, or hopeless, and have felt little interest or pleasure in doing things for 2 weeks straight, talk to your doctor about whether he or she can screen you for depression.
- Sexually Transmitted Diseases: Talk to your doctor to see whether you should be screened for sexually transmitted diseases, such as HIV.
- Prostate Cancer Screening: Talk to your doctor about the possible benefits and harms of prostate cancer screening if you are considering having a prostate–specific antigen (PSA) test or digital rectal examination (DRE).

Should You Take Medicines to Prevent Disease?

- Aspirin: Talk to your doctor about taking aspirin to prevent heart disease if you are older than 40, or if you are younger than 40 and have high blood pressure, high cholesterol, diabetes, or if you smoke.

Immunizations:

- Have a flu shot every year starting at age 50.
- Have a tetanus–diphtheria shot every 10 years.

- Have a pneumonia shot once at age 65 (you may need it earlier if you have certain health problems, such as lung disease).
- Talk to your doctor to see whether you need hepatitis B shots.

Women

Screening tests, what you need and when:

Screening tests, such as mammograms and Pap smears, can find diseases early when they are easier to treat. Some women need certain screening tests earlier, or more often, than others. Talk to your doctor about which of the tests listed below are right for you, when you should have them, and how often.

The Task Force has made the following recommendations, based on scientific evidence, about which screening tests you should have.

- Mammograms: Have a mammogram every 1 to 2 years starting at age 40.
- Pap Smears: Have a Pap smear every 1 to 3 years if you have been sexually active or are older than 21.
- Cholesterol Checks: Have your cholesterol checked regularly starting at age 45. If you smoke, have diabetes, or if heart disease runs in your family, start having your cholesterol checked at age 20.
- Blood Pressure: Have your blood pressure checked at least every 2 years.
- Colorectal Cancer Tests: Begin regular screening for colorectal cancer starting at age 50. Your doctor can help you decide which test is right for you.
- Diabetes Tests: Have a test to screen for diabetes if you have high blood pressure or high cholesterol.

- Depression: If you've felt "down," sad, or hopeless, and have felt little interest or pleasure in doing things for 2 weeks straight, talk to your doctor about whether he or she can screen you for depression.
- Osteoporosis Tests: Have a bone–density test at age 65 to screen for osteoporosis (thinning of the bones). If you are between the ages of 60 and 64 and weigh 154 pounds or less, talk to your doctor about whether you should be tested.
- Chlamydia Tests and Tests for Other Sexually Transmitted Diseases: Have a test for Chlamydia if you are 25 or younger and sexually active. If you are older, talk to your doctor to see whether you should be tested. Also, talk to your doctor to see whether you should be tested for other sexually transmitted diseases.

Should You Take Medicines to Prevent Disease?

- Breast Cancer Drugs: If your mother, sister, or daughter has had breast cancer, talk to your doctor about the risks and benefits of taking medicines to prevent breast cancer.
- Aspirin: Talk to your doctor about taking aspirin to prevent heart disease if you are older than 45 and have high blood pressure, high cholesterol, diabetes, or if you smoke.

Immunizations:

- Have a flu shot every year starting at age 50.
- Have a tetanus–diphtheria shot every 10 years.
- Have a pneumonia shot once at age 65.
- Talk to your doctor to see whether you need hepatitis B shots.

Clinical Preventive Services for Normal–Risk Adults Recommended by the U.S. Preventive Services Task Force

Current as of January 2003

Screening

- Blood Pressure, Height and Weight: Periodically, 18 years and older.
- Cholesterol: Men, Every 5 years, 35 years and older, Women, Every 5 years, 45 years and older.
- Diabetes: Periodically, adults with hypertension or hyperlipidemia.
- Pap Smear: Women, Every 1 to 3 Years, 18–65 years, Chlamydia: 18–25 years.
- Mammography: Every 1 to 2 Years, 40 years and older.
- Colorectal Cancer: Periodically, 50 years and older. Osteoporosis: Women, routinely, > 65 years or > 60 years at increased risk for fractures.
- Alcohol Use: Periodically, 18 years and older.
- Vision, Hearing: Periodically, 65 years and older.

Immunization

- Tetanus–Diphtheria (Td): Every 10 Years, 18 years and older.
- Varicella (VZV): Susceptibles only—Two doses, 18 years and older.
- Measles, Mumps, Rubella (MMR): Women of childbearing age—One dose, 18–50 years.
- Pneumococcal: One dose, 65 years and older.
- Influenza: Yearly, 50 years and older.

Chemoprevention

- Discuss aspirin to prevent cardiovascular events: Men, Periodically, 40 years and older. Women, Periodically, 50 years and older. Discuss breast cancer chemoprevention with women at high risk.

Counseling

- Calcium Intake: Women, Periodically, 18 years and older.
- Folic Acid: Women of childbearing age, 18–50 years.
- Tobacco cessation, drug and alcohol use, STDs and HIV, nutrition, physical activity, sun exposure, oral health, injury prevention, and polypharmacy: Periodically, 18 years and older.

Appendix III

Glycemic Index

Instructions: I have broken down an example Glycemic Index based on the time of day foods can be eaten. This list should be used as a reference only, as it is not all–inclusive. Compare the types of foods listed with others as you make your selection.

Anytime Foods

Slow inducers of insulin secretion

- Most all meats
- Most all cheeses
- Yogurt, low fat, artificially sweet
- Soy-beans (canned)
- Peanuts
- Soya beans
- Rice beans
- Green apples
- Cherries
- Peas, dried
- Grapefruit
- Red lentils
- Spaghetti, protein-enriched
- Milk, full fat

Before 3:00 p.m.

Moderate inducers of insulin secretion

- Kidney beans
- Black beans
- Soymilk
- Apricots, dried
- Milk, skim
- Lima beans, baby frozen
- Fettuccine
- Garbanzo beans
- Pinto beans
- Kellogg's All Bran Fruit 'N Oats
- Mars Snicker bar
- Apple juice
- Spaghetti, white
- Pear, fresh
- Navy beans
- Tomato soup
- Plums

Before Noon

Moderate inducers of insulin secretion

- All-Bran
- Peach, fresh
- Twix Cookie Bar (Caramel)
- Orange
- Pears (canned)
- Sweet potato
- Mars chocolate
- Pinto beans (canned)

- Macaroni
- Linguine
- Instant Rice, boiled 1 minute
- Sponge cake
- Grapes
- Pineapple juice
- Peaches (canned)
- Instant noodles
- Green Peas
- Mixed-grain bread
- Grapefruit juice
- Baked beans
- Muffins
- Potato, canned
- Ice cream
- Oatmeal
- Hamburger bun
- Split-pea soup
- Pizza, cheese
- Pastry
- Rice, vermicelli
- Rice, white
- Bran
- Chex
- Honey
- Apricots, fresh
- Pita bread, white
- Power bar
- Mango

Early Morning

Rapid inducers of insulin secretion

- Kellogg's Mini Wheats
- Shredded Wheat
- Skittles
- Wheat bread, high fiber
- Taco shells
- Stoned Wheat Thins
- Grape Nuts Cereal
- Croissant
- Cake, angel food
- Green pea soup (canned)
- Pineapple
- Nutri-grain Life cereal
- Potato, steamed
- Sucrose
- Black bean soup
- Macaroni and cheese
- Mars bar
- Beets
- Raisins
- Shortbread
- Apricots (canned), syrup
- Tofu frozen desert, non-dairy
- Maltodextrin
- Maltose
- Glucose tablets
- Dates
- Parsnips
- Glucose

- Rice, instant, boiled 6 minutes
- Rice Chex
- Potatoes, microwaved
- Rice Krispies
- Pretzels
- Jellybeans
- Post Flakes
- Rice cakes
- Vanilla Wafers
- Coco Pops
- Total Cereal
- Waffles
- Donuts
- Pumpkins
- Cheerios Cereal
- Puffed Wheat Cereal
- Potato, boiled, mashed
- Rutabaga
- Watermelon
- Bagel, white
- Golden Grahams
- Wheat bread, white
- Potato, mashed
- Cream of Wheat
- Melba toast

Appendix IV

Aerobic/Fat–Burning Program

Instructions:

- Discuss any and all exercise programs with your doctor prior to starting.
- Using this style of exercise, you can walk, run, bike, or swim, inside or outside, with any modality you have available (treadmill, stationary bike, elliptical, etc.)
- Perform your aerobic/fat–burning program at least three times a week.
- Be sure to warm up prior to starting with a slow walk followed by some stretching.
- For maximal fat–burning results, complete this program first thing in the morning, prior to food, and then wait approximately one half to one hour before eating your first meal.
- You will be alternating low intensity with high–intensity exercise, based on the time intervals provided.
- Following your warm–up, do the suggested time interval for the low intensity followed immediately by the suggested time interval for the high intensity. This makes up one cycle. This should be repeated as many times as suggested in the far column titled "Cycles."
- Where it says LSD, meaning Long, Slow Distance, do a moderate–intensity exercise for at least 40 minutes.

- In gauging the intensity of your exercise, utilize the following perceived exertion:
    - Low Intensity – Should be relatively easy without too much strain or work.
    - High Intensity – Really push the envelope on this portion of your program. Go for it hard and fast. If you are on a bike or treadmill, increase the resistance and your speed for the suggested time period.
- *If you experience any dizziness, chest pain, nausea, or shortness of breath, discontinue exercise immediately and consult medical personnel.*

Appendix IV
Exercise Chart:

Exercise Day	Date	High Intensity	Low Intensity	Cycles
Day 1		30	90	5 cycles
Day 2		30	90	5 cycles
Day 3		30	90	5 cycles
Day 4		30	90	5 cycles
Day 5				LSD
Day 6		45	90	5 cycles
Day 7		45	90	5 cycles
Day 8		45	90	5 cycles
Day 9		45	90	5 cycles
Day 10				LSD
Day 11		30	60	6 cycles
Day 12				LSD
Day 13		30	60	6 cycles
Day 14		45	60	6 cycles
Day 15		45	60	6 cycles
Day 16				LSD
Day 17		45	60	4 cycles
Day 18		45	60	4 cycles
Day 19				LSD
Day 20		60	90	4 cycles
Day 21		60	90	5 cycles
Day 22				LSD
Day 23		60	60	4 cycles
Day 24				LSD
Day 25		60	60	5 cycles
Day 26		60	60	6 cycles
Day 27				LSD

Day 28				LSD
Day 29		90	60	4 cycles
Day 30		90	60	4 cycles
Day 31		90	60	4 cycles
Day 32		90	60	4 cycles
Day 33				LSD
Day 34		90	60	5 cycles
Day 35		90	60	5 cycles
Day 36				LSD
Day 37		60	60	6 cycles
Day 38		60	60	6 cycles
Day 39		60	60	6 cycles
Day 40				LSD
Day 41		60	45	5 cycles
Day 42		60	45	5 cycles
Day 43		60	30	4 cycles

Continue exercising in this fashion, by alternating high and low intensity intervals.

Appendix V

Resistance–Training Program

Please consult your personal physician
before starting any exercise program.

Both novice and more advanced weightlifters can use this beginning resistance–training program. I would suggest beginners start with simple soup cans (or equivalent) and work your way up to heavier items found around the home. Regardless of the modalities used (soup cans, dumbbells, etc.), the style is very effective. It is a variation of a weightlifting technique called Timed Sets/Reps, or Time Under Tension. Following the exercise instructions, you will perform 2 sets of each exercise for 40 seconds each, followed by 60 seconds of rest. We are not counting repetitions with this particular technique; we are just doing the repetitions in a slow and controlled fashion for a total of 40 seconds a set. To advance your program, I would suggest one of two things: increase the amount of resistance for the same time period, or keep the resistance the same and increase the time. This should be done when the set becomes too easy, and you no longer feel you are putting forth much effort.

Appendix V

	Body Part	Exercise	Sets	Time
1	Legs	Wall Squats / Stance	2	40 seconds
2	Shoulders	Sitting Shoulder Press	2	40 seconds
3	Biceps	Sitting Curls	2	40 seconds
4	Chest	Wall / Chair Presses	2	40 seconds
5	Back	Seated bent over rows	2	40 seconds
6	Triceps	Seated Kick backs	2	40 seconds
7	Lower Legs	Heel Raises	2	40 seconds

1. Wall Squats/Stance

Standing with your back against a wall, place your feet in front of you so your shoelaces are in front of your knees. Squat down by bending your knees to a comfortable position. Do not exceed a 90–degree angle at the knee. Place a chair or bench under you as a safety measure. Hold this position for (up to) 40 seconds. Rest for 60 seconds and then repeat. Following, move on to exercise #2.

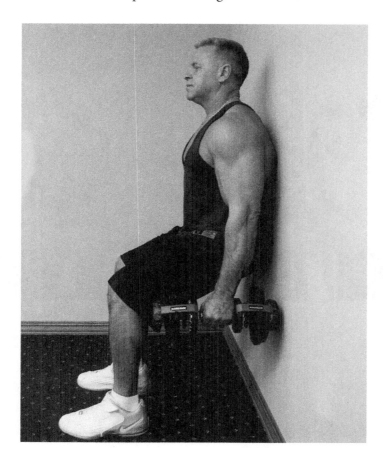

2. Sitting Shoulder Press

Sitting upright with your back firmly against a chair or wall, keep your chest out and bring your elbows to your side as pictured above. Using slow and controlled movements, press up to bring your hands over your head. Slowly lower your arms to the starting position. Repeat this movement for 40 seconds. Rest for 60 seconds and then repeat. Following, move on to exercise #3.

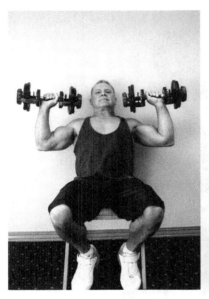 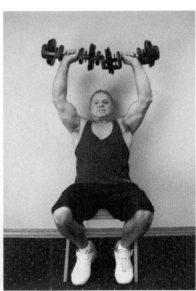

3. Bicep Curl

Sitting upright with your back firmly against a chair or wall, keep your chest out and bring your elbows to your side. Starting with your arms straight and to your side and keeping your elbows stationary, using slow and controlled movements, bring your hand to your shoulder. Slowly lower your arms to the starting position. Repeat this movement for 40 seconds. Rest for 60 seconds and then repeat. Following, move on to exercise #4.

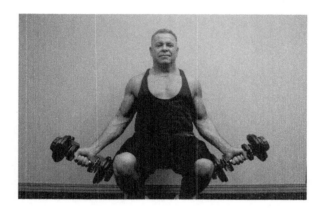

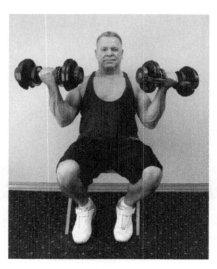

4. Wall/Chair Presses

Leaning against a chair or wall and keeping your chest out in front of you and your elbows slightly off your side, lower yourself to the chair or wall by bending at the elbows. Go as far as you can comfortably using slow and controlled movements. Repeat this movement for 40 seconds. The farther your feet are from the chair or wall, the harder the movement will be. Rest for 60 seconds and then repeat. Following, move on to exercise #5.

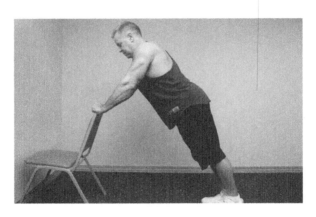

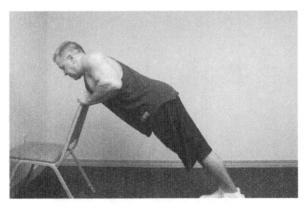

5. Seated Bent–Over Rows

Sitting upright with your chest slightly forward and lower back arched (as shown above), start with your arms to your side and, using slow and controlled movements, pull your elbow up and behind you (by bending at the elbow joint). At the same time, shrug your shoulders up and squeeze your shoulder blades together. Slowly lower your arms to the starting position. Repeat this movement for 40 seconds. Rest for 60 seconds and then repeat. Following, move on to exercise #6.

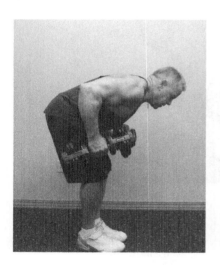 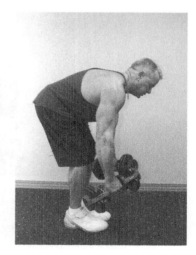

6. Triceps Kick Backs

Sitting upright with your chest slightly forward and lower back arched (as shown), keep your elbows behind you and stationary. Using slow and controlled movements and your upper arms motionless, straighten your forearm behind you until your elbow is fully extended. Slowly lower your arms to the starting position. Repeat this movement for 40 seconds. Rest for 60 seconds and then repeat. Following, move on to exercise #7.

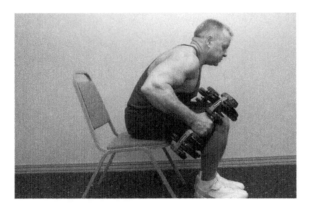

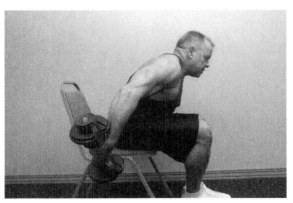

7. Heel Raises

Standing with your hands on the back of a chair or table, keeping your chest out and back straight, slowly raise your heel off the ground by placing all of your weight on your toes. Slowly lower your heels to their starting position. Repeat this movement for 40 seconds. Rest for 60 seconds and then repeat. Following, take some time to stretch and go for a brisk walk as a cool down.

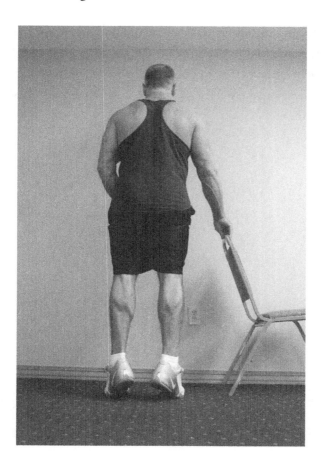

Appendix VI

Supplement Recommendations

The following recommendations are only a suggestion. We all have different needs and indications for supplements. Before taking any supplement, discuss it with your doctor to ensure that you have no contraindications or potential interactions with other medications or supplements.

Time	Supplement	What they do
Before Exercise	1 cup of coffee 81 mg aspirin	Great fat-burning combination. Aspirin is also used to prevent heart disease and colon cancer.
After Exercise	400 IU Vitamin E 1000 mg Vitamin C 1000 - 3000 mg Glutamine	Vitamin C and E are excellent anti-oxidants to help you recover from exercise. Glutamine helps to increase protein in your muscles.
Meal One	Multivitamin 200 mcg Chromium Picoilinate 500 mg Calcium 500 mg Magnesium Digestive Enzymes 2000 IU Vitamin D	According to recent studies, we all need a multivitamin. Chromium acts to help sugar go to the right place after eating. Calcium and Magnesium are essential elements for weight loss, bone protection, and a number of other processes.
Meal Two	B-Complex Vitamin	Energy Booster!
Between Meals	1000 - 3000 mg Glutamine	Protects lean mass and reduces sugar cravings.
Meal Three	200 mcg Chromium Picoilinate 100 mg Alpha Lipoic Acid Digestive Enzymes	Alpha Lipoic Acid is a great anti-oxidant and sugar modifier. Digestive enzymes ensure proper digestion and utilization of foods.
Between Meals	1000 - 3000 mg Glutamine	Protects lean mass and reduces sugar cravings.
Meal Five	500 mg Calcium 500 mg Magnesium Omega 3 fatty acids Digestive Enzymes	Omega Three fatty Acids are essential fats that aid with fat loss, heart protection, and a number of other physiological functions.
Bedtime	Fiber replacement: Sugar Free Metamucil - 1 or 2 Tablespoons.	Assists in proper colon functioning, lowering cholesterol, and helps with the late-night sugar cravings.

The table is headed: **Exercise first thing in the morning BEFORE FOOD!**

Appendix VII

Optimal Style of Eating

The following set of "rules" should be applied to any and all eating programs, diets, and lifestyle choices you make. It is a basic summary of the book and has been instrumental in helping people achieve their goals!

- Biggest Meal in the a.m., Smallest in the evening (last meal)
- Eat smaller, more frequent meals (every 2.5–3 hours)
- Eat majority of carbohydrates in the a.m. (moderate carbs post–workout)
- Drink at least 12–8 oz. glasses of water a day (generalization)
- Eat an adequate amount of protein everyday (dairy, meats, beans, etc.)
- Move as often as possible!
- Eat "naked foods," like fruit, dairy, vegetables, etc.
- Avoid processed foods (canned foods, breads, etc.)
- Avoid high–glycemic carbohydrates (sugar, cornflakes, instant potatoes, etc.)
- Bring your own food to dinner (i.e. *know* what you are eating. *Know* how many calories are in your food.)
- Do not eat within two to three hours of going to bed
- When scheduled, schedule!
- If you fail to plan, plan to fail!

Food Types (Examples)

- *Good protein sources:* egg white, whole egg, low fat/fat–free cottage cheese, low fat/fat–free cheese, tofu, whey protein powder, bass, flounder, haddock, halibut, hamburger (10% fat), perch, salmon, steak/eye round, steak/top round, steak/round tip, steak/top loin, steak/top sirloin, trout, skim mozzarella string cheese, chicken breast (skinless), shrimp, cod, crab, lobster, orange roughy, turkey breast (skinless), canned tuna
- *Fibrous carbohydrates:* zucchini, green beans, squash, broccoli, spinach, red peppers, green peppers, mushrooms, cauliflower, lettuce, cucumber, pickles
- *Starchy carbohydrates:* barley, yams, oatmeal, red beans, tomatoes, black–eyed peas, corn, sweet potatoes, long–grain rice, potatoes, popcorn, lentils, pasta, peas, whole–meal flour

Appendix VIII

Frequently Asked Questions

I have included and answered a list of questions I get on a regular basis from my clients and people who have read this book to date. If you have others, please do not hesitate to contact me (see Appendix X).

- *What is the average weight loss with this type of eating and how long does it take?*

    First, let's change the question to: What is the average *fat* loss? as we no longer care about scale weight! The scale, in some cases like Vicky's in Chapter 9, will not necessarily change that quickly, if at all. If this is the case, you need to track your lean versus fat mass, as these will be changing if you are following the program. That is also why we use subjective and objective measures to track progress. The average fat loss is quite variable due to exercise, daily activities, etc., so it is very hard, if not impossible, to give you an accurate guess. The way the program is designed, with the eating variable, the free window, and the advice on breaking through walls, and the fact that you are now armed with the information for accomplishment, you will succeed!

- *Why do you use raw almonds for meal number two in all the eating plans? Can I use other forms of nuts, such as peanuts or baked almonds?*

    Raw almonds are full of the essential fat called monounsaturated fat. This fat, as we discussed in Chapter 13, is an absolutely essential part of anyone's diet, especially those after optimal health and fat loss. They have also been proven to increase the amount of weight loss as compared to diets that do not contain them. In a study in the *International Journal of Obesity* (2003) 27, 1365–1372, entitled "Almonds vs. complex carbohydrates in a weight reduction program," it was demonstrated in the almond group that there was a 62% greater reduction in weight/BMI (body mass index), a 50% greater reduction in waist circumference, and 56% greater reduction in fat mass as compared to the complex carbohydrate group. I have put this powerful tool to use in my own clients and had wonderful results, which is why I added it to all the diets! As far as using other forms of nuts? It should be okay, but the studies and my experience dictate that raw almonds are your best bet!

- *After I have made use of the eating variable and changed my diet a few times with it, will I find an amount that I can maintain my progress with?*

    Yes! Once you have made some progress and get to a stage you are happy with, you will find a caloric amount that will work well with your given free windows and lifestyle. As some of us have a hard time finding a place where we are happy with our bodies, start using the suggestions in Chapter 18 on a regular basis, not just when you hit a wall. This will allow you to continually shock the system and stay one step ahead of your body.

- *How does this program differ from that used by clients you have personally worked with?*

  All of the theory and thought put into this book has been utilized with my personal clients and is a large part of the reason for their success. I also write all of my personal clients' diets for them as often as they need and based on their subjective and objective changes. The biggest difference, however, would be the one–on–one accountability I have with my clients. That is why I encourage you to get a partner (or two or three) who will help you with accountability.

  There is another powerful reason for success I have observed in my practice: the *financial accountability*. This liability comes in the form of (as the words indicate) finances. People who spent money on their programs always did better than those who did not. This is very apparent with my employees. They never do as well as clients, and they have me around all the time for questions, changes to their eating programs, etc. I truly believe this is due to the fact they did not lay out any cash in the process. To make up for this I would do the following: give one thousand dollars to a friend or loved one, fully intending to let them keep it unless you start meeting your goals. As goals are met, for example, the changing of a dress size, you get fifty dollars to one hundred dollars back as a reward. When you meet your final goal, you get the whole sum back. For some reason, nothing motivates us like money…

- What is your next book, *Better than Steroids,* about?

  Better than Steroids is the secret to a breathtaking physique! It is loaded with specifics on training, cardio routines, and, most importantly, how to set up the most successful eating plans to optimize your muscle mass and burn fat! With information on the pre– and post–workout meal and glycogen supercompensation, this book is a must–have for anyone who wants to look good!

- *Are the eating plan and caloric determinants in this book for people of all sizes?*

  The way the eating plan is designed, with the ratios of protein, carbohydrates, and fats, as well as the calculation of calories using the eating variable, it will work for everyone, no matter their size. I would suggest, however, that people who weigh more than 280 pounds (scale weight) get their body composition determined and use their lean mass in the caloric calculations. For example: If you weighed 325 pounds scale weight and determined your lean mass to weigh 210 pounds, divide 210 pounds by 2.2, then multiply that number by your eating variable.

  210/2.2 = 95.5 x Eating Variable (24) = 2290

  Round your calories to the nearest 100 and use the 2,300–calorie eating plan.

  If you have no way of determining your lean mass, please use Appendix IX to order a skin caliper and how–to book. If you cannot do this either, use the following sliding scale in your calculations.

  To use the sliding scale, determine your scale weight and subtract that number from the number in the right column. For example: If you weighed 325 pounds scale weight, subtract 85 from 325 (off the chart below) to get 240. Then divide 240 by 2.2, and then multiply that number by your eating variable.

$$240/2.2 = 109 \times \text{Eating Variable (24)} = 2{,}618$$

Round your calories to the nearest 100 and use the 2,600–calorie eating plan.

Obviously, determining your lean mass will be most accurate, but the sliding scale shown below works very well.

Appendix VIII:

If your scale weight is:	Subtract the following number (in the column below) from your scale weight and use that number in your determination of caloric amounts.
280 - 350	85
351 - 380	115
381 - 400	135
401 - 425	160
426 - 450	185
451 - 500	235
501 +	300

• *Can I drink alcohol while obtaining optimal health?*

As I stated in the book, I do not believe there is a bad food, alcohol included. However, like all food, too much can be bad for you. Alcohol, in moderation, can be beneficial. It is known to increase the good cholesterol, HDL, and the benefits of certain kinds of alcohol, red wine for example, continue to appear in the medical literature. One must recall that alcohol has calories, seven calories per gram to be exact. Therefore, one must weight the benefits of the extra calories versus the risks. In general, a glass or two of red wine a week is encouraged in my practice.

- *Can I follow the suggested eating and exercise program while I am pregnant or breastfeeding?*

    While both the exercise and eating programs are simple and well tolerated by anyone in any condition, I would encourage all current and future mothers to consult with their physicians before attempting any diet or exercise program.

Appendix IX

How to Contact Dr. Willey

Dr. Willey is an osteopathic physician, board certified with the American Board of Family Practice and the American Board of Holistic Medicine. His areas of expertise include nutritional and exercise medicine with an emphasis in preventive medicine.

While completing pre–med requirements at Colorado State University, Dr. Willey often felt disheartened that most health care providers did *not* discuss the impact of diet and exercise with their patients. Most medical care resulted in a prescription for medications while avoiding the topics of nutrition and an exercise program. When asking a physician colleague about the importance of nutrition and exercise, he replied, "There is no time for that, and besides, no one listens if you do."

Dr. Willey was dumbfounded. He found that if he was not careful, he would fall into the trap of being a *disease care* provider versus a *health care* provider (focusing more on a disease state than a healthy state). This focused his practice to be primarily centered on diet and exercise: teaching people how to eat, not just to "diet."

Following graduation from medical school, Dr. Willey went on to the Mayo Clinic for a 36–month residency in family medicine. At the completion of his residency, he started the Fitness Medicine Clinic in Colorado, a full–service weight loss and age–management clinic. Wanting to offer his optimal health program to more people, he left the private–pay clinic to move to an urgent–care format where he can see a larger variety and number of clients.

Dr. Willey is the medical director at Physicians Immediate Care Center, where he supervises the provision of walk–in family medicine, a growing occupational medicine service, urgent care, and Southeast Idaho's most successful weight–loss program. He serves as a consultant to several nutritional companies, he is a freelance author for many fitness magazines, and he has spoken at several engagements about nutrition, exercise, and health management.

Dr. Willey's lectures are engaging and speak to people in virtually every stage of life. Viewers come away with nutritional tips and insights that will help them feel better, live longer, and embrace life. Dr. Willey is an expert at mingling solid, researched medical facts with humor, and he keeps his audiences engaged and listening for more. He is adept at reading audiences and giving them the information that will benefit them nutritionally and medically, and audience members frequently comment that he inspires them to change their habits and lifestyle.

Dr. Willey uses his knowledge about nutrition and exercise in pursuit of one of his favorite activities, competing in bodybuilding contests. He has won numerous awards and is recognized in many different venues.

Dr. Willey is the author of three books, a medical text book, and a self–help book: "What Does Your Doctor Look Like Naked? Your Guide to Optimal Health" and "Better than Steroids."

To contact Dr. Willey for an appointment or to set up a speaking engagement, please e–mail him at doc@pocatllopicc.com or visit his web site at www.eatright4u.com.

Index

Chapter 1

1. http://www.americanheart.org/downloadable/heart/
   461207852142003HDSStatsBook.pdf

Chapter 3

1. Gates, Thomas. Screening for Cancer: Evaluating the
   Evidence. Am Fam Physician 2001; 63:513-22.

Chapter 5

1. An Introduction to the Science of Anti-Aging Medicine.
   Klatz, Ronald. Lecture presented at the 9th International
   Congress on Anti-Aging & Biomedical Technologies.
   December 14-16, 2001.

2. Aging and exercise. Buckwalter JA. Decreasing Mobility in
   the Elderly. Physician Sportsmed Sep 1997; 25 (9): 12733.

3. Antioxidants. J Appl Psychology 1993: 74 (2):968-69.

4. Longevity/fitness. Lee CD Blair SN, Jackson AS.
   Cardiorespiratory fitness, body composition, and all-cause
   and cardiovascular disease mortality in men. AM J Clin
   Nutr 1999 Mar: 69(3):373-80.

5. Longevity/grip strength. Rantanen T, Guralnik JM, Foley D et al. Midlife hand grip strength as a predictor of old age disability. JAMA 1999 Feb 10; 281(6):558-60.

6. Longevity/predictors. Leveille SG et al. Aging successfully until death in old age: opportunities for increasing active life expectancy. Am J Epidemiol 1999 Apr 1; 149(7): 654-64.

7. Mortality exercise. Kujala UM, Kaprio J, Sarna S, Koskenvivo M. Relationship of Leisure-Time Physical Activity and Mortality JAMA Feb 11 1998; 279(6): 440-44.

8. Mortality/walking. Hakim AA et al. Effects of Walking on Mortality among Nonsmoking Retired Men. N Engl J Med Jan 8 1998; 338(2): 94-99.

9. Mortality/actual causes. McGinnis JM, Foege WH. Actual Causes of Death in the U.S. JAMA Nov 10; 270(18): 2207-11.

10. Coronary artery disease/exercise frequency. Chae CU. Brigham and Women's Hospital, Boston. American Heart Association annual meeting. Fam Pract News Jan 15, 1998: 28(2): 18.

11. Hyperlipidermia. Boreham CAG it al. Effects of a Stair-Climbing Programme on Physical Fitness and Blood Lipids in Young Females. Med Sci Sports Exer June 6, 1998; 30(5suppl): S297.

12. Hypertension/sedentary risk. Blair SN et al. Physical Fitness and Incidence of Hypertension in Health Normotensive Men and Women. JAMA Jul 27, 1984; 252(4):487-90.

13. Hypertension/exercise. Kokkinos PF, Narayan P, Colleran JA et al. Effects of regular exercise on blood pressure and left ventricular hypertrophy in African-American men with severe hypertension. N Engl J Med 1995 Nov 30; 333(22): 1462-7.

14. Stroke exercise. Lee IM, Paffenbarger RS Jr. Physical activity and stroke incidence: the Harvard Alumni Health Study. Stroke 1998 Oct: 29(10):2049-54.

15. Stroke/exercise. Lee IM, Hennekens CH, Berger K et al. Exercise and risk of stroke in male physicians. Stroke 1999 Jan; 30(1):1-6.

16. Diabetes incidence. Manson JE et al. A prospective study of exercise and incidence of diabetes among U.S. male physicians JAMA Jul 1, 1992: 268(1): 63-67.

17. Exercise prevalence obesity. Crespo CS et al. Leisure-Time Physical Activity among U.S. Adults. Arch Int Med Jan 8, 1996; 165(1): 93-98.

18. Obesity/exercise. Jakicic JM, Wing RR, Butler BA, Robertson RJ. Prescribing exercise in multiple short bouts versus one continuous bout: effects on adherence, cardiorespriatory fitness, and weight loss in overweight women. Int J Obes Relat Metab Disord 1995 Dec; 10(12): 893-901.

19. Cancer/exercise. Kampert JB, Blair SN, Barlow CE, Kohl HW 3rd. Physical activity, physical fitness, and all-cause and cancer mortality: a prospective study of men and women. Ann Epidemiol 1996 Sep; 6(5): 452-57.

20. Cancer-colon/walking exercise. Martinez ME, Giovannucci E, Spiegelman D et al. Leisure Rime Physical Activity, Body-Size and Colon Cancer in Women. J Natl Cancer Inst Jul 2, 1997; 89(13): 948-55.

21. Cancer-breast/exercise. Thune I et al. Physical Activity and the Risk of Breast Cancer. N Engl J Med May 1, 1997; 336(18): 1269-75.

22. Cancer-prostate/exercise. Oliveria SA, Kohl HW III, Trichopoulos D, Blair SN. The association between cardiorespiratory fitness and prostate cancer. Med Sci Sports Exerc 1996 Jan; 28(1): 97-104.

23. Glaucoma. Passeo MS et al. Exercise training reduces intraocular pressure among subjects suspected of having glaucoma. Arch Ophthalmol 1991 Aug; 109(8): 1096-98

24. Osteoporosis/dancing. Kudlacek S et al. The impact of a senior dancing program on spinal and peripheral bone mass. Am J Phys Med Rehabil 1997 Nov-Dec; 76(6):477-81.

25. Osteoporosis/strength training. Nelson ME et al. Effects of High-Intensity Strength Training on Multiple Risk Factors for Osteoporotic Fractures. JAMA Dec 28, 1994; 272(24):1909-14.

26. Low back pain/exercise. BMJ Jan 21, 1995; 310(6973): 151-54. Creativity/aerobic exercise. Steinberg H et al. Exercise Enhancers Creativity Independently of Mood. Br J Sports Med Sep 1997; 31 (3): 240-45.

27. Depression. Weyerer S. Physical inactivity and depression in the community. Evidence from the Upper Bavarian field Study. Int J Sports Med 1992 Aug; 13(6): 492-96.

28. Chronic obstructive pulmonary disease. Reardon J, Awad E, Normandin E et al. The Effect of Comprehensive Outpatient Pulmonary Rehabilitation on Dyspnea. Chest Apr 1994; 105(4): 1046-52.

29. Health/exercise interventions. Dunn AL et al. Comparison of lifestyle and structured interventions to increase physical activity and cardiorespiratory fitness: a randomized trial. JAMA 1999 Jan 27; 281 (4): 327-34.

30. Sexual Behavior. White JR et al. Enhanced sexual behavior in exercising men. Arch Sex Behav 1990 Jun; 19(3): 193-209.

31. Mortality/fruit. Key TJ et al. Dietary habits and mortality in 11,000 vegetarians and health-conscious people: results of a 17-year follow up. BMJ 1996 Sep 28; 313(7060): 775-79.

32. Calcium. Lipids Mar 1972; 7(3): 202-06.

33. Cholesterol, triglycerides/a-3 oils. Phillipson BE et al. Reduction of plasma lipids, lipoproteins, and apoproteins by dietary fish oils in patients with hypertriglyceridemia. N Engl J Med 1985 May 9; 312(19): 1210-16.

34. Coronary artery disease. N Engl J Med Feb 4 1993; 328(5): 313-18.

35. Fiber. Jenkins DJ et al. Effect on blood lipids of very high intakes of fiber in diets low in saturated fat and cholesterol. N Engl J Med 1993 Jul 1; 329(1): 21-26.

36. High density lipoprotein/magnesium. Curr Ther Res. Aug 1984; 36(2): 341-46.

37. High density lipoprotein/vitamin C. Int J Sport Nutrition Sep 1992; 2(3):260-71.

38. Low density lipoprotein/red wine. Lancet Feb 20 1993; 341(8843):454-57.

39. Lycopene. Agarwal S, Tao AV. Tomato Lycopene and Low Density Lipoprotein Oxidation: A Human Dietary Intervention Study. Lipids 1998 Oct; 33(10): 981-84.

40. Niacin. Am J Med Oct 1994; 97(4): 323-31.

41. Psyllium. Anderson JW et al. Long-term cholesterol-lowering effects of psyllium as an adjunct to diet therapy in the treatment of hypercholesterolemia. Am J Clin Nutr 2000 Jun; 71(6): 1433-8.

42. Sucrose. Br Med J 1980 Nov 22; 281(6252): 1396.

43. Coronary artery disease/fibrinogen, omega-3 oils. Am J Cardiol Jul 15 1994; 74(2): 189-91.

44. Coronary artery disease/flavonoids. Hertog MG et al. Flavonoid intake and long-term risk of coronary heart disease and cancer in the seven countries study. Arch Intern Med 1995 Feb 27; 155(4):381-86.

45. Coronary artery disease/lipoprotein [a]. JAMA Apr 6 1994; 271(13):999-1003.

46. Coronary artery disease/magnesium. Elwood PC et al. Dietary magnesium and prediction of heart disease. Lancet 1992 Aug 22; 340(8817):483.

47. Coronary artery disease/nuts. N Engl J Med Mar 4 1993; 328(9): 603-07.

48. Coronary artery disease/obesity. Texrode KM et al. Abdominal Adiposity and Coronary Artery Disease in Women. JAMA 1998 Dec 2; 280(21): 1843-48.

49. Coronary artery disease/reversal. Ornish D et al. Can lifestyle changes reverse coronary disease? The Lifestyle Heart Trial. Lancet 1990 Jul 21; 336(8704): 129-33.

50. Coronary artery disease/risk factors. J Chronic Dis Aug 1965; 18(8): 515-16.

51. Coronary artery disease/selenium. Atherosclerosis Sep 1992; 96(1): 33-44.

52. Surwit RS, Schneider MS: Role of stress in the etiology and treatment of diabetes mellitus. Psychosom Med 55:380-393, 1993

53. Viner R, McGrath M, Trudinger P: Family stress and metabolic control in diabetes. Arch Dis Child 74:418-421, 1996

54. Graham J, et al. Stressful life experiences and risk of relapse of breast cancer: observational cohort study. BMJ June 15, 2002; 324:1420-2.

55. Vedhara K, et al. Chronic stress in elderly carers of demented patients and antibody response to influenza vaccination. Lancet February 20, 1999; 353:627-31.

56. Lillberg K, Verkasalo PK, Kaprio J, Teppo L, Helenius H, Koskenvuo M. Stressful life events and risk of breast cancer in 10,808 women: a cohort study. Am J Epidemiol 2003 Mar 1; 157(5):415-23.

57. Chang PP, Ford DE, Meoni LA, Wang NY, Klag MJ. Anger in young men and subsequent premature cardiovascular disease: the precursors study. Arch Intern Med 2002 Apr 22; 162(8):901-6.

58. Fauvel JP, Quelin P, Ducher M, Rakotomalala H, Laville M. Perceived job stress but not individual cardiovascular reactivity to stress is related to higher blood pressure at work. Hypertension 2001 Jul; 38(1)71-5.

59. Gates, Thomas. Screening for Cancer: Evaluating the Evidence. Am Fam Physician 2001; 63:513-22.

Chapter 8

1. Journal of Clinical Endocrinology and Metabolism, August 2001, Vol. 86 No. 8 3604

2. Journal of Clinical Endocrinology and Metabolism, October 1997, Vol. 82 No. 10 3203

3. Journal of American Epidemiology October 15, 1997, Vol. 146 No. 8 609

4. Reuters Health. July 17, 2001, Vol.57, pg 80-88

5. Journal of Hypertension, April 1988, Vol. 6 No. 4 329

6. International Journal of Obesity-Related Metabolic Disorders, December 1992, Vol. 16, No. 12 pg 991

7. Journal of American Epidemiology May 1, 1996, Vol. 143 No. 9 889

8. Journal of Epidemiology September 1992, Vol. 2 No. 5 675

9. Journal of Clinical Endocrinology and Metabolism November 1997, Vol. 82 No. 2 407

10. Mayo Clinic Proceedings January, 2000, Vol. 75 (Suppl) J. Lisa Tenover, M.D., Ph.D.

11. Morley J. Longitudinal changes in testosterone, LH, FSH in healthy older men. Metabolism 1997, April;46(4):410-3

12. Annewieke W et al. Measures of bioavailable serum testosterone and estradiol and their relationships with muscle strength, bone density, and body composisiton in elderly men. The Journal of Clinical Endocrinology & Metabolism. Vol. 85, No. 9 3276-3282, 2000

13. Nankin HR et al. Decreased bioavailable testosterone in aging normal and impotent men. J Clin Endocrinol Metab. 1986 Dec; 63(6):1418-20.PMID:3782425; UI:87057957

14. Korenman SG, Morley JE, Mooradian AD, et al. 1990 Secondary hypogonadism in older men: its relationship to impotence. J Clin Endocrinol Metab. 71:963-969

15. JAMA 1944; 126[8]: 472-477. Androgen deficiency in the aging male: benefits and risks of androgen supplementation.J Steroid Biochem Mol Biol. 2003 Jun; 85(2-5):349-55.

16. Rhoden EL, and Abraham Morgentaler A. Risks of Testosterone-Replacement Therapy and Recommendations for Monitoring. N Engl J Med. 2004;350:482-92

17. Feldman HA, Longcope C, Derby CA, et al. Age Trends in the Level of Serum Testosterone and other Hormones in Middle-Aged Men: Longitudinal Results from the Massachusetts Male Aging Study. J Clin Endocrinol Metab 2000; 287: 589–598.

18. Haren MT, Kim MJ, Tariq SH, et al. Andropause: A Quality-of-Life Issue in Older Males. Med Clin N Am. 2006; 90:1005–1023.

19. Kapoor D, Malkin CJ, Channert and Jones TH. Androgens, insulin resistance and vascular disease in men. *Clin End* 2005; 63:239-250.

20. Laaksonen DE, Niskanen L, Punnonen K, et al. Sex hormones, inflammation and the metabolic syndrome. *European J of End*. 2003; 149:601-608.

21. Svartberg J. Epidemiology: testosterone and the metabolic syndrome. *Int J of Imp Research*. 2007; 19:124-128.

22. Selvin E, Feinleib M, Lei Z, et al. Androgens and Diabetes in men. Diabetes Care. 2007; 30(2):234-23.

Chapter 15

1. Westrate JA, Hautvast JG. The effects of short-term carbohydrate overfeeding and prior exercise on resting metabolic rate and diet-induced thermogenesis. Metabolism. 1990 Dec; 39(12):1232-9.

Chapter 18

1. Kohl HW, Blair SN, Paffenbarger RS, Macera CA, Kronenfeld JJ. A mall survey of physical activity habits as related to measured physical fitness. Am J Epidemiol. 1988; 127:1228-1239.

2. Taylor HL, Jacobs DR, Schucker B, Knudsen J, Leon AS, Debacker G. A questionnaire for the assessment of leisure time physical activities. J Chronic Dis. 1978; 31:741-755.

3. American College of Sports Medicine. Position stand on the recommended quantity and quality of exercise for developing and maintaining cardiorespiratory and muscular fitness in healthy adults. Med Sci Sports Exert. 1990; 22:265-274.

4. Paffenbarger RS, Hyde RT, Wing AL, Hsieh C-C. Physical activity, all-cause mortality, and longevity of college alumni. N Engl J Med. 1986; 314:605-613.

5. Morris JN, Clayton DG, Everitt MG, Semmence AM, Burgess EH. Exercise in leisure time: coronary attack and death rates. Br Heart J. 1990; 63:325-334.

6. Powell KE, Thompson PD, Caspersen CJ, Ford ES.

7. Physical activity and the incidence of coronary heart disease. Annu Rev Public Health. 1987; 8:253-287.

8. Leon AS, Connett J, Jacobs DR Jr, Rauramaa R. Leisure-time physical activity levels and risk of coronary heart disease and death: the Multiple Risk Factor Intervention trial. JAMA. 1987; 258:2388-2395.

9. Morris JN, Kagan A, Pattison DC, Chave SPW, Semmence AM. Incidence and prediction of ischemic heart disease in London busman. Lancet. 1966; 2:533-559.

10. Hagberg JM. Exercise, fitness, and hypertension. In: Bouchard C, Shephard RJ, Stephens T, Sutton JR, McPherson BD, eds. Exercise, Fitness, and Health. Champaign, Ill: Human Kinetics Publishers; 1990:455-566.

11. Blair SN, Goodyear NN, Gibbons LW, Cooper KH. Physical fitness and incidence of hypertension in healthy normotensive men and women. JAMA. 1984; 252:487-490.

12. Paffenbarger RS. Wing AL, Hyde RT, Jung DL. Physical activity and incidence of hypertension in college alumni. Am J Epidemiol. 1983; 117:245-257.

13. American College of Sports Medicine. Position stand: physical activity, physical fitness, and hypertension. Med Sci Sports Exerc. 1993; 10:i-x.

14. Helmrich SP, Ragland DR, Leung RW, Paffenbarger RS. Physical activity and reduced occurrence of non-insulin-dependent diabetes mellitus. N Engl J Med. 1991; 325:147-152.

15. Manson JE, Nathan DM, Krolewski AS, Stampfer M J, Willett WC, Hennekens CH. A prospective study of exercise and incidence of diabetes among US male physicians. JAMA. 1992; 268:63-67.

16. Manson JE, Rimm EB, Stampfer MJ, et al. Physical activity and incidence of non-insulin-dependent diabetes mellitus in women. Lancet. 1991; 338:774-778.

17. Cummings SR, Kelsey JL, Nevitt MD, O'Dowd KJ. Epidemiology of osteoporosis and osteoporotic fractures. Epidemiol Rev. 1985; 7:178-208.

18. Marcus R, Drinkwater B, Dalsky G, et al. Osteoporosis and exercise in women. Med Sci Sports Exerc.1992; 24 (suppl):S301-S307.

19. Snow-Harter C, Marcus R. Exercise, bone mineral density, and osteoporosis. Exerc Sport Sci Rev. 1991; 19:351-388.

20. Lee I, Paffenbarger RS, Hsieh C. Physical activity and risk of developing colorectal cancer among college alumni. J Natl Cancer Inst. 1991; 83:1324-1329.

21. King AC, Taylor CB, Haskell WL, DeBusk RF. Influence of regular aerobic exercise on psychological health. Health Psychol. 1989; 8:305-324.

22. Taylor CB, Sallis JF, Needle R. The relationship of physical activity and exercise to mental health. Public Health Rep. 1985; 100:195-201.

23. Blair SN, Kohl HW, Paffenbarger RS, Clark DG,

24. Cooper KH, Gibbons LW. Physical fitness and all-cause mortality. JAMA. 1989; 262:2395-2401.

25. Paffenbarger RS, Hyde RT, Wing AL, Lee I, Jung DL, Kampert JB. The association of changes in physical-activity level and other lifestyle characteristics with mortality among men. N Engl J Med. 1993; 328:538-545.

26. Hahn RA, Teutsch SM, Rothenberg RB, Marks JS. Excess deaths from nine chronic diseases in the United States. JAMA. 1986; 264:2654-2659.

27. McGinnis JM, Foege WH. Actual causes of death in the United States. JAMA. 1993; 270:2207-2212.

28. Haskell WL. The influence of exercise training on plasma lipids and lipoproteins in health and disease. Acta Med Scand. 1986; 711 (suppl): 25-37.

29. Duncan JJ, Farr JE, Upton SJ, Hagan RD, Oglesby ME, Blair SN. The effects of aerobic exercise on plasma catecholamines and blood pressure in patients with mild essential hypertension. JAMA. 1985; 254:2609-2613.

30. Hagberg JM, Montain S J, Martin WH, et al. Effect of exercise training on 60-69-year-old persons with essential hypertension. Am J Cardiol. 1989; 64:348-353.

31. Tipton CM. Exercise training and hypertension: an update. Exerc Sports Sci Rev. 1991; 19:447-505.

32. Bouchard C, Depres JP, Tremblay A. Exercise and obesity. Obesity Res. 1993; 1:133-147.

33. Pavlou K, Krey S, Steffee WP. Exercise as an adjunct to weight loss and maintenance in moderately obese subjects. Am J Clin Nutr. 1989; 49: 1115-1123.

34. Wood PD. Stefanick ML, Williams PT, Haskell WL. The effects on plasma lipoproteins of prudent weight-reducing diet, with or without exercise, in overweight men and women. N Engl J Med. 1991; 325: 461-466.

35. Ivy JL. The insulin-like effect of muscle contraction. Exerc Sports Sci Rev. 1987; 15:29-51.

36. Koivisto VA, Yki-Jarvinen H, DeFronzo RA. Physical training and insulin sensitivity. Diabetes Metab Rev. 1986; 1:445-481.

37. Dalsky GP, Stoke KS, Ehsani AA, Slatopolsky E, Lee WC, Birge SJ. Weight-bearing exercise training and lumbar bone mineral content in postmenopausal women. Ann Intern Med. 1988; 108:824-828.

38. Nehlsen-Cannarella SL, Niemann DC, Balk-Lamberton AJ, et al. The effects of moderate exercise training on immune response. Med Sci Sports Exerc. 1991; 23:64-70.

39. Nieman DC. Physical activity, fitness, and infection. In: Bouchard C, Shephard R J, Stephens T, eds. Physical Activity, Fitness, and Health. Champaign, Ill: Human Kinetics Publishers; 1994; 796-813.

40. King AC, Taylor CB, Haskell WL. Effects of differing intensities and formats of 12 months of exercise training on psychological outcomes in older adults. Health Psychol. 1993; 12:292-300.

41. Hill AB. The environment and disease: association or causation? Proc R Soc Med. 1965; 58:295-300.

42. Centers for Disease Control and Prevention. Public health focus: physical activity and the prevention of coronary heart disease. MMWR Morb Mortal Wkly Rep. 1993; 42:669-672.

43. Rauramaa R, Salonen JT. Physical activity, fibrinolysis, and platelet aggregability. In: Bouchard C, Shephard

R J, Stephens T, eds. Physical Activity, Fitness, and Health. Champaign, Ill: Human Kinetics Publishers; 1994:471-479.

44. Moore S. Physical activity, fitness, and atherosclerosis. In: Bouchard C, Shephard R J, Stephens T, eds. Physical Activity, Fitness, and Health. Champaign, Ill: Human Kinetics Publishers; 1994:570-578.

45. Parsons D, Foster V, Harman F, Dickinson A, Westerlind K. Balance and strength changes in elderly subjects after heavy-resistance strength training. Med Sci Sports Exerc. 1992; 24 (suppl):S21.

CPSIA information can be obtained at www.ICGtesting.com
Printed in the USA
LVOW04s2358131014

408538LV00025B/992/P